CURRENT TOPICS IN SALMONELLA AND SALMONELLOSIS

Edited by **Mihai Mareș**

Current Topics in Salmonella and Salmonellosis
http://dx.doi.org/10.5772/63008
Edited by Mihai Mareş

Contributors
Niki Mouttotou, Shakeel Ahmad, Zahid Kamran, Konstantinos C. Koutoulis, Fathalla A. Rihan, Karine Dufresne, France Daigle, Yasuhiko Suzuki, Nammalwar Sriranganathan, Rachel Rezende, Bianca Maciel, Samuel Ajoseh, Kabiru Olusegun Akinyemi, Lingwen Zeng, Wei Wu, Rebeca Zamora, Andrea Molina, Luma Akil, Hafiz Anwar Ahmad, David Ussery, Trudy Wassenaar, Małgorzata Szczawińska, Rachida Mimouni, Eva Fornefeld, Jasper Schierstaedt, Sven Jechalke, Rita Grosch, Kornelia Smalla, Adam Schikora, Shrikant Pawar, Md. Izhar Ashraf, K. M. Mehata, Chandrajit Lahiri

Published by InTech
Janeza Trdine 9, 51000 Rijeka, Croatia

Publishing Process Manager Dajana Pemac
Technical Editor SPi Global
Cover InTech Design team

First published April, 2017
Printed in Croatia
Legal deposit, Croatia: National and University Library in Zagreb

Additional hard copies can be obtained from orders@intechopen.com

Current Topics in Salmonella and Salmonellosis, Edited by Mihai Mareş
p. cm.
Print ISBN 978-953-51-3065-9
Online ISBN 978-953-51-3066-6

For EU product safety concerns:
IN TECH d.o.o., Prolaz Marije Krucifikse Kozulić 3, 51000 Rijeka, Croatia,
info@intechopen.com or visit our website at intechopen.com.

Meet the editor

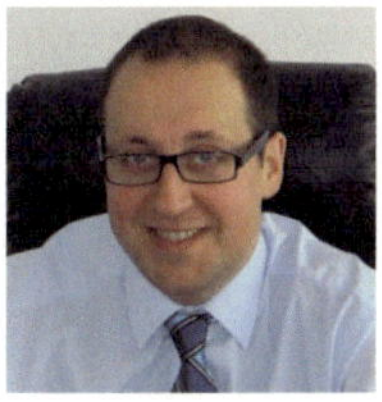

Dr. Mihai Mareş received his PhD degree in Microbiology at "Gr. T. Popa" University of Medicine and Pharmacy from Iaşi, Romania (2005), and had the postgraduate training at the University VII Denis-Diderot, Pasteur Institute, Pitié-Salpêtrière Hospital, and École du Val-de-Grâce, Paris (France); Complutense University of Madrid (Spain); Instituto de Salud Global, Barcelona (Spain); Karolinska Institute, Stockholm (Sweden); and Danish Technical University, Lyngby (Denmark). His areas of interest are medical mycology, antimicrobial resistance, mycobacteria, food microbiology, biofilms and biomedical applications of plasma discharges, and cold plasma–activated water. Currently, Dr. Mareş is a professor of Microbiology and the head of the Antimicrobial Chemotherapy Laboratory at the Ion Ionescu de la Brad University, Iaşi (Romania). He has served as consultant for several pharmaceutical companies during the past few years.

Contents

Preface

The genus *Salmonella* comprises an important number of bacterial species able to colonize and infect numerous animal species and humans. Although more than a hundred years passed since its discovery, *Salmonella* still represents a redoubtable and successful microorganism, difficult to deal with. Whether we discuss about typhoid fever or food poisoning, the public health and financial consequences are practically incalculable. The costs attributable to *Salmonella* contamination of meat, eggs, and vegetables are also very high worldwide. Antimicrobial resistance in *Salmonella* isolates is an emerging threat not only in humans, and special measures should be addressed to this global problem.

The book *Current Topics in Salmonella and Salmonellosis* contains a series of reviews about all-important issues concerning these subjects. It comprises 14 chapters grouped in 4 sections emphasizing new insights into pathogenesis, bacterial detection and antibiotic resistance, infections in animals, risk factors, and control strategies. The new genomic data and the exhaustive presentation of molecular pathogenesis bring novelty to the book and can help to improve our knowledge about *Salmonella*-induced diseases.

More than 40 international specialists have contributed as coauthors to this book, resulting in an interdisciplinary view on the topic. I would like to express my gratitude and appreciation to all of them and, last but not least, to all those who assisted me in this editorial project.

Mihai Mareş, PhD
Professor of Microbiology, Department of Public Health
Head, Laboratory of Antimicrobial Chemotherapy
Ion Ionescu de la Brad University
Iasi, Romania

Section 1

New Insights in Pathogenesis

Chapter 1

Insights from Comparative Genomics of the Genus *Salmonella*

Trudy M. Wassenaar, Se-Ran Jun, Visanu Wanchai,
Preecha Patumcharoenpol, Intawat Nookaew,
Katrina Schlum, Michael R. Leuze and
David W. Ussery

Additional information is available at the end of the chapter

http://dx.doi.org/10.5772/67131

Abstract

Comparative genomics have become a standard approach to gain insights into the interrelationships of microorganisms. Here, we have applied variable bioinformatic techniques to compare over 200 *Salmonella* genomes. First, we present a tree of all sequenced different members of the *Enterobacteriaceae* family, based on comparison of average amino acid identities. This technique was also applied to zoom in on the genomes of the genus *Salmonella*. The pan and core genomes of this genus were established and compared to experimental data available on the literature that identified essential genes. Difficulties and shortcomings of both approaches are discussed. Metabolic pathways unique for *Salmonella* were identified. Finally, we present an analysis of genes coding for small RNAs, an important part of the genetic repertoire of bacteria that is often ignored. The findings reported here are discussed and compared with available literature.

Keywords: comparative genomics, *Salmonella*, core genome, small RNA, AAI tree

1. Introduction

The genus *Salmonella* belongs to the *Enterobacteriaceae*, a large family within the gamma-proteobacteria to which *E. coli* also belongs. Since its first characterization in 1884 from diseased pigs by scientists working in the group of Daniel Salmon (after whom the genus is named), *Salmonella* species have been known to cause disease, notably typhoid fever and food poisoning. Pathogenic *Salmonella* types can be found in a wide range of animal hosts and often infect humans via contaminated food; they are responsible for more than a million infections in the

United States every year. Infections vary from (long-term) asymptomatic carriage and self-limiting salmonellosis to life-threatening conditions and fatal typhoidal fever [1].

Historically, many species of this genus were recognized, at first based on the clinical symptoms typical for their infections and it was soon recognized that these correlated with their serotype. However, based on sequence analysis, in 1973, it was proposed that all these *Salmonella* serotypes belonged to the same species [2]. This resulted, in 2005, to the designation of *Salmonella enterica* as the type species for the genus, as described by the International Committee on Systematics of Procaryotes [3]. Only one other species is currently formally recognized within the genus: *Salmonella bongori*, which lives in cold-blooded reptiles. *S. enterica* is further divided into six subspecies, of which *S. enterica* subsp. *enterica* is clinically most relevant. The names originally used to describe clinically distinct 'species' live on as serovars or serotypes. All *Salmonella* bacteria are none spore-forming, chemotrophic, facultative anaerobes, which survive in their host intracellularly [1].

The number of *Salmonella* genome sequences available in GenBank is constantly increasing. At the time of writing their number reached five thousand, the vast majority of which were obtained from *S. enterica*. As of September 15, 2016, there were 4934 genomes of this species in GenBank, with three additional genomes from *S. bongori*. Only a small fraction of these genomes are submitted as complete sequences without gaps and fulfilling all criteria set by GenBank for a genome to be listed as 'complete' (201 genomes at the time of writing, corresponding to 4% of the total). In this chapter, we employ whole-genome methods to compare complete *Salmonella* genomes in order to produce insights into the genomic diversity of this genus.

2. *Salmonella* comparative genome analyses

2.1. Genome-based trees

The first approach was aimed to show the overall relatedness of all species belonging to the *Enterobacteriaceae* family, based on their (completely sequenced) genomes. For this, we collected up to ten genome sequences per species, as far as these were available, which led to 255 genome sequences to be compared. The comparison was based on average amino acid identity (AAI) comparison, a method that uses all annotated protein genes in a given genome, producing more robust trees than methods based on direct alignments or concatenated protein sequence alignments [4]. The resulting tree is presented with collapsed branches for redundant species (**Figure 1**). The *Salmonella* genus, shown in red, is positioned on a cluster together with *Citrobacter*, with *Escherichia/Shigella* as the closest neighbors. These genera are supposed to have been separated for tens of millions of years [5]. The close relationship between *Citrobacter* and *Salmonella* has been observed before, and it was proposed that recombination between these and to a lesser extent with *Escherichia*, has been frequent in the past, during a process of fragmented speciation [5].

Next, we extracted all 201 complete genomes from the *Salmonella* genus (in May 2016), combined with 164 'nearly completed' genomes. The latter were extracted from GenBank as good quality draft sequences only, retrieved from GenBank when selecting for genomes of 'chromosome' quality; all contained one contiguous sequence, without gaps. These 365 *Salmonella* genomes represent only a tiny fraction of what is available. Apart from the nearly 5000 *Salmonella* genomes available in GenBank, there are currently more than 62,000 *Salmonella enterica* genomes stored in the Sequence Read Archive. However, in principle, the complete genome sequences should be of high quality and reliable in terms of annotation; therefore, we restricted the analysis to complete genomes.

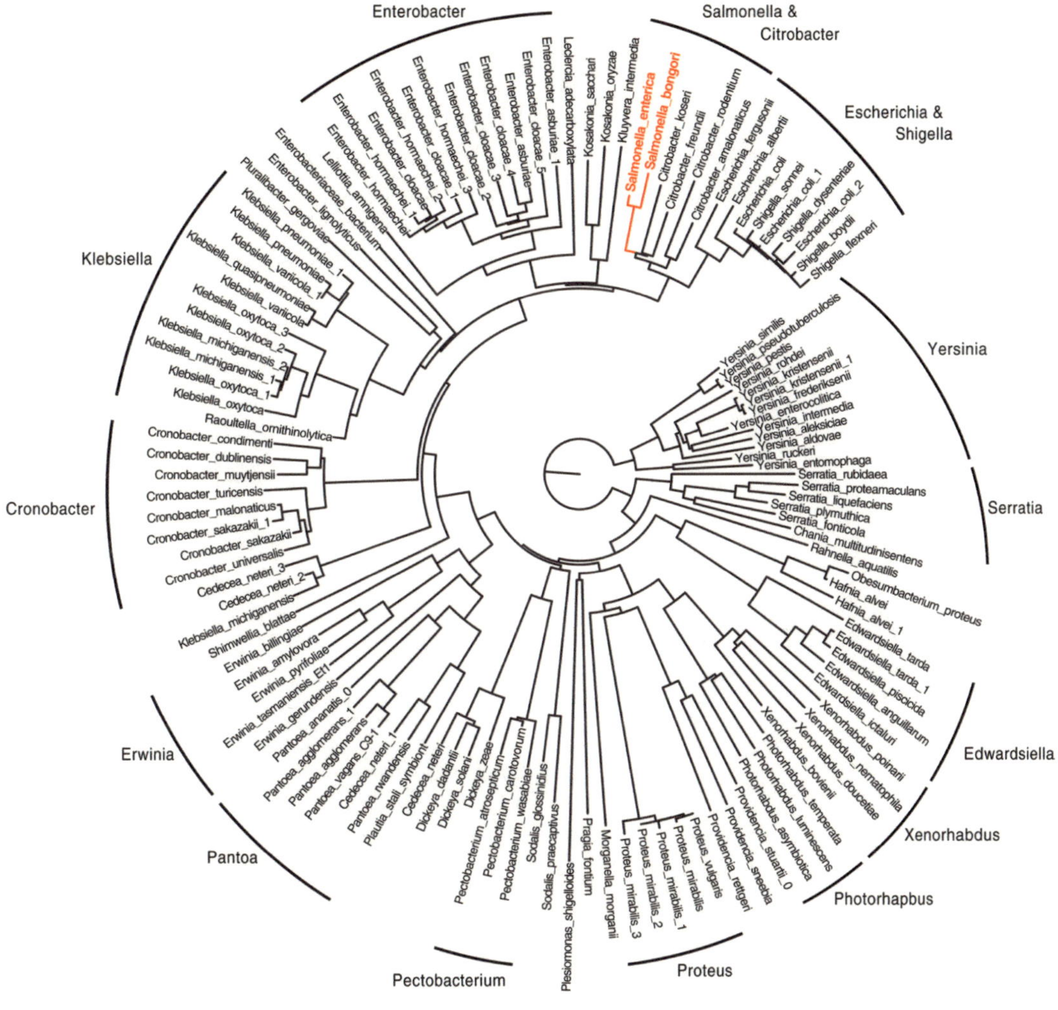

Figure 1. Tree based on average amino acid identity (AAI) of 255 genomes from members of the *Enterobacteraceae*. Branches were collapsed at the species level. The branch with the two *Salmonella* species is colored and some distinct genus clusters are labeled.

An AAI tree was constructed to establish the interrelationship of the 365 complete genomes, representing 33 different serovars including 36 Typhimurium and 6 Typhi genomes. The branches of the AAI tree were collapsed at serovar level. This produced a tree with 62 branches, as shown in **Figure 2**. As can be observed, by and large the tree clustered the genomes according to serovars, though the separation is not absolute and some serovars end up in mixed clusters. This was to be expected, as the analysis is based on the complete annotated proteome (capturing all protein-coded sequences), while the phenotypic characteristics that determine a serovar are determined by a limited number of genes only, that produce the surface antigens captured by serotyping. Of the 36 *S. enterica* sv. Typhimurium genomes (represented on 13 branches, blue in the figure), 32 cluster together on 10 branches (together with four branches of non-specified serovars), while four are placed on three branches outside the Typhimurium cluster. A distinct cluster is also observed containing the serovars Enteritidis, Pullorum, Gallinarum and Dublin (colored green in the figure) which together are known as 'group D *Salmonella*' [6]. The first three of these are adapted to the chicken host, but serovar Dublin is mostly colonizing cattle, and other serovars frequently found in chickens are placed outside the group D cluster. It has been suggested that the serovars Paratyphi and Choleraesuis, both with a narrow host range (for humans and pigs, respectively) are phylogenetically related, a conclusion that was based on SNP analysis [6]. Indeed, we observe that one Paratyphi genome clusters with a Choleraesuis, but two other Paratyphi and another Choleraesuis genome are more distinct (colored red in **Figure 2**).

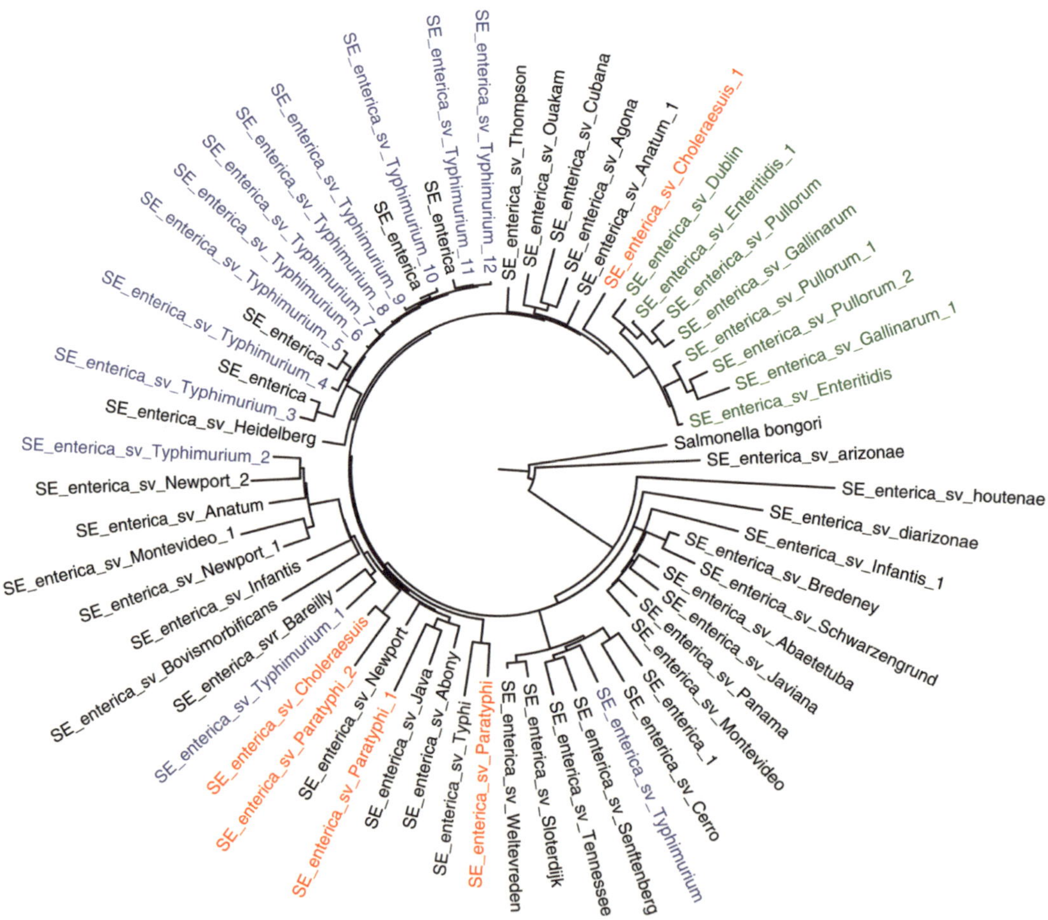

Figure 2. AAI tree of 365 *Salmonella* genomes representing 33 serovars of *S. enterica* (abbreviated as 'SE') subsp *enterica*. Indentical branches were collapsed per serotype. For explanation of the colors, see text.

http://dx.doi.org/10.5772/67131

2.2. Essential genes based on published gene inactivation studies

What makes a *Salmonella* a *Salmonella*? There are of course particular biochemical characteristics that can be used for identification, but can we recognize a set of genes that are always conserved, required and necessary for a *Salmonella* to be called that? And how many of those genes would be essential for growth and survival of the bacteria? These questions are addressed in this and the next session. Here, we start with genes proposed to be essential for survival under laboratory conditions, based on experimental data.

Traditionally, targeted mutagenesis has been used to determine if a gene from a given *Salmonella* strain were essential for infection, an approach that restricted the analyses to low numbers of genes only. An alternative approach was published in 2004 (based on previously developed techniques) to identify larger numbers of essential genes, by insertion of conditional lethal mutations into random gene fragments in a *S. typhimurium* strain [7]. The conditional switch used here was growth temperature, while tetracycline-dependent expression was used by others [8], although they only reported findings for four essential genes. A few years later, transposon (Tn) mutagenesis combined with high-throughput sequencing became available and this was applied to *S. enterica* strains [9–12]. Typically, in this approach mutants are screened for growth in LB broth. With a sufficiently high density of transposon insertions, genes that have not received insertions can be considered essential, as their inactivation had resulted in mutants unable to multiply under the conditions applied. Yet another approach was followed by Thiele and coworkers, who used metabolic reconstruction (MR) to extract a list of essential genes in *S*. Typhimurium that could be possible drug targets [13].

The experimental approaches reported in the literature are not without difficulties, as realized by their authors. For instance, polarity of transposon insertions in operons containing multiple genes can result in genes being scored as essential only because they are positioned downstream of an inactivated essential gene; attempts have been made to correct for this. Gene orthologs can further complicate findings, whereby one copy of an essential gene can be inactivated as long as a second copy remains intact. When an obtained mutant library is cultured for several generations, some mutants that originally survived will be removed from the population because their deletions are disadvantageous though not directly lethal. Such genes are typically scored as being under strong selection, an analysis that has been performed for *S*. Typhimurium strain ATCC 14028 and *S*. Thyphi strain Ty2 [11].

That experimental wet-laboratory data can be controversial is demonstrated by the fact that 26 of the 28 genes in *S*. Typhimurium strain ATCC 14028 that Knuth and coworkers reported as essential [7] could nevertheless be inactivated by site-directed mutagenesis [14].

Some research groups selected for conditions more closely resembling natural conditions of infection, for instance growth at 42°C instead of 37°C, to resemble the body temperature of mice that *S*. Typhimurium would typically encounter, or in the presence of bile acid ([10], work conducted with strain ATCC 14028). Exposure to low pH has also been tested [8]. Moreover, even 'essential' genes can often endure a transposon insertion without complete loss of function. If only those genes would be scored as essential that were truly resistant to Tn insertions from high-throughput mutagenesis, the essential gene pool would be very small indeed: only 96 genes from *S*. Typhi strain Ty2 and 57 genes from *S*. Typhimurium strain SL3261 remained free of Tn insertions under conditions that were considered to have reached Tn saturation [12]. Thus, a small number of insertions can be permitted, even in genes considered essential for life in laboratory medium. Since the chance to receive a Tn insertion depends on gene length, a highly variable parameter, the number of observed insertions needs to be corrected for gene length [9]. This produces an insertion index, where the number of observed insertions is divided by gene length. In addition, a likelihood can be calculated from the ratio of observed versus expected number of Tn insertions, to predict the chance of a gene being essential [9, 12]. For this approach, a cutoff value is required, to bin genes as either essential or not. The problem with this is that the used parameter (likelihood P value, Tn-insertion index or both) is a continuously increasing value. This makes the choice of the cutoff inevitably arbitrarily: There is no biological reason why genes bordering this cutoff would or would not be essential.

To illustrate the difficulty, we plotted the P value reported by Barquist and colleagues [12], who provided the most elaborate list of Tn mutants available to date (**Figure 3**). Panel A of the figure shows how the P value of all genes of *S.* Typhimurium steadily increases. Similar results are obtained for *S.* Typhi (not shown), and even for those genes that have very low P values, there is a continuous increase, as shown in Panel B. Note that in this figure, the log10 value was plotted for clarity, and the cutoff value corresponding to a P value of <0.05 is indicated by the red line. Clearly, this value is artificial, since there is no noticeable increment around this value.

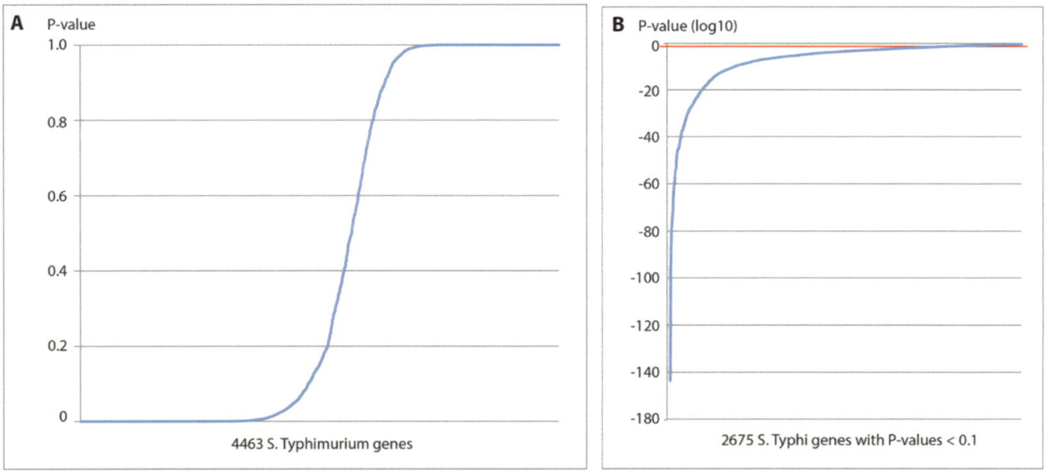

Figure 3. The continuous increase of P values of Tn insertions. In Panel A, P values of all 4463 genes of *S.* Typhimurium are plotted. In Panel B, a selection of 2675 *S.* Typhimurium genes is shown with P values >0 but <0.1, plotted for the exponent (log10) of the P values for clarity. The red line indicates the cutoff of $P < 0.05$, corresponding with a log10 value of −1.3 that was used by the authors. Data after Ref. [12].

A slightly different picture emerges when the Tn-insertion index is plotted, as shown in **Figure 4**. Although the increase in this index is also continuous, the shape of the obtained curve is slightly sigmoidal at the beginning, suggesting a trend toward saturation of the index value around 0.03, before it increases again. This trend is stronger for *S.* Typhi (Panel 4A) than for

S. Typhimurium (Panel 4B). Based on these findings, a cutoff value of 0.25 and 0.03 for the Tn index, respectively, might be appropriate for these species. We therefore recorded genes with a Tn index <0.25 for *S.* Typhi (n = 545 genes) and with a Tn index <0.30 for *S.* Typhimurium (n = 445), based on the data from Barquist and coworkers [12]. The Tn index of these genes is shown in Panels C and D of **Figure 4**. We further recorded the genes that Barquist and colleagues had originally selected (301 genes from *S.* Typhi and 299 for *S.* Typhimurium) which contained a reanalysis of the data from Langridge [9], as well as all genes previously identified as 'essential' by Knuth [7], Khatiwari [10], Canals [11] and Thiele [13], regardless of whether such genes were successfully inactivated by others. This produced an 'all inclusive' list of 847 genes putatively essential for growth and survival, or under strong selection, in LB medium. Relatively few genes were consistently recorded as essential by all or most authors; most genes were found in two independent approaches or were single findings (results not shown).

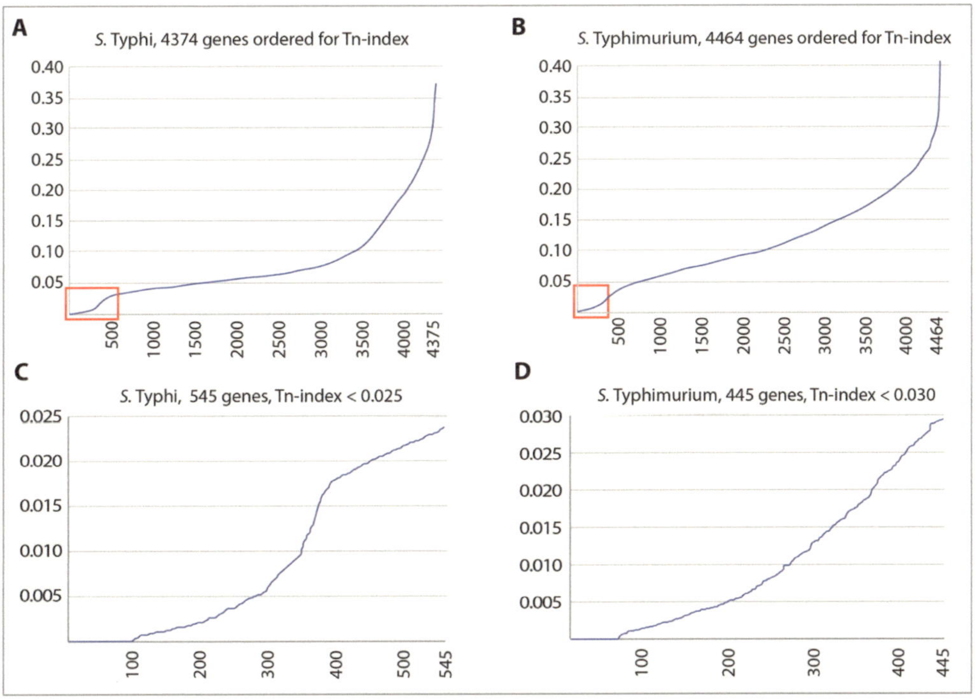

Figure 4. Analysis of transposon insertion frequency for genes of *S.* Typhi (left) and *S.* Typhimurium (right), based on data published by [12]. In Panels A and B, all genes are sorted for Tn index. The bottom Panels C and D show an enlargement of the part in the red square of A and B, respectively. For more explanation, see text.

A word of caution is needed here. It turned out to be rather cumbersome to identify the genes mentioned in the original published data (mostly using the supplementary tables provided with the publications) and to compare the findings with those of others, because genes were mostly described by gene names, which are by no means suitable as unique identifiers. For instance, the large operon for LPS-biosynthesis is called *waa* in *S.* Typhi but *rfb* in

S. Typhimurium; the essential gene *mrdA* of *E. coli* is called that in S. typhimurium, but it is *pbpA* in S. Typhimurium. The gene that is called *ribE* in both *Salmonella* genomes is essential, but it is called *ribC* in *E. coli*, while *ribE* in the latter species is called *ribH* in *Salmonella* (also essential). This makes it very risky to assume two genes are the same if they have the same name, or different if they do not. In most reports, a short protein functional description is provided, which can assist in correct identification, but many genes have very general functional characteristics, or are of unknown function. In such cases, the only way to identify which gene was meant is to use the gene location, but even that information does not always prove to be sufficient, for instance, when authors have re-annotated a genome but did not make this annotation public.

In conclusion, it is tedious and sometimes impossible to connect the findings from one study to those of another. Genes scored as 'essential' by one group can be inactivated without consequences on viability by another group. Moreover, most so-called essential genes endure a low number of transposon insertions without the loss of viability.

2.3. Conserved genes found in the core genome of *Salmonella enterica*

The second approach to identify essential genes in *Salmonella* is based on bioinformatical analysis of published genome sequences. If a gene is essential for growth, one can expect it to be strictly conserved between genomes, so a comparison on gene conservation can identify possible candidates. This is also not a completely unambiguous approach and depends on a number of choices that have to be made. For instance, one must define homologs between genomes in order to assess if genes are conserved, but this requires a defined percentage of homology that must be allowed and required for genes to be combined into a gene family. In addition, how should one deal with very short open reading frames, in other words, what is the minimum length of genes included, without adding too many artificial short open reading frames? And should one use original gene annotations, which is a transparent procedure that is easily reproducible, or is it better to re-annotate genomes using a standardized procedure to reduce variation? The latter approach produces more robust data as it no longer depends on variable gene calling, but it is less transparent when the used re-annotations are not made public. When core genomes are being defined from a set of highly different organisms, it may be required to allow for genes that are missing in a low number of analyzed genomes. However, when dealing with a single species, one could apply a strict requirement of presence in all genomes to produce a realistic core, especially if only fully sequenced genomes, re-annotated with a standardized algorithm, are included.

For this chapter, we decided to use publically available annotations, to aim for maximum transparency, and we further illustrate the effect of different core genome definitions. The core genome was established based on the annotations of the 362 completely sequenced *Salmonella enterica* genomes that were used to construct **Figure 2**, complemented with the three *S. bongori* genomes. Protein-coding genes were binned into gene families by the use of the program USEARCH [15] such that members of each family have at least 50% sequence identity and at least 50% alignment length of the best hit against the centroid of the family. Using a strict definition of required presence in all analyzed genomes, a so-called 100% core genome could be identified that consisted of 1061 gene families. Although this seems an impressive number, it is lower than expected, probably because of variations in the used gene annotations. Based on our experience with core-genome determination from many bacterial genera, we were expecting the core genome of *S. enterica* to be larger, as the species contains relatively closely related organisms. Thus, we relaxed the requirement to allow gene presence in 344 or 95% of the investigated genomes. This produced a core genome of 3499 gene families, a size that is comparable with the preliminary core established for thousands of sequenced *Salmonella* genomes (S-R Jun and DW Ussery, unpublished data). We also constructed the core genome for *S. bongori*, but with only three genomes available, this core is relatively large, as a core genome usually decreases with an increasing number of included genomes. For the core genome of the complete *Salmonella* genus, these two datasets were combined. The results are summarized in **Table 1**.

Table 1 further lists that 11 genes from the 95% core were not annotated in the reference genome of the species typestrain *S. enterica* subsp *enterica* Typhimurium LT2. Originally, this number was much higher: There appeared to be 141 of the 3499 core genes missing in the annotated *S.* Typhimurium LT2 genome. However, when the DNA sequences of these genes were checked against the reference genome, 130 were actually present but not annotated. Thus, only 11 core genes remained that appear to be truly missing in the reference genome. This number did not change for core gene families based on *S. enterica* or the complete *Salmonella* genome (**Table 1**).

Dataset	Core genome size in 100% of dataset	Core genome size in 95% of dataset	Number of core genes missing in reference genome
362 *S. enterica* genomes	1061 gene families	3499 gene families	11 core genes out of 3499 are missing in *S.* Typhimurium LT2
3 *S. bongori* genomes	3368 gene families	3368 gene families	n.a.
365 *Salmonella* genomes	1009 gene families	3470 gene families	11 core genes out of 3470 are missing in *S.* Typhimurium LT2

Table 1. Core genome analysis based on 365 *Salmonella* genome sequences.

It was further checked if core gene families in the reference genome contained multiple entries, in other words, whether those core gene families contained orthologs or paralogs. This was the case for 120 gene families. When the function of these gene copies is interchangeable, these orthologs can be considered as 'back-up' copies, possibly maintained in the genome to protect against loss of essential function; alternatively, the genome can contain orthologs to allow for a higher production of the gene product. The multiple copies of the ribosomal RNA genes would be a nice example of the latter, though they are not captured in our core genome analysis, which was restricted to protein-coding genes only. To give another example, multiple copies of ferric enterobactin (enterochelin) transporters were found. Such orthologs of essential genes can complicate the outcome of in vitro mutagenesis analyses, as discussed above. However, not all orthologous genes are duplicated because they are essential, so it is not a predictive characteristic.

The genomes used for **Table 1** were not only used to select conserved core genomes, but also to define the pan genome, containing all gene families of the *Salmonella* genus. This is visually represented in **Figure 5**. The pan genome increases in size until approximately 180 genomes have been added, at which stage it reaches a plateau and is hardly affected by addition of further *S. enterica* genomes. It increases again when *S. enterica* Infantis and especially when *S. bongori* genomes are added, as these introduce novel gene families to the pan genome. Panel B of **Figure 5** illustrates the validity of defining a 95% core, instead of applying the strict requirement of presence in 100% of all genomes. The 100% core genome steadily decreases with the cumulative addition of the genomes analyzed here (the order of the genomes is the same as for Panel A) and decreases sharply to approximately 1000 gene families after addition of the *S. bongori* genomes. Instead, in the 95%, core genome is quite robust and remains more or less constant at around 3470 gene families (**Figure 5**).

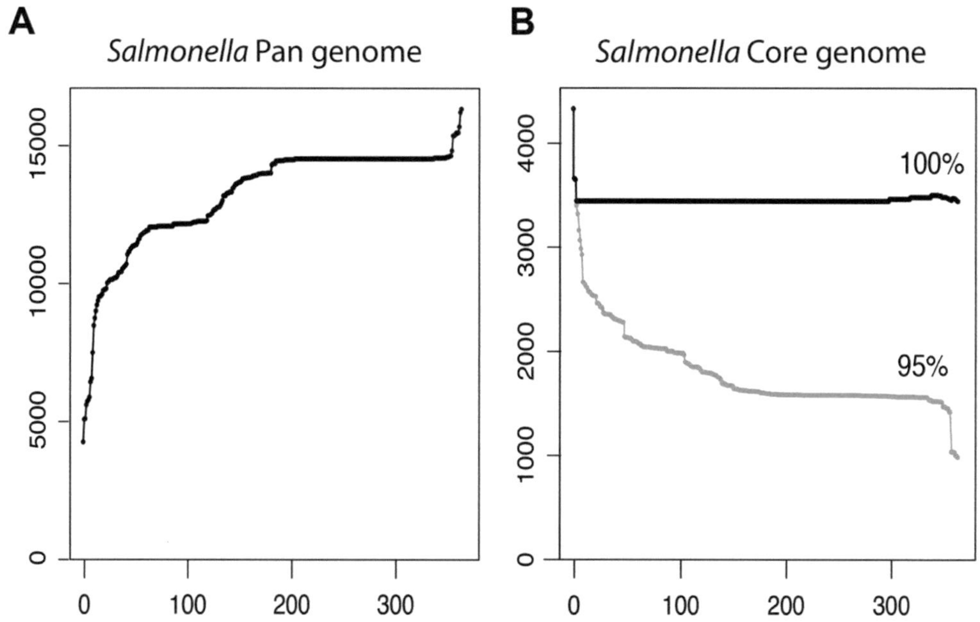

Figure 5. Pan-core plots based on 365 *Salmonella* genomes. Panel A shows the pan genome of *Salmonella,* with *S. bongori* added last. Panel B shows the core genome of the 365 *Salmonella* genomes with 95 and 100% conservation.

As was discussed in the previous section, the literature findings on essential genes are often controversial, for reasons discussed, while core genome determination is also not without caveats. Importantly, one can assume that all genes required for growth in LB medium must be conserved in all genomes and thus be part of the core, though the reverse may not be true: Not all core genes will be essential for growth and survival under these laboratory conditions. Therefore, we checked which of the essential genes reported in the literature were actually present in the core genome. For this, we used the 95% core genome, though core genes missing in the original annotation of the reference genome of *S.* Typhimurium LT2 were added manually. A total of 683 core genes could with reasonable confidence be identified that at least by one approach was found as putatively essential (results not shown). Conversely, of the

870 genes that were identified as essential by any of the methods discussed in the previous section, 694 were identified as part of the 95% core. The least reliable prediction of 'essential' genes turned out to be a low P value of Tn insertion, as this contained the highest fraction of genes that were not part of the core.

2.4. How close is *S.* Typhimurium to *E. coli*?

This chapter started with a comparison of all *Enterobacteriaceae,* to illustrate the close relationship between *Salmonella, Citrobacter* and *Escherichia*. But how close are *Salmonella* and *Escherichia,* in terms of conserved proteins? To address this question, the core genes of *S. enterica* Typhimurium LT2 (the type strain of the species) were compared to the core genes recently defined for *E. coli* (using the same definitions and parameters) [16], which we applied to the species typestrain *E. coli* DSM 30083. As reported in **Table 1**, the 95% core genome of all *Salmonella* comprises 3470 gene families, of which 11 are missing in Typhimurium LT2. This strain thus contains 3459 core gene families, while the *E. coli* typestrain contains 3100 core gene families. When these were compared, it was found that 2615 of these are shared, which corresponds to 75.6% of the *S.* Typhimurium LT2 core gene families, 84.4% of *E. coli* DSM 30083 and 66.3% of the total gene families assessed for these two species. This is illustrated in Panel A of **Figure 6**. The definition for gene families applied here is the same as for **Table 1** and **Figure 5**, but as explained above, this requires a defined cutoff for sequence similarity. The biological function of proteins is mostly defined by their functional domains, which is sometimes only a fraction of the total protein sequence. Thus, we narrowed this analysis down, to define the common core genome based on functional domains only, using Pfam domains. Since a Pfam domain is not described for all core genes, there were fewer domains captured in this comparison (2416 for *S.* typhimurium LT2 and 2263 for *E. coli* DSM 30083). Panel B of **Figure 6** shows that there are 2142 shared protein domains, corresponding to 88.7% of the *S.* Typhimurium LT2 core proteins, 94.7% of the *E. coli* DSM 30083 core proteins, and 84.4% of the total number of functional domains captured here. Interestingly, the fractions of shared core genes and shared functional domains are larger for the *E. coli* typestrain than for the *Salmonella enterica* typestrain. We believe this is caused by the larger diversity of the *E. coli* species, compared to *S. enterica*. As a consequence, the core genome of *E. coli* is smaller, even at 95%, which means a larger fraction of these is shared with *S. enterica*.

We further investigated the functions of the *Salmonella* core gene families in *S. Typhimurium* LT2 and found that most of them related to cellular metabolism. The core genome of *S. Typhimurium* LT2 was mapped to the genome-scale metabolic model SMT_v1.0 [13], which resulted in a total of 1271 genes and 2545 metabolic reactions. As shown in Panel C of **Figure 6**, 1012 genes from the *S. Typhimurium* LT2 core genome have a metabolic function (~80% of total genes in the model) and these account for 2358 metabolic reactions (93% of total reactions in the model). When comparing this with the *E. coli* core genome, *S. Typhimurium* LT2 has 156 unique metabolic genes, responsible for 452 metabolic reactions. The unique metabolic reactions that were identified here are mostly involved in transport systems across the inner membrane as well as the outer membrane (porins), specific transport of inorganic ions, and the recycling of lipopolysaccharide biosynthesis components. Such analyses can share light on the biochemical and metabolic properties that *Salmonella* is specialized in, related to its intracellular lifestyle.

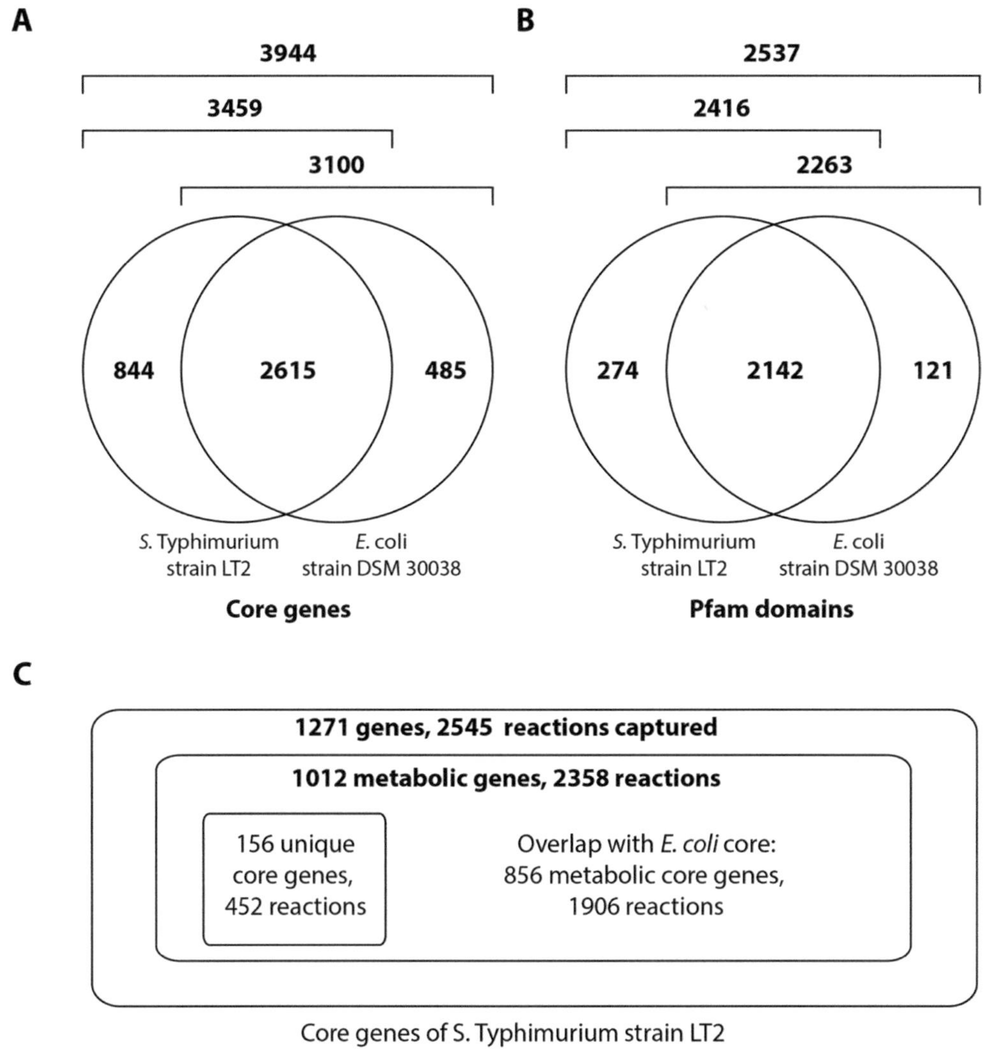

Figure 6. Comparison of *Salmonella* and *E. coli* core genes, using the type strains for both species. Panel A shows the size and overlap of the core gene families. Panel B shows the comparison using PfamA domains. Panel C summarizes how many metabolic pathways are shared in the *Salmonella* and *E. coli* cores.

2.5. Conserved RNAs across 201 *Salmonella* genomes

So far, all analyses were based on the annotated proteomes of the *Salmonella* genomes, but genes that code for RNA as the final product should not be ignored. A genome annotation would not be complete without its ribosomal RNA genes, coding for 5S, 16S and 23S RNA, as well as the tRNA genes. *Salmonella enterica* contains 7 *rrn* operons, which is more than can be found in many bacterial species but certainly is not a maximum, as some soil bacteria can contain up to 15 copies of the rRNA genes. The number of *rrn* copies of bacterial species has been related to their capacity to change their metabolism to use available resources [17]. Although it is often assumed that these gene duplications are all identical, in fact some degree of sequence variation can be observed, even within a genome. For *Salmonella*, it was reported that the gene encoding 16S rRNA (which is typically used for taxonomic description) is conserved for 97% only [18]. The gene coding for 23S rRNA is also not strictly conserved in *Salmonella*, as it contains both point mutations and indels [19].

The number of tRNA genes present in the *Salmonella* reference genome is 85, representing 47 different tRNA molecules that together cover the 40 required anticodons [20]. These numbers can vary between genomes and serovars. But these are not the only bacterial genes that are never translated into protein. In addition to essential RNA genes such as the gene coding for tmRNA (transfer-messenger RNA, required for correct protein translation), it is now recognized that bacterial genomes contain a large number of small RNA genes (sRNA) that are not always annotated. These are often involved in post-transcriptional regulation of gene expression [21]. As a final analysis, we decided to assess the conservation of these, incorrectly neglected, RNA genes.

The bioinformatic analysis performed was based on a publication where transcription start sites were identified from 31 *Salmonella* genomes [22]. We analyzed those 113 RNA genes in the 201 completely sequenced genomes. For this analysis, we excluded the nearly completed sequences that had been included in the analyses resulting in **Figures 2** and **5**, because genome assembly is biased toward protein-coding regions, so that regions on which sRNA genes may reside are likely to be missed, unless a genome is truly completed. For comparison, eight other *Enterobacteriaceae* were included. The results are presented in a matrix heat map (**Figure 7**). Based on their sRNA content, most of the genomes neatly clustered according to their serotype, with only few exceptions. Interestingly, the genomes of strains FORC-015 and FORC-020, which are annotated as Typhimurium, are placed outside the Typhimurium cluster in **Figure 7**, and these were also placed outside the main Typhimurium cluster in the AAI tree of **Figure 2**. Thus, it can be questioned if the serotype of these two strains was correctly identified. That most of the *Salmonella* genomes are nicely clustered according to their serotype in **Figure 7** is surprising, as the nonprotein coding sRNA genes analyzed here do not have a specific role in expression of surface antigens. The correlation identified here is in line with a publication that sRNA genes can be used as targets for serotype-specific PCR detection of Typhi and Paratyphi [23]. It was recently described that some sRNA genes of *S.* Typhimurium are under regulation of Sigma 28, and there is extensive cross talk between genes of the *Salmonella* pathogenicity pathways SPI1 and SPI2 and particular sRNA genes [24]. In this context, it is surprising that the sRNA genes are so strongly conserved throughout the *Salmonella* genomes (illustrated by the dominant red in **Figure 7**), whereas the presence of SPIs widely varies across serotypes [24]. This suggests that sRNA genes are strongly conserved and may well belong to the collection of essential genes, though this has not yet been experimentally demonstrated. The analysis further showed that the sRNA genes are specific for the *Salmonella* genus, and bear relatively little resemblance with the other *Enterobacteriacea* members included at the bottom of the figure.

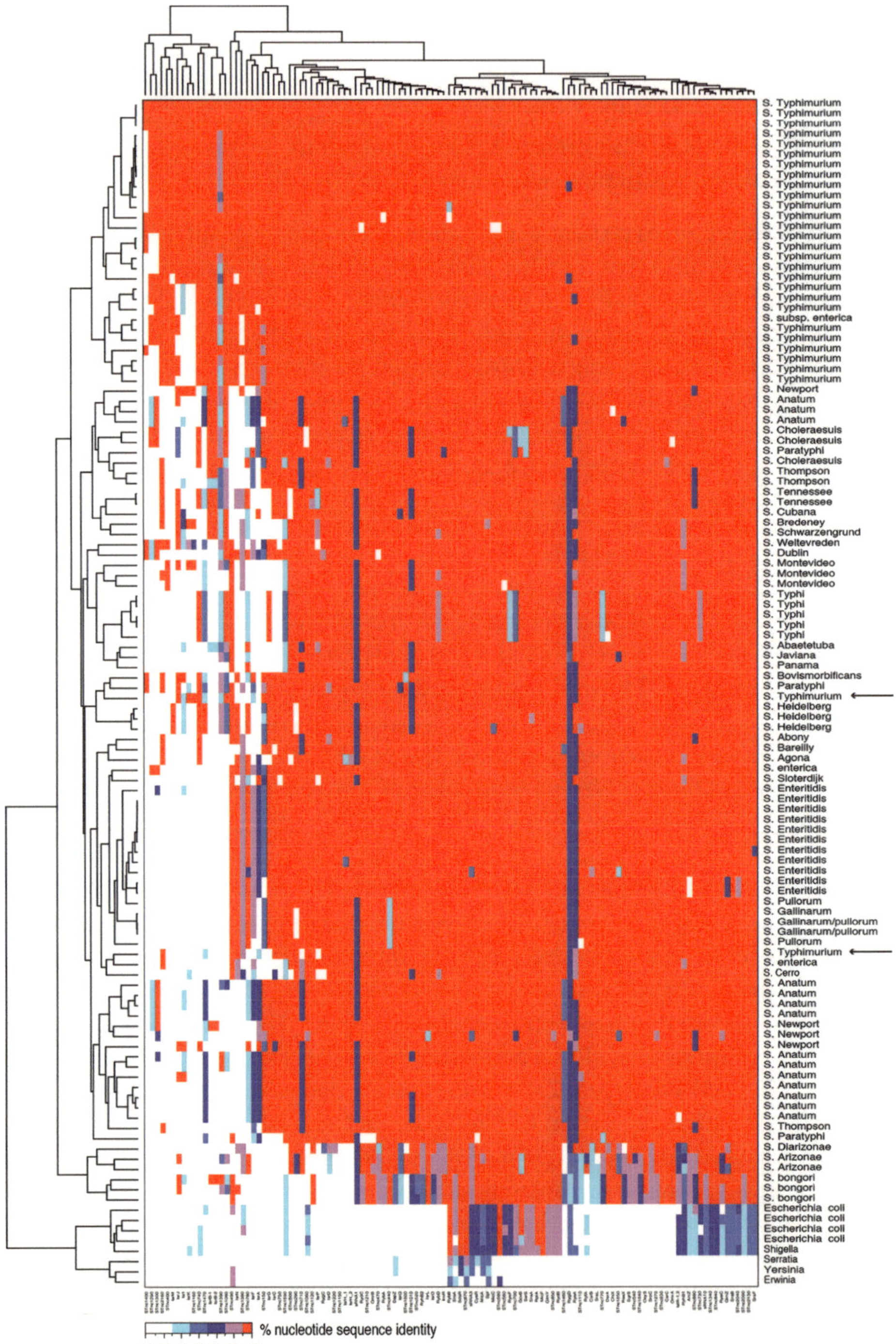

Figure 7. Conserved sRNAs across 201 *Salmonella* genomes. The tree to the left mostly clusters serotypes together, based on their sRNA genes. Two wrongly placed *S.* Typhimurium genomes are pointed out by the arrows to the right. The tree at the top identifies clusters of related sRNA genes. The eight genomes at the bottom are from other *Enterobacteriaceae*.

3. Conclusions

Based on genomic average amino acid identity (AAI), *Salmonella* genomes appear as a distinct clade within the enterics, closely related to the *Citrobacter* genus. The serovars of *S. enterica* subsp. *enterica* generally cluster together when analyzed for AAI. There is a stable core set of about 3400 gene families, found in nearly all *Salmonella enterica* genomes, and these genes are on average 99% or more identical to each other across all the *Salmonella* genomes. Further, many of these genes seem to be involved in metabolic processes, and the core genes account for about 80% of the total genes of the *Salmonella* genome-scale metabolic model. Finally, we examined small RNA conservation and found the same clustering of outlier genomes (e.g., particular *S.* Typhimurium strains) that were observed in the AAI analysis.

Acknowledgements

This work has been funded in part by The Arkansas Research Alliance and UAMS.

Author details

Trudy M. Wassenaar[1*], Se-Ran Jun[2], Visanu Wanchai[2], Preecha Patumcharoenpol[2], Intawat Nookaew[2], Katrina Schlum[3], Michael R. Leuze[3] and David W. Ussery[2]

*Address all correspondence to: trudy@mmgc.eu

1 Molecular Microbiology and Genomics Consultants, Zotzenheim, Germany

2 Department of BioMedical Informatics, University of Arkansas for Medical Sciences, Little Rock, AR, USA

3 Computing Science and Mathematics Division, Oak Ridge National Labs, Oak Ridge, Tennessee, USA

References

[1] Dekker JP, Frank KM. *Salmonella, Shigella* and *Yersinia*. Clin Lab Med. 2015;**35**:225–246. doi:10.1016/j.cll.2015.02.002

[2] Crosa JH, Brenner DJ, Ewing WH, Falkow S. Molecular relationships among the *Salmonelleae*. J Bacteriol. 1973;**115**:307–315.

[3] International Committee on Systematics of Prokaryotes. The type species of the genus *Salmonella Lignieres* 1900 is *Salmonella enterica* (ex Kauffmann and Edwards 1952) Le Minor and Popoff 1987, with the type strain LT2T and conservation of the epithet *enterica* in *Salmonella enterica* over all earlier epithets that may be applied to this species. Opinion 80. Int J Syst Evol Microbiol. 2005;**55**:519–520. doi:10.1099/ijs.0.63579-0

[4] Konstantinidis KT, Tiedje JM. Towards a genome-based taxonomy for prokaryotes. J Bacteriol. 2005;**187**:6258–6264. doi:10.1128/JB.187.18.6258-6264.2005

[5] Retchless AC, Lawrence JG. Phylogenetic incongruence arising from fragmented speciation in enteric bacteria. Proc Natl Acad Sci USA. 2010;**107**:11453–11458. doi:10.1073/pnas.1001291107

[6] Foley SL, Johnson TJ, Ricke SC, Nayak R, Danzeisen J. *Salmonella* pathogenicity and host adaptation in chicken-associated serovars. Microbiol Mol Biol Rev. 2013;**77**:582–607. doi:10.1128/MMBR.00015-13

[7] Knuth K, Niesalla H, Hueck CJ, Fuchs TM. Large-scale identification of essential *Salmonella* genes by trapping lethal insertions. Mol Microbiol. 2004;**51**:1729–1744.

[8] Hidalgo AA, Trombert AN, Castro-Alonso JC, Santiviago CA, Tesser BR, Youderian P, Mora GC. Insertions of mini-Tn10 transposon T-POP in *Salmonella enterica* sv. typhi. Genetics. 2004;**167**:1069–1077. doi:10.1534/genetics.104.026682

[9] Langridge GC, Phan MD, Turner DJ, Perkins TT, Parts L, Haase J, Charles I, Maskell DJ, Peters SE, Dougan G, Wain J, Parkhill J, Turner AK. Simultaneous assay of every *Salmonella* Typhi gene using one million transposon mutants. Genome Res. 2009; **19**:2308–2316. doi:10.1101/gr.097097.109

[10] Khatiwara A, Jiang T, Sung SS, Dawoud T, Kim JN, Bhattacharya D, Kim HB, Ricke SC, Kwon YM. Genome scanning for conditionally essential genes in *Salmonella enterica* Serotype Typhimurium. Appl Environ Microbiol. 2012;**78**:3098–3107. doi:10.1128/AEM.06865-11

[11] Canals R, Xia XQ, Fronick C, Clifton SW, Ahmer BM, Andrews-Polymenis HL, Porwollik S, McClelland M. High-throughput comparison of gene fitness among related bacteria. BMC Genomics. 2012;**13**:212. doi:10.1186/1471-2164-13-212

[12] Barquist L, Langridge GC, Turner DJ, Phan MD, Turner AK, Bateman A, Parkhill J, Wain J, Gardner PP. A comparison of dense transposon insertion libraries in the *Salmonella* serovars Typhi and Typhimurium. Nucleic Acids Res; 2013;**41**:4549–4564. doi:10.1093/nar/gkt148

[13] Thiele I, Hyduke DR, Steeb B, Fankam G, Allen DK, Bazzani S, Charusanti P, Chen FC, Fleming RM, Hsiung CA, De Keersmaecker SC, Liao YC, Marchal K, Mo ML, Özdemir E, Raghunathan A, Reed JL, Shin SI, Sigurbjörnsdóttir S, Steinmann J, Sudarsan S, Swainston N, Thijs IM, Zengler K, Palsson BO, Adkins JN, Bumann D. A community effort towards a knowledge-base and mathematical model of the human pathogen *Salmonella Typhimurium* LT2. BMC Syst Biol. 2011;**5**:8. doi:10.1186/1752-0509-5-8

[14] Santiviago CA, Reynolds MM, Porwollik S, Choi SH, Long F, Andrews-Polymenis HL, McClelland M. Analysis of pools of targeted *Salmonella* deletion mutants identifies novel genes affecting fitness during competitive infection in mice. PLoS Pathog. 2009;**5**(7):e1000477. doi:10.1371/journal.ppat.1000477

[15] Edgar RC. Search and clustering orders of magnitude faster than BLAST. Bioinformatics. 2010;**26**:2460–2461. doi:10.1093/bioinformatics/btq461

[16] Land M, Hauser L, Jun SR, Nookaew I, Leuze MR, Ahn TH, Karpinets T, Lund O, Kora G, Wassenaar T, Poudel S, Ussery DW. Insights from 20 years of bacterial genome sequencing. Funct Integr Genomics. 2015;**15**:141–161. doi:10.1007/s10142-015-0433-4

[17] Klappenbach JA, Dunbar JM, Schmidt TM. rRNA operon copy number reflects ecological strategies of bacteria. Appl Environ Microbiol. 2000;**66**:1328–1333.

[18] Větrovský T, Baldrian P. The variability of the 16S rRNA gene in bacterial genomes and its consequences for bacterial community analyses. PLoS One. 2013;**8**(2):e57923. doi:10.1371/journal.pone.0057923

[19] Pei A, Nossa CW, Chokshi P, Blaser MJ, Yang L, Rosmarin DM, Pei Z. Diversity of 23S rRNA genes within individual prokaryotic genomes. PLoS One 2009;**4**(5):e5437. doi:10.1371/journal.pone.0005437

[20] Withers M, Wernisch L, dos Reis M. Archaeology and evolution of transfer RNA genes in the *Escherichia coli* genome. RNA. 2006;**12**:933–942. doi:10.1261/rna.2272306

[21] Papenfort K, Vogel J. Regulatory RNA in bacterial pathogens. Cell Host Microbe. 2010;**8**:116–127. doi:10.1016/j.chom.2010.06.008

[22] Kröger C, Dillon SC, Cameron AD, Papenfort K, Sivasankaran SK, Hokamp K, Chao Y, Sittka A, Hébrard M, Händler K, Colgan A, Leekitcharoenphon P, Langridge GC, Lohan AJ, Loftus B, Lucchini S, Ussery DW, Dorman CJ, Thomson NR, Vogel J, Hinton JC. The transcriptional landscape and small RNAs of *Salmonella enterica* serovar Typhimurium. Proc Natl Acad Sci USA. 2012;**109**:1277–1286. doi:10.1073/pnas.1201061109

[23] Nithya R, Ahmed SA, Hoe CH, Gopinath SC, Citartan M, Chinni SV, Lee LP, Rozhdestvensky TS, Tang TH. Non-protein coding RNA genes as the novel diagnostic markers for the discrimination of *Salmonella* species using PCR. PLoS One. 2015;**10**(3):e0118668. doi:10.1371/journal.pone.0118668

[24] Blondel CJ, Jiménez JC, Contreras I, Santiviago CA. Comparative genomic analysis uncovers 3 novel loci encoding type six secretion systems differentially distributed in *Salmonella* serotypes. BMC Genomics. 2009;**10**:354. doi:10.1186/1471-2164-10-354

Computational Identification of Indispensable Virulence Proteins of *Salmonella* Typhi CT18

Shrikant Pawar, Izhar Ashraf,
Kondamudi Manobhai Mehata and
Chandrajit Lahiri

Additional information is available at the end of the chapter

http://dx.doi.org/10.5772/66489

Abstract

Typhoid infections have become an alarming concern with the increase of multidrug resistant strains of *Salmonella* serovars. The new pathogenic Gram-negative strains are resistant to most antibiotics such as chloramphenicol, ampicillin, trimethoprim, ciprofloxacin and even co-trimoxazole and their derivatives thereby causing numerous outbreaks in the Indian subcontinent, Southeast Asian and African countries. Conventional and modern methods of typing had been adopted to differentiate outbreak strains. However, identifying the most indispensable proteins from the complete set of proteins of the whole genome of *Salmonella* sp., comprising the *Salmonella* pathogenicity islands (SPI) responsible for virulence, has remained an ever challenging task. We have adopted a network-based method to figure out, albeit theoretically, the most significant proteins which might be involved in the resistance to antibiotics of the *Salmonella* sp. An understanding of the above will provide insight into conditions that are encountered by this pathogen during the course of infection, which will further contribute in identifying new targets for antimicrobial agents.

Keywords: *Salmonella*, *Salmonella* pathogenicity island, SicA, eigen vector centrality, k-core analysis

1. Introduction

Food-borne infections are quite common and widely distributed worldwide, though there can be several sources of such diseases. Human Salmonellosis or typhoid, causing systemic infection of the human gastrointestinal tract and diarrhoea, is one such common disease caused by *Salmonella enterica* serovar Typhi. With a prevalence of probably 10 millions of cases and hundreds of thousands of deaths every year [1], the disease has turned out to be a major cause for concern with the emergence of multidrug-resistant (MDR) *Salmonella* strains [2]. Such new strains are resistant to chloramphenicol, ampicillin, trimethoprim, ciprofloxacin and even co-trimoxazole and their derivatives, thereby causing numerous outbreaks in the Indian subcontinent, Southeast Asian and African countries [3, 4]. Thus, newer drugs like cephalosporins and quinolone derivatives needed to be explored to combat the situation [5].

To deal with the threats of multidrug resistance, several health intervention strategies have been undertaken. However, the prospects for finding new antibiotics for several classes of Gram-negative pathogens are especially poor due to the blockades provided by their outer membrane to the entry of some existing antibiotics and expulsion of many of the remainder by their efflux pumps [6]. It has become imperative that the conventional strategies for dealing with such pathogens are less effective or even at times, ineffective completely, to emerge victorious against the strategies for the war waged out by them. In such cases, the complexities posed can be solved by adopting some non-conventional approaches of finding the drug targets for these pathogens. Proteins, being the functional unit of the cell of any living organism, have always been good targets for combating diseases. Diseases, on the other hand, serve as interesting examples of complex protein interactions among several other heterogeneous entities of and between organisms. However, understanding the complexity of such interacting protein partners, especially with respect to the combat against the pathogens, has always been elusive. Thus, analyses of the mosaic mesh or network of interacting proteins, commonly known as protein interaction networks (PINs) can provide sufficient insight to reveal the indispensable virulent proteins for valuable drug targets [7].

Analyses of a PIN, to highlight important and/or indispensable proteins, can be as simple as centrality measurements with respect to the biological scenario. These can start by determining the number of interacting partners of a particular protein to identify its *degree* centrality (DC) which correlates with its biological importance. Thus, high-degree proteins (or hubs) are known to correspond to proteins that are essential [8]. As a protein can be affected locally while interacting with its other partners in the global network, other centrality measures are also given importance based on their relevance. Thus, we have discussed the importance of the measures like *closeness centrality* (CC), *betweenness centrality* (BC) and *eigenvector centrality* (EC) [8] parameters for PIN comprising the *Salmonella* pathogenicity islands (SPI) harbouring the specialized virulent proteins characterized by the type III secretion system (T3SS) among others. Till date, 17 such discrete sets have been reported for *S. Typhi* [9] along with the five SPI (1 till 5) characterized experimentally [10] among which SicA has been identified as the indispensable one in the phylogenetically closest neighbour, *S. enterica* serovar Typhimurium strain LT2 [11].

Again, extracting knowledge of the most indispensable virulence proteins from among the stipulated sets of SPI proteins could be quite insufficient. Thus, we have carried out further analyses of the whole genome of S. Typhi CT18 encompassing the decomposition of the whole genome protein interactome to a core of highly interacting proteins through the k-core analysis approach [12]. We have performed cartographic analyses further to identify the functional modules in the network [13] and predicted the indispensability of certain sets of proteins, which have been shown to be sharing similar functional modules empirically important for drug targets.

2. Approach

2.1. Dataset collection

Proteins for 17 *Salmonella* pathogenicity islands (SPIs) were collected from an in silico study of SPI for *S. enterica* serovar Typhi strain CT18 [9]. The locus tag of all the proteins of SPI for *S*. Typhi CT18 was fed as queries to the STRING 10.0 biological meta-database [14] to get all the possible interactions of a particular protein (date and time of access: Jul 28 2016 13:07:15). Detailed protein links file under the accession number 220341 in STRING was used to collect all the interactions of the whole genome proteins of *S*. Typhi.

The number of proteins from the different genomic islands starting from SPI-1 till -13 and -15 till -18 were 54, 43, 8, 7, 10, 55, 144, 12, 4, 23, 16, 4, 14, 9, 7, 2 and 97, respectively, with all the combined SPI amounting to a total of 502. The total number of protein interactions obtained from STRING v10 were 334, 339, 3, 21, 9, 192, 1193, 12, 6, 69, 19, 1, 19, 5, 3, 1, 343, for the 17 SPI loci mentioned above and 2570 interactions for all of these combined together. The whole genome of *S*. Typhi had 1041274 interaction information arising out of 4529 unique proteins.

2.2. Interactome construction

All individual protein interaction data, with medium confidence values obtained by default from String 10.0, were imported into Cytoscape version 3.3.0 [15] to integrate and build the interactomes of network comprising SPI-1 till -13 and -15 till -18, individually and all these 17 SPI collectively (AS). The interaction information, weighted by their strength as per STRING, of all the proteins of *S*. Typhi genome was imported into Gephi 0.9.1 [16] to construct and visualize the interactome of the whole genome. An interactome of proteins can be perceived as the protein interaction network (PIN) and can be represented as an undirected graph $G = (V, E)$ consisting of a finite set of V vertices (or nodes) and E edges. An edge $e = (u, v)$ connects two vertices (nodes) u and v. Each protein in the above PIN is represented as a vertex/node. The number of connections/interactions/associations/links a node has with other nodes comprises its degree $d(v)$ [17].

2.3. Network analyses

2.3.1. SPI-PIN

All the interactomes of SPI-PIN have been viewed by Cytoscape version 3.3.0 in the form of graphs of aforementioned interconnected proteins. The networks were subsequently analysed via the Cytoscape integrated java plugin CytoNCA [18] to compute values for the network centrality parameters namely EC, DC, CC and BC. Combined scores from different parameters considered in STRING were taken as edge weights for computing CytoNCA scores. Top 20 proteins for each of the centrality measures were taken for drawing Venn diagrams to find common proteins from each measure.

2.3.2. WhoG-PIN

As few (21) nodes out of the whole genome were isolated from the major part of network, these were considered to have less impact on the overall topology and thus ignored. Further analyses were based on the large connected component (LCC) of network comprising 4508 protein partners having 1041182 interactions. The analytical study has been done by using MATLAB version 7.11, a programming language developed by MathWorks [19].

For the primary understanding of the network, the distributions of network degree (k) were plotted by Complementary Cumulative Distribution Function (CCDF). To extract significant information from the topology of the large and complex Whole Genome Protein Interaction Network (WhoG-PIN), knowledge of the role of each protein was derived from the cartographic representation of within-module degree z-score of the protein versus its participation coefficient as per the methodology described by Guimera et al. [20]. Participation of each protein reflected its positioning within own module and with respect to other modules, where modules were calculated based on Rosvall method [21]. To have an idea of the core group of the very specific proteins which might have variety of role to play in the whole genome context, a k-core analysis was performed following the network decomposition (pruning) techniques to produce a sequence of subgraph of gradually increasing cohesion [12].

3. Features of the 17 SPIs

The virulence proteins of *Salmonella* are spread across the 17 *Salmonella* pathogenicity islands (SPIs) in *S.* Typhi as implied by Ong et al. [9]. Among these, five have been well characterized and reported to have SicA as the most indispensable one as identified computationally by Lahiri et al. [11]. A detailed insight into these SPI proteins would reveal SPI-1 and -2 to encode the proteins of the type III secretion systems (T3SSs), while SPI-4 encodes those of type I secretion system (T1SS) mediated by a giant non-fimbrial adhesin, which is co-regulated by the invasion genes encoded by the SPI-1 [22]. The *sit* gene cluster proteins of SPI-1 T3SS, encoding an iron uptake system, are involved in the invasion into the eukaryotic host non-phagocytic cells mediated by the delivery of effectors that directly engage host cell signalling pathways [10]. For the systemic phase of infection, proteins of the SPI-2 cluster are essential for the survival and replication in eukaryotic host cells [23], which are aided by the high-affinity magnesium uptake system encoded by *mgtCB*, harboured by SPI-3 [24]. The effector proteins of enteropathogenesis are harboured by SPI-5 and are induced by distinct regulatory cues and targeted to different TTSS, namely, SopB, secreted by SPI1 T3SS and PipB, translocated by SPI-2 T3SS to the *Salmonella*-containing vacuole and *Salmonella*-induced filaments.

The 59 kb SPI-6 consists of a type VI secretion system (T6SS), the *safABCD* fimbrial gene cluster, the invasin *pagN*, two pseudogenes as transposase remnants (*STY0343* and *STY0344*), the fimbrial operon *tcfABCD* and the genes *tinR* and *tioA* [25–29]. The largest SPI identified till date is that of SPI-7 with 134 kb size [25, 30, 31] and 150 genes inserted between duplicated *pheU* tRNA sequences [30, 32] containing the Vi capsule biosynthesis genes [33], a type IVB pilus operon [34] and the *SopE* prophage (*ST44*) [35]. SPI-9 is a 16 kb locus containing three genes encoding for a T1SS and one for a large protein [36]. SPI-10 is an island found next to the *leuX* tRNA gene at centisome 93. It is a 33 kb fragment [25] carrying a full P4-related prophage, termed *ST46* [37–39]. ST46 harbours the *prpZ* cluster as cargo genes encoding eukaryotic-type Ser/Thr protein kinases and phosphatases involved in *S.* Typhi survival in macrophages [40]. SPI-11 is a 10 kb fragment in *S.* Typhi and includes phoP-activated genes *pagD* and *pagC* involved in intramacrophage survival [41, 42]. The 6.3 kb SPI-12 contains the effector *SspH2* [43] along with the three ORFs are pseudogenes (*STY2466a, STY2468* and *STY2469*). SPI-13 was initially identified in serovar Gallinarum [44]. In *S.* Typhi, it is a 25-kb gene cluster found next to the *pheV* tRNA gene on centrosome 67. The 8-kb portion of this island corresponds to SPI-8 whose virulence function is unknown, and it harbours two bacteriocin immunity proteins (*STY3281* and *STY3283*) and four pseudogenes [25]. SPI-14 is absent in *S.* Typhi [36, 44]. SPI-15 in *S.* Typhi is a 6.5 kb island of five ORFs encoding hypothetical proteins [44]. SPI-16 is a 4.5 kb fragment inserted next to an *argU* tRNA site, and encodes five or seven Open reading frames (ORFs), four of which are pseudogenes, the three remaining ORFs show a high level of identity with P22 phage genes involved in seroconversion [45]. SPI-17 is a 5-kb island encoding six ORFs inserted next to an *argW* tRNA site [45]. SPI-18 was recently identified in *S.* Typhi as a 2.3 kb fragment harbouring only two ORFs: *STY1498* (*clyA*) and *STY1499* [46] of which the former encodes a 34 kDa pore-forming secreted cytolysin [46, 47].

4. The individual and the combined SPI-PINs

To focus upon the most indispensable proteins of the highly complex virulent phenotype as that of *Salmonella*, an integrated picture comprising the involvement of all the SPI and the connected associated proteins must be taken into account. Thus, with an ultimate goal to identify the indispensable virulent proteins for potential candidates of therapeutic targets, we have constructed the PINs or interactomes of the 17 individual SPI mentioned above, along with and a combined network of all of these SPI-PINs (AS). These were then analysed to identify the most important proteins among a group of highest number of interacting partners. This was done by utilizing the four important concepts of centrality applied to biological networks, namely eigenvector centrality (EC), degree centrality (DC), closeness centrality (CC) and betweenness centrality (BC) [48–50].

Amongst the four centrality measures being mentioned above, DC is the most basic as it brings out the involvement of the protein in a large number of interactions in a network. However, in a biological scenario of *Salmonella* infection, having the primary stages as attachment and invasion, the interactions of those proteins may not be in a sequential order so as to carry out a particular function as reflected through DC parametric analyses. In such cases, analyses of CC could be a good measure, which would reveal the close proximities of the proteins expected to communicate sequentially with other network proteins essential for a particular function. Again, a one-to-many type simultaneous interaction of a protein, rendering different functions, is imperative from the complexities of biological phenotype like virulence. Thus, the protein with a high proportion of interactions lying 'in between' and thereby connecting many other proteins in the network would be revealed through BC measures. This could have reflected to be quite an important protein, though it lacks the idea of connecting other important proteins in the network. EC measures the last concept and reflects the indispensable protein connecting other important proteins. A comparative picture of the parametric values of the top 20 rank holders in their descending order have been consolidated and put in a tabular form (**Table 1**). These rankers in either of the cases have the proteins reflected to be important.

There have been three clear trends observed across the topmost rankers of the SPI-PINs for the measures of DC, BC, CC and EC, respectively. In most of the cases, there is a unanimous decision for the top ranking protein showing its utmost importance nearing to indispensability. SPI-PINs of these categories are -1, -3, -4, -5, -7, -8, -9, -10 to -13 and -15 to -17. The other categories have either three or two of the centrality measures conforming to the unanimosity of the top ranking proteins. SPI-2, -18 and the all SPI (AS-PIN) have BC differing in the top ranking position whereas SPI-6 and -10 have segregation of DC and EC against CC and BC for the top ranking positions. The common top ranking proteins across these 17 SPI and the AS has been reflected in **Figure 1** with Venn diagrams.

It has been observed that with SPI-1, protein HilA is ranked highest. HilA is the central regulator in SPI-1, which activates the sip operon that is responsible in encoding secreted proteins, as well as the *inv/spa* and *prg* operons encoding components of the secretion apparatus [51, 52]. SPI-2 till -4 has all the secretion apparatus inner membrane proteins SsaG, FidL and STY4452 as the top rankers, respectively. Among the other top rankers, the inositol phosphate phosphatase, SopB, of SPI-5, an atypical fimbria chaperone protein SafB and ImpA-related N-family protein, STY0286, of SPI-6, the pilin protein, PilL, of SPI-7, bacteriocin immunity protein, STY3281, of SPI-8, a large repetitive protein with six Bacterial_Ig-like domains, t2643, of SPI-9, bacteriophage gene regulatory protein, STY4826, of SPI-10, cytolethal distending toxin protein, CdtB, of SPI-11, uronate isomerase, UxaC, of SPI-13 and the sensory histidine kinase protein, having role in motility and virulence, BarA, of SPI-18 are noteworthy.

With respect to the above analyses of the individual interactomes of the SPI, an idea about the importance of these proteins in their individual SPI and finally across all SPI could be obtained. However, for a drug to be effective, the indispensability issue of these proteins needs to be taken care of. Thus, a broader picture with respect to the whole genome proteins of *S.* Typhi is then delineated to address the concern.

SPI	Degree	Betweenness	Closeness	Eigenvector
1	hilA,iacP,invA,invE,invF, invG,prgH,prgI,prgK,sicA, sipA,sipB,sipC,sipD,spaL, spaO,spaQ,spaR,spaS,sptP,	hilA,invA,invE,invF,invG, prgH,prgI,prgJ,prgK,sicA, sipA,sipB,sipC,sipD,sirC, sitD,spaO,spaR,spaS,sptP,	hilA,invA,invE,invF,invG, prgH,prgI,prgJ,prgK,sicA, sipA,sipB,sipC,sipD,sirC, spaL,spaO,spaR,spaS,sptP,	hilA,iacP,invA,invE,invF, invG,prgH,prgK,sicA,sipA, sipB,sipC,sipD,spaK,spaL, spaO,spaQ,spaR,spaS,sptP,
2	ssaG, sscB, sscA,ssaJ,STY1710, STY1709,ssaL,ssaN,ssaQ,ssaU, ssaS,sseC,sseD,yscR,ssaD,ssaM, ssaT,ssaH,ssaV,ssaI,	ssrA,ssaQ,ttrR,ttrC,STY1710, STY1709,ssaG,sscB,sscA,ssaJ, sseC,ssaD,sseD,ssrB,spiA,ssaL, ssaN,ssaU,STY1730,ssaH,	ssaG,sscB,sscA,ssaJ,ssaQ,ssaN, STY1710,STY1709,ssaL,ssaU, ssaS,yscR,sseC,ssaD,sseD,ssaM, ssaT,ssrA,ssaH,ssaV,	ssaG,ssaJ,sscB,ssaL,sscA,ssaN,ssaS,ssaU,STY1710,STY 1709,ssaQ,yscR,ssaV,ssaT,sseD, ssaM,ssaH,sseC,ssaD,ssaI,
3	fidL,STY4039,slsA,rmbA,mgtC,mgtB,	fidL,STY4039,slsA,rmbA,mgtC,mgtB,	fidL,STY4039,slsA,rmbA,mgtC,mgtB,	fidL,STY4039,slsA,rmbA, mgtC,mgtB,
4	STY4452,STY4453,STY4458, STY4459,STY4460,STY4456, STY4457,	STY4452,STY4453,STY4458, STY4459,STY4460,STY4456, STY4457,	STY4452,STY4453,STY4458, STY4459,STY4460,STY4456, STY4457,	STY4452,STY4453,STY4458,STY4459,STY4460, STY4456, STY4457,
5	sopB,pipB,pipD,STY1124, STY1125,sigE,sicA,pipA,	sopB,pipB,pipD,STY1124, STY1125,sigE,sicA,pipA,	sopB,pipB,pipD,STY1124, STY1125,sigE,sicA,pipA,	sopB,pipB,pipD,STY1124, STY1125,sigE,sicA,pipA,
6	STY0286,STY0287,STY0288, STY0290,STY0291,STY0294, STY0297,STY0302,STY0303, STY0305,STY0313,STY0317, STY0319,STY0320,STY0321, STY0322,STY0323,STY0324, t2582,t2597,	safB,safC,STY0286,STY0294, STY0297,STY0302,STY0313, STY0314,STY0316,STY0317, STY0318,STY0319,STY0320, STY0321,STY0324,STY0352, tcfA,tcfC,tcfD,tinR,	safB,safC,STY0286,STY0287, STY0288,STY0290,STY0291, STY0294,STY0297,STY0302, STY0303,STY0305,STY0317, STY0319,STY0320,STY0321, STY0323,STY0324,t2582,t2597,	STY0286,STY0287,STY0288,STY0290,STY0291, STY0292, STY0294,STY0297,STY0302,STY0303,STY0305, STY0306, STY0307,STY0319,STY0320,STY0321,STY0323, STY0324, t2582,t2597,
7	pilL,STY4521,STY4523, STY4526,STY4528,STY4530, STY4534,STY4562,STY4564, STY4569,STY4571,STY4572, STY4573,STY4575,STY4576, STY4577,STY4579,STY4665, STY4666,t4268,	pilL,pilV,STY4521,STY4523, STY4526,STY4530,STY4561, STY4586,STY4592,STY4618, STY4622,STY4644,STY4645, STY4658,STY4664,STY4666, STY4676,STY4678,t4317, tviD,	pilL,STY4521,STY4523, STY4528,STY4530,STY4534, STY4561,STY4562,STY4564, STY4569,STY4571,STY4572, STY4573,STY4575,STY4576, STY4577,STY4586,STY4665, STY4666,t4268,	pilL,STY4521,STY4523, STY4528,STY4558,STY4559,STY4562,STY4563, STY4564, STY4568,STY4569,STY4571,STY4572,STY4573, STY4575, STY4576,STY4577,STY4579,STY4665,t4268,
8	STY3281,STY3277,STY3278, STY3279,STY3283,STY3287, STY3289,STY3288,STY3285, STY3290,STY3291,	STY3281,STY3277,STY3278, STY3279,STY3283,STY3287, STY3289,STY3288,STY3285, STY3290,STY3291,	STY3281,STY3277,STY3278, STY3279,STY3283,STY3287, STY3289,STY3288,STY3285, STY3290,STY3291,	STY3281,STY3277,STY3278,STY3279, STY3283,STY3287, STY3289,STY3288,STY3285,STY3290,STY3291,

SPI	Degree	Betweenness	Closeness	Eigenvector
9	t2643,STY2876,STY2877, STY2878,	t2643,STY2876,STY2877, STY2878,	t2643,STY2876,STY2877, STY2878,	t2643,STY2876,STY2877, STY2878,
10	STY4826,STY4832,STY4830, STY4822,STY4852,STY4821, STY4849,t4521,STY4834, STY4828,STY4833,STY4829, t2655,STY4851,STY4825, STY4827,STY4823,sefC,sefB,	STY4832,sefC,STY4826, STY4830,STY4843,STY4822, STY4849,STY4852,sefB, STY4821,t4521,STY4834, STY4828,STY4851,STY4833, STY4829,t2655,STY4825, STY4827,STY4823,	STY4832,STY4826,STY4830, STY4822,STY4821,STY4849, STY4834,STY4828,STY4852, t4521,sefC,STY4833,STY4829, t2655,sefB,STY4851,STY4825, STY4827,STY4823,STY4850,	STY4826,STY4830,STY4832,STY4822,STY4852, STY4821, STY4849,STY4834,t4521, STY4828,STY4851,STY4825,STY4827,STY4823, STY4833, STY4829,t2655,STY4850,sefC,sefB,
11	cdtB,pagC,envE,STY1879, STY1880,pagD,STY1889, STY1890,STY1891,cspH, msgA,STY1887,	cdtB,pagC,envE,STY1879, STY1880,pagD,STY1889, STY1890,STY1891,cspH, msgA,TY1887,	cdtB,pagC,envE,STY1879, STY1880,pagD,STY1889, STY1890,STY1891,cspH, msgA,STY1887,	cdtB,pagC,envE,STY1879, STY1880,pagD,STY1889, STY1890,STY1891,cspH, msgA,STY1887,
12	sspH2,STY2468,	sspH2,STY2468,	sspH2,STY2468,	sspH2,STY2468,
13	uxaC,ordL,STY3296,STY3294, STY3295,STY3298,STY3293, uxuA,uxuB,exuT,STY3302, STY3303,	uxaC,ordL,STY3296,STY3294, STY3295,STY3298,STY3293, uxuA,uxuB,exuT,STY3302, STY3303,	uxaC,ordL,STY3296,STY3294, STY3295,STY3298,STY3293, uxuA,uxuB,exuT,STY3302, STY3303,	uxaC,ordL,STY3296, STY3294,STY3295, STY3298,STY3293,uxuA, uxuB,exuT,STY3302, STY3303,
15	STY0605,gtrB,gtrA,STY3188, STY3189,STY3192,STY3193,	STY0605,gtrB,gtrA,STY3188, STY3189,STY3192,STY3193,	STY0605,gtrB,gtrA,STY3188, STY3189,STY3192,STY3193,	STY0605,gtrB,gtrA,STY3188,STY3189,STY3192, STY3193,
16	STY0605, gtrB, gtrA	STY0605, gtrB, gtrA	STY0605, gtrB, gtrA	STY0605, gtrB, gtrA
17	gtrA2,STY2629,	gtrA2,STY2629,	gtrA2,STY2629,	gtrA2,STY2629,
18	barA,cpxR,csrA,flag,flhA,flhB, fliA,fliF,fliH,fliJ,fliP,fliQ,fliR, fliZ,phoQ,rcsB,rcsC,rpoS, STY1297,yojN,	acrR,baeR,barA,clpP,csrA,dnaK, flag,fliA,hns,mgtA,mntH, ompF,phoQ,rcsB,rcsC,rpoN,rpoS,soxS, STY1297,STY1678,	barA,clpP,cpxR,csrA,dnaK,flag, fliA,groL,hns,ompR,phoB,phoQ, rcsB,rcsC,rpoN,rpoS,sirA, STY1297,STY1678,yojN,	barA,flag,flhA,flhB,flhD, fliA,fliF,fliH,fliI,fliJ,fliO, fliP,fliQ,fliR,fliZ,rcsB, rcsC,rpoS,STY1297,yojN,
All SPI	pilL,STY4521,STY4523, STY4526,STY4528,STY4530, STY4534,STY4562,STY4564, STY4569,STY4571,STY4572, STY4573,STY4575,STY4576, STY4577,STY4579,STY4665, STY4666,t4268,	barA,pilL,pilV,rpoS,sicA, STY4521,STY4523,STY4526, STY4561,STY4586,STY4592, STY4618,STY4622,STY4644, STY4645,STY4658,STY4664, STY4666,t4317,tviD,	pilL,STY4521,STY4523, STY4528,STY4530,STY4534, STY4561,STY4562,STY4564, STY4569,STY4571,STY4572, STY4573,STY4575,STY4576, STY4577,STY4586,STY4665, STY4666,t4268,	pilL,STY4521,STY4523, STY4528,STY4558,STY4559,STY4562,STY4563, STY4564, STY4568,STY4569,STY4571,STY4572,STY4573, STY4575, STY4576,STY4577,STY4579,STY4665,t4268,

Table 1. Details of the 17 groups of SPI proteins involved in the network.

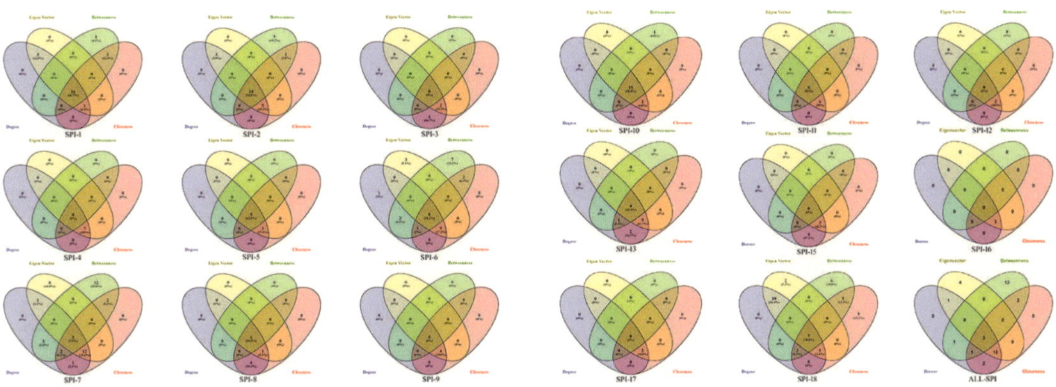

Figure 1. Venn diagram representation for the top rankers of DC, CC, BC and EC parametric analyses of 17 SPI-PINs and AS-PIN.

5. Feature of the WhoG-PIN

It is imperative that the WhoG-PIN, built from the empirical and theoretical results of physical and functional interactions among proteins laid down in STRING, can be random like that

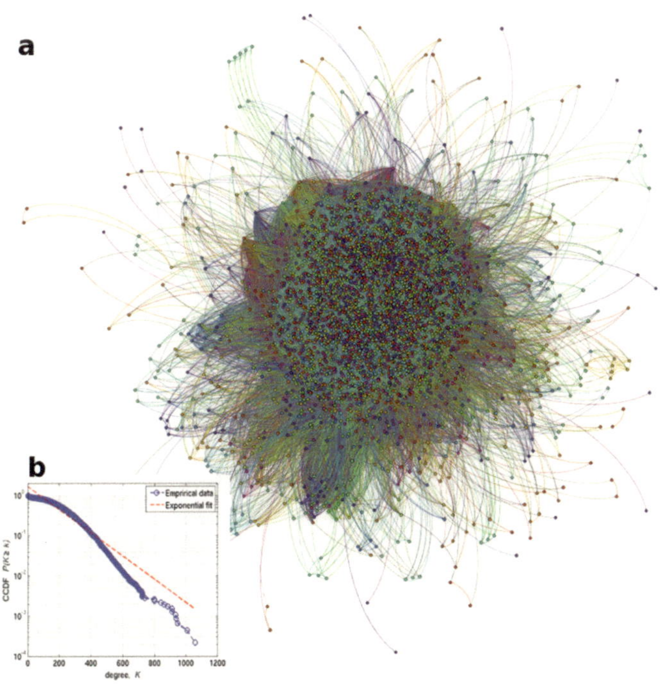

Figure 2. (a) Protein-protein interaction network of the whole genome of Salmonella Typhi CT18 with inset (b) showing degree distribution of the proteins from the large connected component.

proposed by Erdos and Renyi [53] or a small-world type proposed by Watts and Strogatz [54]. The idea was to see if the connectivity distribution, $P(k)$, of a node in a network getting connected to k other nodes, decays exponentially for large values of k. It was observed that the WhoG-PIN roughly follows the power law and is free of a characteristic scale [55] with a tailed degree distribution (**Figure 2**).

6. Decomposition of WhoG-PIN

In order to get an idea of the indispensable ones from the barrage of proteins involved in the individual SPI-PINs and AS, we have performed a k-core analysis for them. A k-core is a subgraph whose nodes have degree at least equal to k. Nodes which are part of k-core, but not in the k+1 core, is called, k-shell. This is able to classify the nodes (proteins, in our study) based on the variety of their interacting partners. Proteins, which belong to outer shell, have lower k value and thus reflect limited number of interacting partner proteins. Moreover, proteins, which belong to inner k-core/shell, are specific ones, highly interacting with each other and thus can be considered to be the most important ones. Decomposition of this core decomposes the network and thus makes this the innermost core.

After decomposition of the WhoG-PIN, we have obtained the inner core member proteins which are highly robust, central and thus highly interactive in nature [56]. We have arrived to the 154th core with a number of 2180 proteins (**Figure 3**; data not shown). An idea was to look in for the rank holder proteins of the AS-PIN obtained through the EC, DC, CC or BC measures. Interestingly, it was found that the top ranker PilL, across EC, DC and CC measures, belong to the 111th core and not the 154th core. On the contrary, the top ranking BC protein, BarA, was in the 154th core along with the closely ranked PilV in the 150th core. The only other protein, amongst the unanimous top rankers of AS-PIN, STY4521 had a position of 145 in k-core measures. Very strikingly, two proteins of BC top rankers were also in the 154th innermost core along with BarA. These were the RNA polymerase sigma factor, RpoS and the chaperone protein, SicA. On a note of comparison among the top ranking proteins of EC and BC analysed for AS-PIN, proteins of the latter group had higher ranks in the whole genome context, with STY4586, STY4644 and STY4664 having the same 154th innermost core measures. On the contrary, those from the former ranking group (EC) mostly moved around the core numbers 56–70. This reflected that proteins from the BC rankers were more important in their interaction with other proteins, forming a bridge amongst those and thereby rendering high betweenness.

In an earlier work by Lahiri et al., SicA was found to be in the group of innermost core of the interactome comprising the five most extensively worked out SPI of *S.* Typhimurium [11]. This core group had IacP, InvA, InvB, InvC, InvE, InvF, InvG, InvI, InvJ, OrgA, OrgB, OrgC, PrgH, PrgI, PrgJ, PrgK, SipA, SipB, SipC, SipD, SpaO, SpaQ, SpaS, SpiC, SptP, SsaJ, SseC, SseD and SseF as other members. Referring to the context of *S.* Typhi, IacP, InvE, invF, InvG, PrgK, SpaL (InvC in *S.*Typhimurium), SpaO, SpaS and SptP all shared the same innermost 154th core with a close contestant SsaJ in the 153rd core. Interestingly, all these proteins belong to the SPI-1 and SPI-2 group, which makes up the needle for injecting the virulence factors as delineated in the **Figure 4** of Lahiri et al. All these take us to the juncture where we

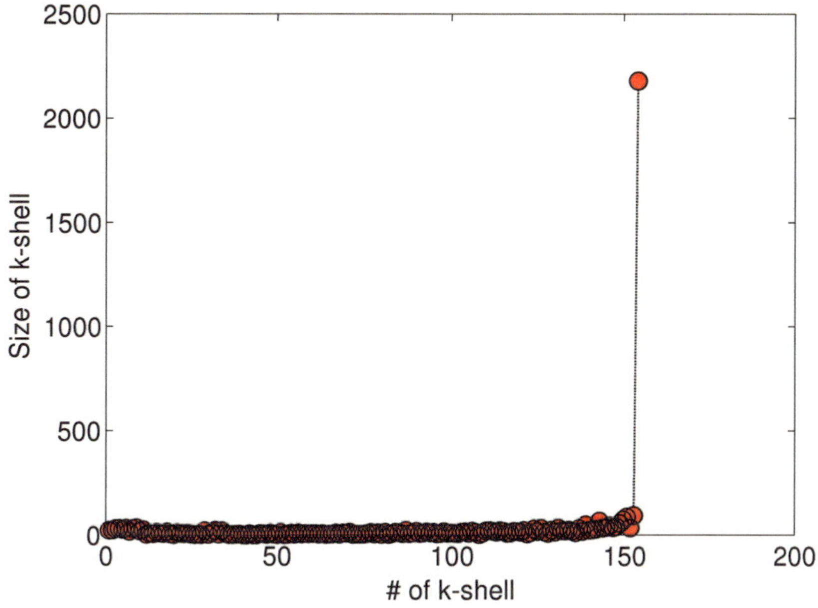

Figure 3. Distribution of the k-shell sizes for the set of proteins from the WhoG-PIN of *S*. Typhi CT18.

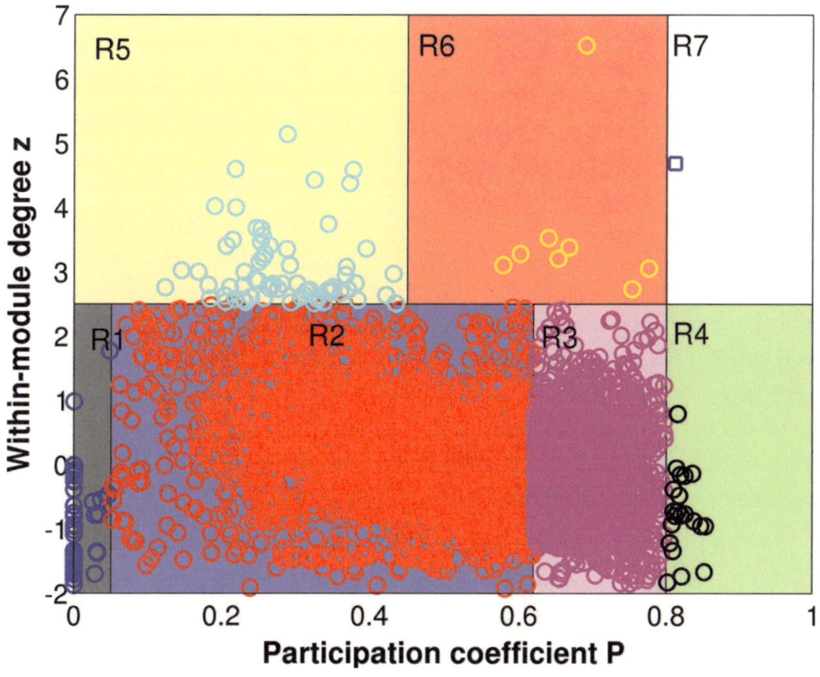

Figure 4. Cartographic representation for classification of proteins from the WhoG-PIN of *S*. Typhi CT18 based on its role and region in network space.

can foresee that the needle proteins are quite important virulence factors when it comes to search targets for drug. To top them all, SicA stands out as being one of the topmost rankers in BC measure of AS-PIN and in the innermost core of the WhoG-PIN. This is quite justified as SicA is a *Salmonella* type III secretion-associated invasin chaperone protein required for the stabilization of SipB and SipC to prevent their premature association which may lead to their targeting for degradation. Along with InvF, SicA is required for transcriptional activation of several virulence genes like *sigDE* (*sopB, pipC*), *sipBCDA* and *sopE*. [57].

7. Cartographic analyses of WhoG-PIN

For the purpose of classification of the proteins of *S*. Typhi CT18, based on their functional role and region in the network space, we have performed a cartographic analyses for the WhoG-PIN. As described earlier here, this is delineated by within module z-score of each node (protein) and its participation coefficient within and between other modules [20]. The within-module degree z-score measures how 'well connected' a node 'i' is to other nodes in the module, while the participation coefficient measures how the node 'i' is positioned in its own module and with respect to other modules. These measures are done based on the modules of the network, which are calculated by Rosval method [21]. The proteins are mainly divided into two major categories namely the hub nodes and the non-hub nodes.

As can be understood from the name itself, a hub is a connection point of many nodes. The category of non-hub nodes can be assigned four different roles namely, R1 comprising ultra-peripheral nodes, R2 of peripheral nodes, R3 of non-hub connector nodes and R4 having the non-hub kinless nodes. Likewise, the hub nodes can be assigned three different roles namely, R5 of provincial hubs, R6 of connector hubs and R7 of kinless hubs (**Figure 4**). The kinless hubs nodes are supposed to be important in terms of functionality, which has high connection within module as well as between modules. Accordingly, the ultra-peripheral nodes occupy the least connecting position in the network followed by the peripheral nodes. These nodes can be pruned easily without much affecting the whole network while decomposing it to reach the core (refer previous section for k-core). The non-hub connectors are expected to take part in only a small but fundamental set of interactions. This is just opposite to those of the provincial hubs class which have many within-module connections. The non-hub kinless nodes are those with links homogeneously distributed among all modules. The most conserved in terms of decomposition as well as evolution would be, however, those from the connector hubs with many links to most of the other modules. The system would try to retain these connections as essential ones for their very survival.

As can be perceived from the above classification of the connectors and the hubs, the proteins belonging to the R4, R6 and R7 role players are very crucial and can be regarded as potential drug targets. In the context of our WhoG-PIN, the only one R7 is a putative transposase, STY0115 and reminds of the Tn5 transposase, the enzyme that helps bacteria to share antibiotic resistance genes [58, 59]. This is closely followed by the plasmid transfer protein, TrhC

Protein name	R	Description of function
STY0115	7	Putative transposase
trhC	6	Plasmid transfer protein
gltB	6	Glutamate synthase (NADPH) large subunit
ptsG	6	PTS system glucose-specific transporter subunit IIBC
hemE	6	Uroporphyrinogen decarboxylase
nagE	6	PTS system N-acetylglucosamine-specific transporter subunit IIABC
STY3507	6	Aerobic respiration control sensor protein
t0287	6	PTS system sucrose-specific transporter subunit IIBC
treB	6	PTS system trehalose-specific transporter subunit IIBC
Cat	4	Chloramphenicol acetyltransferase
pspF	4	Phage shock protein operon transcriptional activator
STY4151	4	Acetyltransferase
STY4518	4	Acetyltransferase
STY4668	4	Hypothetical protein with Acetyltransf domain
STY4678	4	Integrase
STY4680	4	Integrase
STY0326	4	Hypothetical protein
STY3695	4	DNA-invertase
modB	4	Molybdenum transporter permease
STY4017	4	Putative transferase
modA	4	Periplasmic molybdenum-binding protein
sopE	4	Guanine nucleotide exchange factors
STY1020	4	Sequence-specific DNA binding
STY3193	4	Hypothetical protein
ugpB	4	Glycerol-3-phosphate-binding periplasmic protein
tviA	4	Flagellar regulator
hpaG	4	Isomerase/decarboxylase
STY4175	4	Hypothetical protein
ratA	4	CS54 island protein
livG	4	High-affinity branched-chain amino acid transport ATP-binding protein LivG
STY0352	4	Periplasmic protein

Table 2. Functions of the R4, R6 and R7 Proteins from the WhoG-PIN cartographic analysis.

in R6 group. This could very well play a good target for drugs as plasmids are known to be powerhouse of the antibiotic resistance genes [60]. Uncoupling of phosphotransferase system could also be an effective way of getting targets for novel drugs as exemplified by PtsG, TreB, NagE and t0287 [61]. Inhibition of glutamate Synthase, GltB has already been utilized as target for *Mycobacterium tuberculosis* [62] as has been uroporphyrinogen decarboxylase, HemE, *albeit* in a different context [63]. Recently, bacterial GCN5-related N-acetyltransferases of the R4 group have been thought of as essential drug targets as well [64]. All the functions of R7, R6 and R4 are listed in **Table 2**.

8. Conclusion

This work schematically delineates a process of figuring out the most indispensable protein in a system of interacting proteins of *S*. Typhi. It deals with the computational framework of building of the theoretical networks comprising the 17 individual SPI-PINs along with the AS-PIN followed by the conventional parametric approach of identifying the most interacting protein connected to other important proteins in the concerned phenotype of virulence. This is reinforced by the analysis of disintegrating the WhoG-PIN to the innermost core of the proteins, essential for virulence. All these lead to the identification of SicA to be the most indispensable one amongst a group of other virulent proteins being benefitted through network centrality and decomposition analyses. A further investigation of the WhoG-PIN brought forth the proteins of important conserved class, potential enough to be the most important ones and thus indispensable among the barrage of other proteins of the whole genome of *S*. Typhi CT18.

Acknowledgements

The authors wish to acknowledge the support of IMSc, Chennai and Dept. of Computer Applications at BSAU, Chennai for the provision of computational facilities. The personal contribution of Ong Su Yean for the SPI data and of Indrajeet Chakraborty for the formatting are highly appreciated and acknowledged.

Author contributions

CL conceived the concepts, planned and designed the analyses. SP and MIA contributed equally for producing the data analysed by CL. Artwork was done by MIA and SP. CL primarily wrote and edited the manuscript aided by additional help from SP, MIA and KMM.

Conflict of interest

The authors declare that they have no conflict of interest.

Author details

Shrikant Pawar[1#], Izhar Ashraf[2,3#], Kondamudi Manobhai Mehata and Chandrajit Lahiri[4*]

*Address all correspondence to: chandrajitl@sunway.edu.my

1 Department of Biology and Department of Computer Science, Georgia State University, Atlanta, GA, USA

2 The Institute of Mathematical Sciences, Chennai, India

3 B.S. Abdur Rahman University, Vandalur, Chennai, India

4 Department of Biological Sciences, Sunway University, Selangor, Malaysia

#These authors contributed equally to this work.

References

[1] Tacket CO, Levine MM. Human typhoid vaccines - old and new. In: DAA Ala'Aldeen, CE Hormaeche, eds. Molecular and Clinical Aspects of Bacterial Vaccine Development. England: John Wiley and Sons, 1995; 119–78.

[2] *Salmonella* (non-typhoidal) [Internet]. 2013. Available from: http://www.who.int/mediacentre/factsheets/fs139/en/ [Accessed: 2016-08-20].

[3] Rowe B, Ward LR, Threlfall EJ Multidrug-resistant *Salmonella* Typhi: a worldwide epidemic. Clinical Infectious Diseases. 1997; 24:S106–S109.

[4] Senthilkumar B, Prabakaran G. Multidrug resistant *Salmonella* typhi in asymptomatic typhoid carriers among food handlers in Namakkal district, Tamil Nadu. Indian Journal of Medical Microbiology. 2005; 23(2):92.

[5] Chitnis V, Chitnis D, Verma S, Hemvani N. Multidrug resistant *Salmonella* Typhi in India. The Lancet. 1999; 354:514–15.

[6] Eliopoulos GM, Maragakis LL, Perl TM. *Acinetobacter baumannii*: epidemiology, antimicrobial resistance, and treatment options. Clinical Infectious Diseases. 2008; 46(8): 1254–63.

[7] Pan A, Lahiri C, Rajendiran A, Shanmugham B. Computational analysis of protein interaction networks for infectious diseases. Briefings in Bioinformatics. 2016; 17(3):517–26.

[8] Jeong H, Mason SP, Barabási AL, Oltvai ZN. Lethality and centrality in protein networks. Nature. 2001; 411(6833):41–2.

[9] Ong SY, Fui Ling N, Siti SB, Anton Y, Maqsudul A. Analysis and construction of pathogenicity island regulatory pathways in *Salmonella enterica* serovar Typhi. Journal of Integrative Bioinformatics. 2010; 7(1):145.

[10] Schmidt H, Hensel M. Pathogenicity islands in bacterial pathogenesis. Clinical Microbiology Reviews. 2004; 17(1):14–56.

[11] Lahiri C, Pawar S, Sabarinathan R, Ashraf MI, Chand Y, Chakravortty D. Interactome analyses of *Salmonella* pathogenicity islands reveal SicA indispensable for virulence. Journal of Theoretical Biology. 2014; 363:188–97.

[12] Seidman SB. Network structure and minimum degree. Social Networks. 1983; 5(3):269–87.

[13] Guimera R, Amaral LA. Functional cartography of complex metabolic networks. Nature. 2005; 433(7028):895–900.

[14] Szklarczyk D, Franceschini A, Wyder S, Forslund K, Heller D, Huerta-Cepas J, Simonovic M, Roth A, Santos A, Tsafou KP, Kuhn M. STRING v10: protein–protein interaction networks, integrated over the tree of life. Nucleic Acids Research. 2014; 43(D1):D447–52.

[15] Shannon P, Markiel A, Ozier O, Baliga NS, Wang JT, Ramage D, Amin N, Schwikowski B, Ideker T. Cytoscape: a software environment for integrated models of biomolecular interaction networks. Genome Research. 2003; 13(11):2498–504.

[16] Bastian M, Heymann S, Jacomy M. Gephi: an open source software for exploring and manipulating networks. ICWSM. 2009; 8:361–2.

[17] Diestel R. Graph Theory. Berlin and Heidelberg: Springer-Verlag, 2000.

[18] Tang Y, Li M, Wang J, Pan Y, Wu FX. CytoNCA: a cytoscape plugin for centrality analysis and evaluation of protein interaction networks. Biosystems. 2015; 127:67–72.

[19] MATLAB and Statistics Toolbox Release. The MathWorks, Inc., Natick, Massachusetts, United States, 2010.

[20] Guimera R, Amaral LA. Cartography of complex networks: modules and universal roles. Journal of Statistical Mechanics: Theory and Experiment. 2005; (02):P02001.

[21] Rosvall M, Bergstrom CT. Multilevel compression of random walks on networks reveals hierarchical organization in large integrated systems. PloS ONE. 2011; 6(4):e18209.

[22] Gerlach RG, Jäckel D, Stecher B, Wagner C, Lupas A, Hardt WD, Hensel M. *Salmonella* Pathogenicity Island 4 encodes a giant non-fimbrial adhesin and the cognate type 1 secretion system. Cellular Microbiology. 2007; 9(7):1834–50.

[23] Hensel M. *Salmonella* pathogenicity island 2. Molecular Microbiology. 2000; 36(5):1015–23.

[24] Blanc-Potard AB, Solomon F, Kayser J, Groisman EA. The SPI-3 pathogenicity island of *Salmonella enterica*. Journal of Bacteriology. 1999; 181(3):998–1004.

[25] Parkhill J, Dougan G, James KD, Thomson NR, Pickard D, Wain J, Churcher C, Mungall KL, Bentley SD, Holden MT, Sebaihia M. Complete genome sequence of a multiple drug resistant *Salmonella enterica* serovar Typhi CT18. Nature. 2001; 413(6858):848–52.

[26] Lambert MA, Smith SG. The PagN protein of *Salmonella enterica* serovar Typhimurium is an adhesin and invasin. BMC Microbiology. 2008; 8(1):1.

[27] Folkesson A, Advani A, Sukupolvi S, Pfeifer JD, Normark S, Löfdahl S. Multiple insertions of fimbrial operons correlate with the evolution of *Salmonella* serovars responsible for human disease. Molecular Microbiology. 1999; 33(3):612–22.

[28] Townsend SM, Kramer NE, Edwards R, Baker S, Hamlin N, Simmonds M, Stevens K, Maloy S, Parkhill J, Dougan G, Bäumler AJ. *Salmonella enterica* serovar Typhi possesses a unique repertoire of fimbrial gene sequences. Infection and Immunity. 2001; 69(5):2894–901.

[29] Porwollik S, McClelland M. Lateral gene transfer in *Salmonella*. Microbes and Infection. 2003; 5(11):977–89.

[30] Pickard D, Wain J, Baker S, Line A, Chohan S, Fookes M, Barron A, Gaora PÓ, Chabalgoity JA, Thanky N, Scholes C. Composition, acquisition, and distribution of the Vi exopolysaccharide-encoding *Salmonella enterica* pathogenicity island SPI-7. Journal of Bacteriology. 2003; 185(17):5055–65.

[31] Bueno SM, Santiviago CA, Murillo AA, et al. Precise excision of the large pathogenicity island, SPI7, in *Salmonella enterica* serovar Typhi. Journal of Bacteriology. 2004; 186:3202–13.

[32] Hansen-Wester I, Hensel M. Genome-based identification of chromosomal regions specific for *Salmonella* spp. Infection and Immunity. 2002; 70(5):2351–60.

[33] Hashimoto Y, Li N, Yokoyama H, Ezaki T. Complete nucleotide sequence and molecular characterization of ViaB region encoding Vi antigen in *Salmonella* Typhi. Journal of Bacteriology. 1993; 175(14):4456–65.

[34] Zhang XL, Tsui IS, Yip CM, Fung AW, Wong DK, Dai X, Yang Y, Hackett J, Morris C. *Salmonella enterica* serovar Typhi uses type IVB pili to enter human intestinal epithelial cells. Infection and Immunity. 2000; 68(6):3067–73.

[35] Mirold S, Rabsch W, Rohde M, Stender S, Tschäpe H, Rüssmann H, Igwe E, Hardt WD. Isolation of a temperate bacteriophage encoding the type III effector protein SopE from an epidemic *Salmonella* Typhimurium strain. Proceedings of the National Academy of Sciences. 1999; 96(17):9845–50.

[36] Morgan E, Campbell JD, Rowe SC, Bispham J, Stevens MP, Bowen AJ, Barrow PA, Maskell DJ, Wallis TS. Identification of host-specific colonization factors of *Salmonella enterica* serovar Typhimurium. Molecular Microbiology. 2004; 54(4):994–1010.

[37] Edwards RA, Matlock BC, Heffernan BJ, Maloy SR. Genomic analysis and growth-phase-dependent regulation of the SEF14 fimbriae of *Salmonella enterica* serovar Enteritidis. Microbiology. 2001; 147(10):2705–15.

[38] Thomson N, Baker S, Pickard D, Fookes M, Anjum M, Hamlin N, Wain J, House D, Bhutta Z, Chan K, Falkow S. The role of prophage-like elements in the diversity of *Salmonella enterica* serovars. Journal of Molecular Biology. 2004; 339(2):279–300.

[39] Bishop AL, Baker S, Jenks S, Fookes M, Gaora PÓ, Pickard D, Anjum M, Farrar J, Hien TT, Ivens A, Dougan G. Analysis of the hypervariable region of the *Salmonella enterica* genome associated with tRNAleuX. Journal of Bacteriology. 2005; 187(7):2469–82.

[40] Faucher SP, Forest C, Beland M, Daigle F. A novel PhoP-regulated locus encoding the cytolysin ClyA and the secreted invasin TaiA of *Salmonella enterica* serovar Typhi is involved in virulence. Microbiology. 2009; 155(2):477–88.

[41] Miller SI, Kukral AM, Mekalanos JJ. A two-component regulatory system (phoP phoQ) controls *Salmonella* Typhimurium virulence. Proceedings of the National Academy of Sciences. 1989; 86(13):5054–8.

[42] Gunn JS, Alpuche-Aranda CM, Loomis WP, Belden WJ, Miller SI. Characterization of the *Salmonella* Typhimurium pagC/pagD chromosomal region. Journal of Bacteriology. 1995; 177(17):5040–7.

[43] Miao EA, Scherer CA, Tsolis RM, Kingsley RA, Adams LG, Bäumler AJ, Miller SI. *Salmonella* Typhimurium leucine-rich repeat proteins are targeted to the SPI1 and SPI2 type III secretion systems. Molecular Microbiology. 1999; 34(4):850–64.

[44] Shah DH, Lee MJ, Park JH, Lee JH, Eo SK, Kwon JT, Chae JS. Identification of *Salmonella* Gallinarum virulence genes in a chicken infection model using PCR-based signature-tagged mutagenesis. Microbiology. 2005; 151(12):3957–68.

[45] Vernikos GS, Parkhill J. Interpolated variable order motifs for identification of horizontally acquired DNA: revisiting the *Salmonella* pathogenicity islands. Bioinformatics. 2006; 22(18):2196–203.

[46] Fuentes JA, Villagra N, Castillo-Ruiz M, Mora GC. The *Salmonella* Typhi hlyE gene plays a role in invasion of cultured epithelial cells and its functional transfer to S. Typhimurium promotes deep organ infection in mice. Research in Microbiology. 2008; 159(4):279–87.

[47] Green J, Baldwin ML. The molecular basis for the differential regulation of the hlyE-encoded haemolysin of Escherichia coli by FNR and HlyX lies in the improved activating region 1 contact of HlyX. Microbiology. 1997; 143(12):3785–93.

[48] Koschützki D, Schreiber F. Comparison of centralities for biological networks. In: Griegerich, R. Stoye, J. (eds.) Proceedings of the German Conference on Bioinformatics (GCB2004), Lecture Notes in Informatics, 2004; P-53, pp.199–206.

[49] Özgür A, Vu T, Erkan G, Radev DR. Identifying gene-disease associations using centrality on a literature mined gene-interaction network. Bioinformatics. 2008; 24(13):i277–85.

[50] Pavlopoulos GA, Secrier M, Moschopoulos CN, Soldatos TG, Kossida S, Aerts J, Schneider R, Bagos PG. Using graph theory to analyze biological networks. BioData Mining. 2011; 4(1):1.

[51] Altier C. Genetic and environmental control of *Salmonella* invasion. Journal of Microbiology. 2005; 43(Spec No):85–92.

[52] Hueck CJ, Hantman MJ, Bajaj V, Johnston C, Lee CA, Miller SI. *Salmonella* Typhimurium secreted invasion determinants are homologous to Shigella lpa proteins. Molecular Microbiology. 1995; 18(3):479–90.

[53] Erdös P, Rényi A. On the evolution of random graphs. Publications of the Mathematical Institute of the Hungarian Academy of Sciences. 1960; 5:17–61.

[54] Watts DJ, Strogatz SH. Collective dynamics of 'small-world' networks. Nature. 1998; 393:440–2.

[55] Albert R, Jeong H, Barabasi AL. Error and attack tolerance of complex networks. Nature. 2000; 406:378–82.

[56] Alvarez-Hamelin I, Dall'Asta L, Barrat A, Vespignani A. Advances in Neural Information Processing Systems 18. Cambridge, MA: MIT Press, 2006; pp. 41–50.

[57] Darwin KH, Robinson LS, Miller VL. SigE is a chaperone for the *Salmonella enterica* serovar Typhimurium invasion protein SigD. Journal Bacteriology. 2001; 183:1452–4.

[58] Meredith TC, Wang H, Beaulieu P, Gründling A, Roemer T. Harnessing the power of transposon mutagenesis for antibacterial target identification and evaluation. Mobile Genetic Elements. 2012; 2(4):171–8.

[59] Devaud M, Kayser FH, Bächi B. Transposon-mediated multiple antibiotic resistance in Acinetobacter strains. Antimicrobial Agents Chemotherapy. 1982; 22(2):323–9.

[60] Williams JJ, Hergenrother PJ. Exposing plasmids as the Achilles' heel of drug-resistant bacteria. Current Opinion in Chemical Biology. 2008; 12(4):389–99.

[61] Garcia De Gonzalo CV, Denham EL, Mars RAT, Stülke J, van der Donk WA, van Dijl JM. The phosphoenolpyruvate:sugar phosphotransferase system is involved in sensitivity to the glucosylated bacteriocin sublancin. Antimicrobial Agents Chemotherapy. 2015; 59:6844–54.

[62] Mowbray SL, Kathiravan MK, Pandey AA, Odell LR. Inhibition of glutamine synthetase: a potential drug target in *Mycobacterium tuberculosis*. Molecules. 2014; 19:13161–76.

[63] Tsou Y-A, Chen K-C, Lin H-C, Chang S-S, Chen CY-C. Uroporphyrinogen decarboxylase as a potential target for specific components of traditional Chinese medicine: a virtual screening and molecular dynamics study. PLoS ONE. 2012; 7(11), e50087.

[64] Favrot L, Blanchard JS, Vergnolle O. Bacterial GCN5-related N-acetyltransferases: from resistance to regulation. Biochemistry. 2016; 55:989–1002.

Chapter 3

Salmonella enterica: Latency

Bianca Mendes Maciel, Rachel Passos Rezende and
Nammalwar Sriranganathan

Additional information is available at the end of the chapter

http://dx.doi.org/10.5772/67173

Abstract

Infection caused by more than 1500 serotypes of *Salmonella enterica* subsp. *enterica* is one of the most common food-borne diseases, prevalent worldwide. Concerning public health, *Salmonella* latent carrier animals represent an important source of transmission of the disease. They are responsible for silent introduction of the bacteria into the food chain and the environment. Most pathogenesis studies of salmonellosis are focused on events that lead to clinical disease. Researchers have been unable to clearly discern the interaction between intracellular microorganisms and their resistant hosts in latency. However, understanding this interaction is essential for the proper employment of the control and eradication strategies. Thus, the objective of this article is to present an overview of some important events that occur during the infection cycle of *S. enterica* in latent carriers.

Keywords: *Salmonella* asymptomatic carrier animals, pathogen-host interaction, pathogenisis, public health, intracellular bacteria

1. Introduction

The genus *Salmonella* belongs to family Enterobacteriaceae, and its classification follows the Kauffmann-White scheme, which groups serotypes according to their somatic, flagellar and capsular antigens. Serotyping is essential for investigation of outbreaks of salmonellosis, contributing to epidemiological surveillance. Currently, the genus consists of two species, *S. enterica* and *S. bongori*, the first being subdivided into six subspecies, which are designed by Roman numeral, containing more than 2500 antigenically distinct serotypes. Of these serotypes, around 1500 belong to *Salmonella enterica* subspecies *enterica (I)*, which colonizes the intestinal tract of warm-blooded animals and is responsible for 99% of *Salmonella* infections, while the others pertain to other subspecies: *salamae (II), arizonae (IIIa), diarizonae (IIIb), houtenae (IV)* and *indica (VI)*. Although *S. bongori* has been determined to be a separate species, it was originally designated as subspecies V, which is commonly found in cold-blooded animals and in the environment [1–3]. After serotyping by Kauffman-White scheme, characterization by pulsed-field gel electrophoresis (PFGE) pattern and phage typing provides further subtyping [3]. Eventually complete genome sequencing will be the norm as the cost of such analysis has come down basically replacing multiple-locus variable-number tandem repeat analysis (MLVA) [4].

Most outbreaks of salmonellosis in humans and in domestic animals are caused by a few serotypes, which are grouped according to their adaptation to the host. The first group consists of a few *host-specific serotypes*, which typically cause systemic disease in a single animal species or a limited number of phylogenetically-related species. Noteworthy examples are *S. enterica* serotype Typhi and Paratyphi of humans, serotypes Pullorum and Gallinarum of birds and serotype Abortusovis of sheep. The second group consists of *host-adapted serotypes* that are associated with one or two animal species that are related to each other; however, they may occasionally cause disease in other hosts. Noteworthy examples are *S. enterica* serotype Dublin and serotype Choleraesuis, which are usually associated with severe systemic disease in ruminants and pigs, respectively. Finally, the third group consists of a large numbers of *ubiquitous serotypes*, which typically cause gastroenteritis in a wide variety of unrelated host species;among these are *S. enterica* serotype Typhimurium and serotype Enteritidis [5], and these are the two most prevalent serotypes in the world [6].

Epidemiologically, infections caused by *Salmonella enterica* subsp. *enterica* correspond to the most prevalent disease transmitted via food worldwide. This high prevalence is associated with the absence of clinical disease in animals that often silently infect herds, contaminate food, the environment and thus cause disease in humans. However, historically, studies on the pathogenesis of salmonellosis are focused on events leading to clinical manifestations, and a few studies are conducted to clarify the interaction between latent microorganisms and their resistant hosts.

Certain animal species may develop asymptomatic persistent infection with intermittent shedding of *Salmonella* in their feces over long periods. These animals are called *latent carriers*. Their impact on public health is that the carriers are natural reservoirs of different *Salmonella* serotypes and may be resistance to multiple antimicrobials. Latent *Salmonella* infections can occur in humans [7], in farm animals such as cattle, sheep, pigs and poultry [5], in pets such as dogs [8] and in wild animals such as reptiles [9, 10].

Latent carrier animals are therefore natural reservoirs of *Salmonella* and are responsible for the silent intermittent introduction of the pathogen into the food chain and the environment, hindering control strategies. Thus, increasing our knowledge regarding the interaction of intracellular pathogen *Salmonella* with their host is essential for the development of an efficient strategy for control. In this mini-review, we present some important events that occur during the infection cycle of *S. enterica* leading to latent carriers, including the mechanisms of invasion of the host cells, bacterial multiplication and persistence in intracellular compartments, and intermittent shedding of the pathogen in the feces.

2. Pathogenesis of *Salmonella enterica*: the role of *Salmonella* pathogenicity islands (SPIs)

The pathogenesis of salmonellosis depends on a combination of several factors, including the components of bacterial virulence, the infective dose, route of infection, the genetic makeup and the immune status of the host [11]. All of these variables can influence the immunological responses of the host, resulting in different degrees of inflammation that confer an acute, moderate, chronic or even asymptomatic nature to the disease [12].

Infection by *S. enterica* has the following characteristics: the ability to interact with enterocytes leading to diarrhea (*Salmonella*-induced enteritis), the invasion of non-phagocytic cells and the ability to survive and proliferate within the phagocytes, resulting in systemic disease [13]. These characteristics are determined by multiple virulence factors encoded in *Salmonella* pathogenicity islands (SPIs) comprising large and unstable segments of the bacterial genome of pathogenic organisms. These SPIs are absent in related non-pathogenic organisms and that were acquired by horizontal gene transfer as SPIs G + C content is lower than *Salmonella* genes [14]. SPIs are conserved in several strains; differences may have implications in host specificity [15]. Currently, 16 pathogenicity island of *Salmonella* encoding distinct virulence factors are described, according to pathogenicity island database, PAI DB (http://www.paidb.re.kr), with different distributions among the various *Salmonella* species, subspecies and serotypes. SPI-1 and SPI-2 (both are about 40 kb in length) are the most studied and are present in all subspecies of *S. enterica* [13, 14, 16]. SPI-1 contains the genes responsible for the bacterial invasion of the host epithelium [17, 18], whereas SPI-2 is responsible for bacterial survival and multiplication within eukaryotic cells, including macrophages [19, 20].

Studies of SPIs help in understanding the mechanisms of bacterial virulence, and they may also be useful to clarify the phylogenetic relationships among species [21, 22]. Phylogenetic studies indicated that the gene sequences present in SPI-1 were acquired by lateral gene transfer before the diversification between *S. enterica* and *S. bongori*. In turn, the acquisition of the SPI-2 genes present in *S. enterica* occurred after speciation but before the diversification of the groups (I, II, IIIa, IIIb, IV, VI and VII); therefore, SPI-2 is present in all *S. enterica* subspecies but is absent in *S. bongori* species [22].

The virulence mechanisms of *Salmonella* serotypes are studied in different animal models, depending on the type of clinical manifestation. To study the pathogenesis of typhoid fever (a systemic disease), strains of susceptible mice (*e.g.*, Balb/c) experimentally infected with serotype Typhimurium are used. However, in this experimental model, the mice do not develop diarrhea, and therefore, mice are not used to study the pathogenesis of enteritis. In contrast, the experimental infection of calves with the same serotype results in enteric disease, and therefore, this experimental model is used to study *Salmonella*-induced enteritis [23].

According to the animal model, the virulence genes required for systemic infection differ from those genes responsible for the enteritis caused by *Salmonella*. This result is observed by analyzing mutant phenotypes of serotype Typhimurium in experimental infection of mice and calves, which are used to study systemic and enteric infections, respectively. Mutations in

SPI-2 result in a significant attenuation of systemic disease in mice, while in calves, the severity of intestinal lesions shows only modest attenuation. In contrast, mutations that prevent the expression of the SPI-1 type III secretion system (T3SS) or of effector proteins translocated by the system result in an avirulent strain with consequent the absence of diarrhea in calves [23].

2.1. SPI-1-mediated invasion of host cells

After oral infection, a proportion of the *Salmonella* organisms survives the low stomach pH and reaches the distal ileum and cecum, where they invade the epithelial cells and M cells, mediated by a T3SS encoded by the SPI-1 [24, 25]. The T3SS allows some of the enteropathogenic bacteria to adhere to the epithelial surface and inject effector proteins that cross the membrane of the host cells, causing cellular injury [26]. Through this system, *Salmonella* translocates effector proteins encoded by genes present in the SPI-1 as well as genes in independent *loci* of the SPI-1 that promote a chain of events in the host cell to allow pathogen invasion [13]. Another function of the SPI-1 is related to hydroelectrolyte imbalance caused by the effector protein SopB, which stimulates the secretion of chloride ions (Cl^-) through its inositol phosphatase activity, thereby leading to loss of fluid into the intestinal lumen [27] (**Figure 1**).

Once in contact with the intestinal epithelium, the effector proteins SopE, SopE2 and SopB (encoded by genes outside of SPI-1) are translocated to the interiors of enterocytes and M cells via the SPI-1 T3SS. These proteins activate certain GTPases within the host cell, such as Cdc42, Rac-1 and Rho, causing a rearrangement of the actin cytoskeleton called membrane ruffling [28], which is stabilized by the SipA and SipC effector proteins. Furthermore, they also activate the MAP kinase (mitogen-activated protein kinase) pathway, thereby destabilizing tight junctions. Consequently, bacteria can penetrate into the host cell through the apical membrane in a process called macropinocytosis or cross the intercellular space until reaching the lamina propria. This destabilization of tight junctions also allows for the transmigration of polymorphonuclear cells (PMNs) from the basolateral space to the apical surface. However, this transmigration can occur independently from the destabilization of tight junctions when mediated by the bacterial protein SopA [29]. Once inside the cell, the effector protein SptP modulates the inactivation of the GTPases Cdc42 and Rac-1, thus resulting in the end of the membrane ruffling [30].

Signaling via MAP kinase, in addition to promoting the destabilization of tight junctions, also activates the transcription factors AP-1 (activator protein-1) and NF-κB (nuclear factor- κB), which leads to the synthesis of pro-inflammatory interleukin (IL)-8 by PMN leukocytes, thus acting as a chemotactic factor for neutrophils [29].

During the invasion of macrophages, the bacterium injects the effector protein SipB, which is encoded by SPI-1, inducing the intracellular activation of caspase-1 by resident macrophages. Caspase-1 induces apoptosis of infected macrophages resulting in *Salmonella* escape from these cells. Caspase-1 also cleaves the pro-inflammatory cytokines IL-1β and IL-18 to produce bioactive cytokines that further enhance the local inflammatory response, causing infiltration by PMN phagocytes and internalization of the bacterium by these cells [31, 32]. The intracellular medium provides a favorable environment for the bacteria to multiply [33], and once the invasion process is concluded, the bacteria are transported from the gastrointestinal tract to systemic organs.

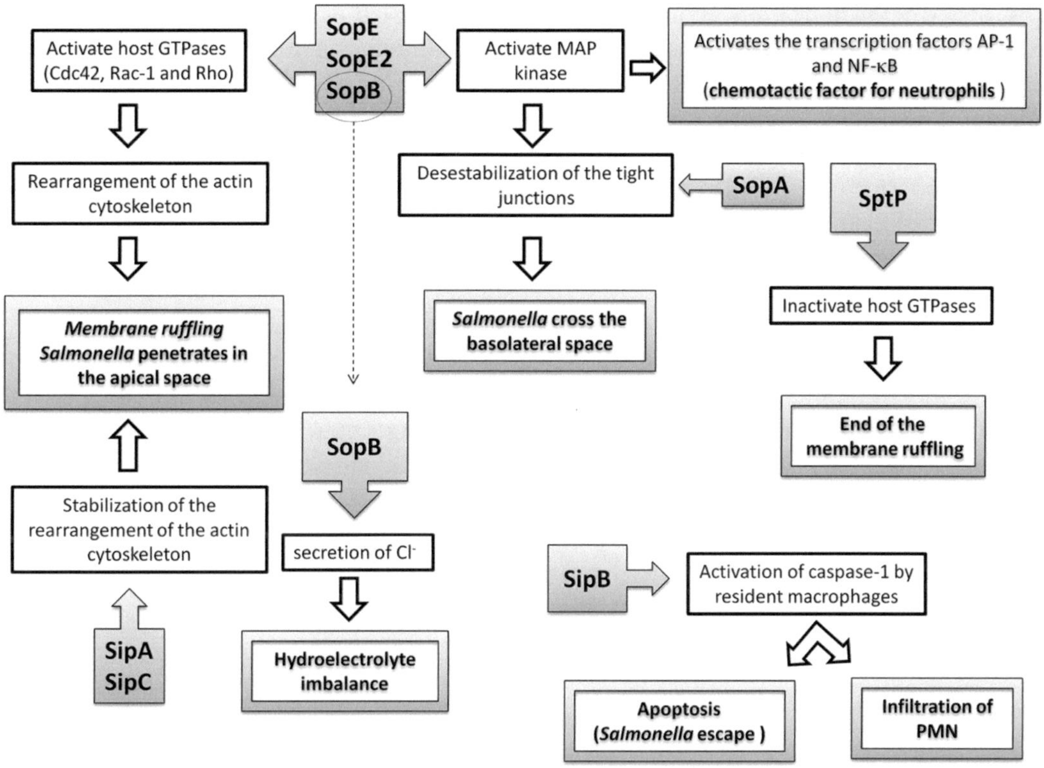

Figure 1. Effector proteins (gray arrows) ejected by type III secretion system encoded in SPI-1 and their actions for *Salmonella* invasion of host cells. *Salmonella* penetrates at the apical space causing the membrane ruffling. It is mediated by SopE, SopE2 and SopB proteins, which promote activation of host GTPases, causing a rearrangement of the actin cytoskeleton that is stabilized by SipA and SipC proteins. *Salmonella* can also cross the basolateral space through destabilization of the tight junctions, also mediated by SopE, SopE2 and SopB proteins (by activation of MAP kinase pathway) and by SopA protein. These events contribute to the activation of chemotactic factors of neutrophils. Once inside the cell, *Salmonella* promotes the end of the membrane ruffling by inactivation of host GTPases by SptP protein. During the invasion of resident macrophages, SipB protein induces the intracellular activation of caspase-1, causing apoptosis and enhancing the local inflammatory response. This event contributes to the escape of *Salmonella* from the macrophages and internalization of the bacteria in PMN phagocytes. The hydroelectrolyte imbalance is caused by SopB protein through inositol phosphatase activity which stimulates the secretion of chloride ions (Cl^-).

There is an alternative SPI-1-independent invasion mechanism in which *S. enterica* does not interact with M cells but is engulfed by dendritic cells that open the tight junctions between epithelial cells, thereby carrying the bacteria to systemic organs [34].

2.2. SPI-2-mediated intracellular multiplication

The ability of *S. enterica* to survive inside phagocytes and to replicate in *Salmonella*-containing vacuoles (SCV) in a variety of eukaryotic cells is dependent on another T3SS that is encoded by SPI-2 [22, 35, 36]. This characteristic can lead to systemic infection [20].

Soon after entry by means of macropinocytosis, *Salmonella* is internalized into a phagosome formed by the membrane ruffling that later fuses with lysosomes, thereby originating the SCV

[29]. Inside of the SCV, the T3SS encoded by SPI-2 is activated using luminal acid pH, translocating the effector proteins across the phagosome membrane (**Figure 2**). The effector protein SipC prevents the fusion of the SCV with vesicles containing NADPH oxidase (nicotinamide adenine dinucleotide phosphate-oxidase) and inducible nitric oxide synthase (iNOS), hindering the action of reactive oxygen intermediates (ROS) and reactive nitrogen intermediates (RNS) [13]. The effector proteins SifA and PipB2 contribute to the formation of *Salmonella*-induced filaments (SIF) along microtubules, while the effector proteins SseF and SseG aggregate the SCV-adjacent microtubules. In addition, an accumulation of actin occurs around the SCV that is mediated by the SspH2, SpvB and SseI proteins. These events contribute to the maturation and stabilization of SCV [29]. As a consequence, *S. enterica* becomes even more protected against RNS and ROS and against the potent antimicrobial activity of peroxynitrite, which is generated by the RNS and ROS reactions. These mechanisms represent a specific adaptation of *S. enterica* to the intracellular environment, especially phagocytes. Thus, the bacteria can multiply inside the phagocytic cells, transported via circulation and cause systemic infection [14].

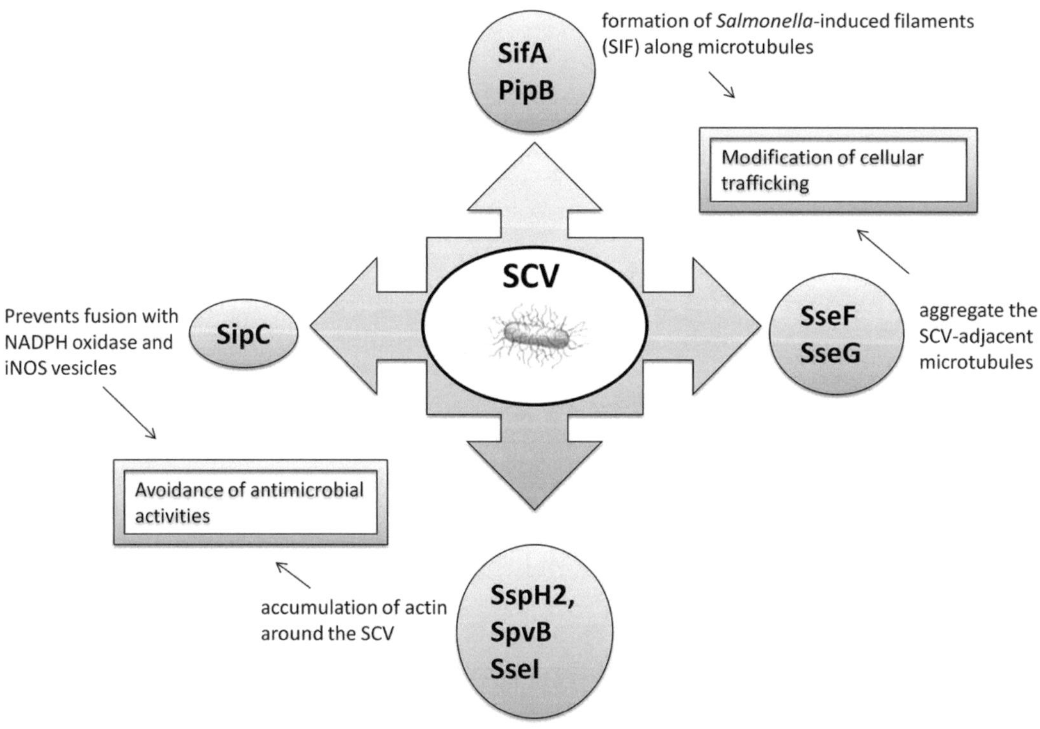

Figure 2. Effector proteins (gray circles) ejected by type III secretion system encoded in SPI-2 and their actions for *Salmonella* survival inside of phagocytes and its replication in *Salmonella*-containing vacuoles (SCV). The translocation of SipC protein avoids the antimicrobial activities of reactive oxygen intermediates and reactive nitrogen intermediates by prevention of fusion of NADPH oxidase and iNOS vesicles. This antimicrobial activity by the host cell is stronger but prevented by the accumulation of actin around the SCV promoted by SspH2, SpvB and Ssel proteins. These events contribute to maturation of SCV. SifA and PipA proteins contribute to the tubular structures known as *Salmoniella*-induced filaments formed along the microtubule motors; in addition, SseF and SseG cause microtubules aggregation adjacent to SCV. These events interfere the molecular motors that drive the cellular trafficking, which transport vesicles and organelles within the cell.

3. Natural resistance mechanism to infection by *S. enterica*: the role of Nramp1 glycoprotein

The resistance mechanisms of host to infection by *S. enterica* are multigenic. Studies in mice have emphasized the *locus* encoding glycoprotein natural resistance-associated macrophage protein-1 (Nramp1), which has been considered the key for the innate host response to intracellular pathogens [37]. This protein belongs to a family of proteins highly conserved in evolution, with homology among mammals, insects and bacteria suggesting an important role in all living organisms [38].

Nramp1 is a transmembrane glycoprotein and divalent metal ion symporter that deprives intracellular pathogens of these metals by removing mainly Fe^{++} and Mn^{++} from the luminal space of the phagosomal and lysosomal vesicles. Because iron and other divalent cations are cofactors for vital enzymes, *S. enterica* expresses a series of carriers that compete with the host cell for traces of these divalent metals within the phagosomes [39]. This Nramp1 glycoprotein is encoded by the gene *Slc11a1* (*Solute carrier family 11 member 1*, first named as *Ity* gene), on chromosome 1 in mice [37]. A single substitution of glycine for aspartate at position 169 results in susceptibility to systemic infection by *S. enterica* in the mice [40]. Consequently, mice that have two *Slc11a1* $^{Asp\ 169}$ alleles are significantly more susceptible to lethal *Salmonella* infections and are therefore being used in studies to clarify the host-pathogen relationships in acute systemic infection. In turn, mice carrying the wild-type *locus* *Slc11a1*$^{+/+}$ can be used to study the pathogenesis of chronic infections that are often asymptomatic [41].

The interaction between the surface receptors of macrophages and microbial ligands results in the internalization of the microorganism into a phagosome. However, this young phagosome is not able to digest its contents, thus requiring a maturation process involving fusion and fission events with endosomes and lysosomes. During the maturation process, phagosomes containing *S. enterica* acquire vacuolar ATPases that acidify the phagosome lumen. In an acidic pH, Nramp1 removes Fe^{++} and other divalent cations from the inside of phagosomes. Concomitantly, in the presence of functional protein Nramp1, the host cell expresses the mannose-6-phosphate receptor (M6PR), which is responsible for interacting with vesicles containing NADPH oxidase and iNOS. This interaction generates positive feedback for the transcription of high levels of iNOS mRNA [39]. In susceptible mice (*Slc11a1*$^{Asp\ 169}$), the phagosomes containing *S. enterica* are negative for M6PR receptors, and therefore, the production of iNOS is lower than in hosts that have the wild-type *locus* *Slc11a1*$^{+/+}$ [36]. Thus, Nramp1 has proven to be very important to control the exponential growth of *Salmonella* during the early stages of systemic infection [23, 42].

4. Infection cycle of *S. enterica* in latent carriers

In asymptomatic carrier animals, the study of the infection cycle of *Salmonella* was described using C57Bl/6-Bcgr (*Slc11a1*$^{+/+}$) mice as a resistant mouse model inoculated orally with a high dose of *Salmonella* serotype Enteritidis [43]. The animals developed an intermittent infection cycle in the gastrointestinal tract during 4 weeks of study, with interspersed periods of intra- and extracellular spread of the infection, which featured three distinct stages over the course of the cycle (**Figure 3**): *(I) the initial stage* represented by intracellular invasion and bacterial multiplication in the intestine, inducing transient damage to the intestinal mucosa and shedding of the pathogen in the feces. A rapid clearance of a large fraction of the inoculums was observed during the first 48 h postinoculation (PI); *(II) the intermediate stage*, the initial period of bacterial sequestration by the mononuclear phagocyte system (MPS) in which the pathogen was detected only within intracellular compartments. In this period, a transient exponential growth of the remaining intracellular bacteria occurred 2–4 d PI followed by a suppression of bacterial growth, establishing a plateau phase until 15 d PI. The intracellular multiplication in the MPS coincided with the IFNγ production; and finally *(III) the intermittent shedding stage*, the *Salmonella* persists sub-clinically in the tissues (spleen and cecum) with recurrence of intracellular bacterial growth that coincided with the intermittent excretion in feces, characterizing a latent infection.

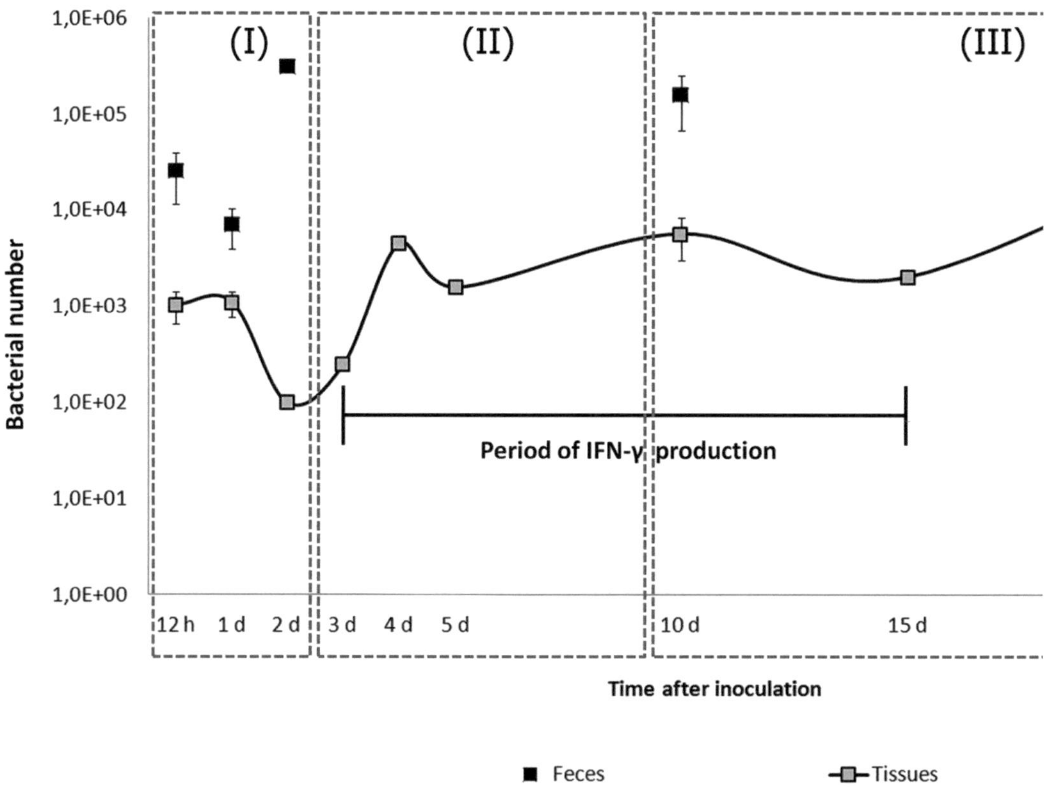

Figure 3. Distribution of *S. enteritidis* in feces (fecal and ileo-cecal content) and tissues (blood, spleen, liver, mesenteric lymph nodes and different parts of the intestine—jejunum, ileum and cecum) at different times after intragastric inoculation with 5 × 108 cfu in C57Bl/6-Bcgr (Slc11a1$^{+/+}$) mice as a resistant mouse model. These numbers are represented as mean ± SD of three animals (in duplicate). (I) Initial stage of infection, when *Salmonella* invades the intestinal mucosa and it is also eliminated in feces. (II) Intermediate stage marks the initial period of mononuclear phagocyte system (MPS) sequestration. *Salmonella* is found intracellular in the intestine but it is not being eliminated to the environment through feces. (III) Intermittent elimination stage of *Salmonella*, common in a resistant animal model, based on [43].

In pigs, by applying a Markov statistical model, Ivanek et al. [44] were able to distinguish different stages during the dynamic shedding of *Salmonella* in feces and their immune response. In this model, the intermittent shedding of the pathogen was clear. The authors characterized the following stages: (i) *latency*, when pigs were negative for the shedding of *Salmonella* immediately after the challenge; (ii) *continuous shedding*, with continuous shedding of the pathogen in the feces; (iii) *non-intermittent shedding*—when *Salmonella* was not being shed in the feces; (iv) *intermittent shedding*—when the bacteria were again shed in the feces; and (v) *recovery*. The authors observed that the stages could vary depending on the infecting dose and the serotype involved in the infection.

Thus, independent of the animal model, in latent carriers, there is a period during which *Salmonella* stays hidden in an intracellular compartment, and it is not being eliminated. It can mask the diagnosis of the positive animals. This "*Salmonella*'s hiding-place" may function as a strategic site of bacteria multiplication and, consequently, elimination of high numbers of pathogens in the environment. So, it is very important to identify the sites of bacterial colonization in different latent carriers.

The site of bacterial colonization in persistent infections varies according to serotype and host species. In humans, serotype Typhi expresses proteins encoded by SPI-7 that inhibit the detection of pathogens by the innate immune system of the host. Thus, the bacteria can spread systemically, colonizing macrophages in the liver, spleen and bone marrow. In the liver, *Salmonella* serotype Typhi can be found latent in the gallbladder, making the host an asymptomatic carrier. Intermittently, the bacteria are transported from the gallbladder into the small intestine through the bile and excreted in the feces [7]. In mice, the mesenteric lymph nodes are the colonization site of serotype Typhimurium [41]. In birds, *Salmonella* serotype Pullorum can be found latent in the spleen, ovary and oviduct of chickens [45], and *S*. Enteritidis can infect the ovaries of healthy hens, contaminating the eggs prior to shell formation [46]. In snakes, there is strong evidence that different serotypes of *Salmonella* also colonize the ovary, spreading bacteria to their offspring vertically [47].

In asymptomatic animals, the cecum plays an important role as a reservoir for longer periods of shedding [48–51]. Research using resistant mice orally challenged with high doses of *Salmonella* serotype Enteritidis [43], and we demonstrate that bacteria reach the cecum in the early stages of infection (12 h to 2 days PI) and remain for long periods from 5 days PI, functioning as a reservoir of bacterial multiplication, causing the shedding of *Salmonella* in the intestinal lumen intermittently. The small intestine does not have this reservoir role, since the bacterial colonization in jejune and ileum occurred only in 1–4 days PI. Spleen is another site of *Salmonella* reservoir; from the moment that bacteria reached the MPS, they stayed in spleen for long periods (**Figure 4**).

In chickens, the cecum is also a site for long-lasting carriage of *S*. Enteritidis, both in susceptible and resistant animals [52]. In asymptomatic carriers, it represents a public health and food protection concerns because the cecum may function as a "strategic site" of *Salmonella* proliferation, releasing bacteria to the environment intermittently.

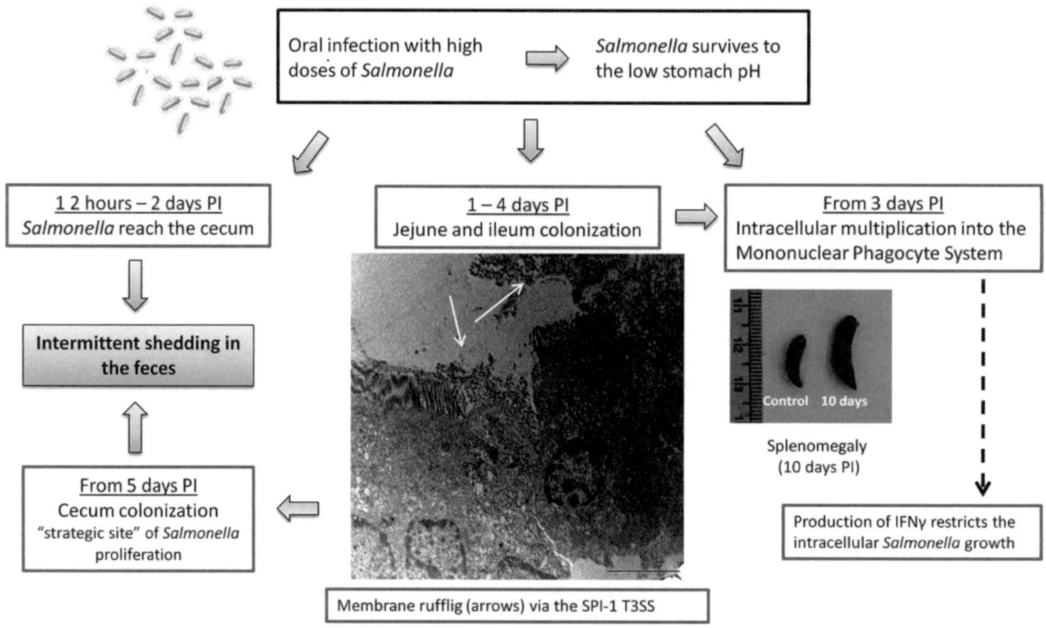

Figure 4. Course of *S. enteritidis* in C57Bl/6-Bcgr (Slc11a1$^{+/+}$), a resistant mouse model. *Salmonella* rapidly reaches the cecum in the early stage of the infection between 12 and 48 h postinoculation (PI) and remains in this organ as an important reservoir for 5 days PI, with increasing bacteria multiplication. The presence of bacteria in the cecum seems to be associated with its extracellular multiplication in the intestinal content and intermittent shedding in the feces. The colonization of the small intestine occurs during the first 4 days PI. In this period, *Salmonella* penetrates the intestinal mucosa, causing different degrees of degeneration of the microvilli, which is reversible (membrane ruffling). This mechanism is mediated by effector proteins translocated by T3SS encoded in SPI-1. Intracellular multiplication of the bacteria in mononuclear phagocyte system (MPS) occurs from 3 days PI. The exact route of *Salmonella* dissemination from intestine to MPS is unclear, but from the moment that bacteria reach the MPS, they remain in spleen, causing splenomegaly by 10 days PI. The intracellular multiplication in MPS coincides with the production of IFN_{γ}, which restricts the replication of intracellular *Salmonella*.

The mechanism of persistence of *Salmonella* in the cecum is not well established. Probably, it is associated with the physiological environment and less peristalsis of this part of the intestine. Upon entry into the large intestine, the bacteria remain longer in the cecum due to fewer peristaltic movements. Despite the production of short-chain fatty acids by resident microbiota due to the intense local fermentation, the pH in the cecal environment remains above 6.3, higher than the inhibitory level for *Salmonella* multiplication [53].

5. Role of IFNγ in controlling of *S. enterica* growth

During intestinal infection, *Salmonella*-host interactions result in different degrees of inflammation related to the levels of cytokines produced [12], which may trigger changes in the composition of the intestinal microbiota. A reduction in symbionts or an increase in pathobionts is usually observed during inflammatory processes, reflecting the diversity of the intestinal microbiota [54]. In gastroenteritis caused by *Salmonella* in susceptible hosts, the production of interferon gamma (IFNγ) in the early stage of intestinal inflammation may alter the lumen conditions, causing an imbalance in the ecology of the resident microbiota that favors competition for pathogen growth and intestinal colonization [55–57]. In latent carriers, however, *S. enterica* can invade the intestinal mucosa and colonize the intestine without triggering a strong immune response, remaining in equilibrium with the resident microbiota [58].

IFNγ plays a crucial role in resistance to systemic infection by *S. enterica*. This cytokine controls the growth of pathogens both in the initial [59, 60] and late stages of the disease [41], and its absence results in septicemia. High levels of IFNγ as well as of its mediator IL-12 contribute to resistance to infection in different animal species [61]. Mice with chronic asymptomatic infection by *Salmonella* serotype Typhimurium develop symptoms after treatment with anti-IFNγ antibodies [41]. In birds, the IFNγ gene expression is lower in susceptible animals than in resistant animals [61].

IFNγ is produced specifically in response to systemic infection and correlates with bacteremia and pathogen invasion of the cells of the mononuclear phagocyte system, such as the lymphoid tissue associated with the intestine (mesenteric lymph nodes and Peyer's patches), spleen and liver. Its production is essential to restrict bacterial intracellular multiplication, thereby contributing to the establishment of a plateau phase during the growth cycle of *Salmonella* serotype Enteritidis in asymptomatic mice [43].

When antigen-specific acquired immunity is triggered, the IFNγ titer in serum begins to decrease [11]. However, even in the presence of high titers of specific circulating antibodies, some *Salmonella* serotypes are capable of causing persistent infections in a host for long periods. This adaptive immune response seems to be important to reduce the number of extracellular bacteria; however, bacteria that are present within macrophages survive both the innate and adaptive immune responses, and the host ultimately becomes a latent carrier [41].

6. Gene expression in latent *Salmonella*

Zoonotic intracellular pathogens that can cause latent carriers pose a unique public health problem. The ability of such carrier animals to shed pathogens without showing any clinical signs of infection can make outbreak control challenging and the potential of transmission to humans a serious public health concern. Before identifying these carriers, we need to understand the mechanism of bacterial invasion of the host cells and follow the process of establishing a persistent state of infection. SPI 1 encodes for genes *hil*A and *inv*F, which allow the bacteria to enter, survive, and replicate within the host cells [62]. Once the pathogen enters the host cells, glycine cleavage protein subunit P (*gcv*P) has been shown to be a potential key player in the transition from acute to chronic infection [63–65]. The activity of *gcv*P has been shown to increase dramatically in other important zoonotic infections like tuberculosis [66, 67] and leishmaniasis [68]. Understanding the pathogenesis of the invasion, intracellular replication, and the transition to latent carrier state in *Salmonella* would potentially lay the groundwork for the development of a control, treatment and eventual eradication strategies. We are just starting to understand potential genes involved in the transition from active to latent stage of infection in case of intracellular pathogens. There is very little information in case of *Salmonella*, but in case of *M. tuberculosis*, glycine dehydrogenase activity increases tenfold upon entering a state of persistence. Another indicator that its metabolism is vital to persistence is the fact that mutants that are deficient in isocitrate lyase, an enzyme involved in the glyoxylate pathway, cannot cause chronic latent infections [67]. We have some preliminary results from our long-term cell culture *Salmonella* infection model (unpublished personal communication). It shows that *Ace*A the gene that codes for isocitrate lyase, which is the first step in the glyoxylate shunt, is over expressed. Even on day 1, the expression levels are elevated, but not significantly more than any of the other genes. However, on day 10 and day 30 post infection,. *Ace*A expression level on day 30 goes up dramatically. This has biological plausibility since it is the first step in the glyoxylate pathway. Such gene expression studies of lymph node biopsies on a herd basis or at slaughter might allow us to detect chronic/persistent *Salmonella* infections.

7. Conclusions

Despite host's activation of anti-inflammatory and antimicrobial responses, *Salmonella* can establish asymptomatic persistent infections, leading to intermittent high-level shedding of the bacteria in feces. This host-pathogen balance leads to serious problems for public health because asymptomatic animals latently carry the infection for long periods with intermittent cycles of shedding of the pathogen in feces. This outcome is epidemiologically important because false-negative *Salmonella* isolation results can be generated if the diagnostic test is performed during the period when the animal is not shedding the pathogen.

Acknowledgements

The authors thank Universidade Estadual de Santa Cruz-UESC (Bahia State, Brazil) and Fundação de Amparo à Pesquisa do Estado da Bahia-FAPESB (Bahia State, Brazil).

Author details

Bianca Mendes Maciel[1]*, Rachel Passos Rezende[1] and Nammalwar Sriranganathan[2]

*Address all correspondence to: caimbi@uol.com.br

1 Department of Biological Sciences, Santa Cruz State University, Ilhéus, BA, Brazil

2 Virginia-Maryland College of Veterinary Medicine, Virginia Teach, Blacksburg, VA, USA

References

[1] Popoff, M.Y.; Bockemuhl, J.; Gheesling, L.L. Supplement 2001 (no. 45) to the Kauffamann-White scheme. Research in Microbiology. 2013;**154**:173–174. doi:10.1016/S0923-2508(03)00025-1

[2] Ellermeier, C.D.; Slauch, J.M. The genus *Salmonella*. In: Dworkin, M. Falkow, S., Rosenberg, E., Schleifer, K.H. and Stackebrandt, E., editors. The Prokaryotes. 3rd ed. vol. 6. New York: Springer; 2006. pp. 123–158. doi:10.1007/0-387-30746-x_7

[3] CDC. National Enteric Disease Surveillance: *Salmonella* Surveillance Overview [Internet]. July, 2011 [Updated: July, 2011]. Available from: http://www.cdc.gov/nationalsurveillance/pdfs/nationalsalmsurveilloverview_508.pdf [Accessed: July 2016].

[4] CDC. PulseNet. Multiple Locus Variable-number Tandem Repeat Analysis (MLVA). [Internet]. February 16, 2016 [Updated: February 16, 2016]. Available from: http://www.cdc.gov/pulsenet/pathogens/mlva.html [Accessed: July, 2016].

[5] Wallis, S.T. Host-specificity of *Salmonella* infections in animal species. In: Mastroeni P. and Maskell D, editors. *Salmonella* Infections – Clinical, Immunological and Molecular Aspects. Cambridge: Cambridge University Press; 2006. pp. 57–88. doi:10.1017/CBO9780511525360.004

[6] Vieira, A.; Jensen, A.R.; Pires, S.M.; Karlsmose, S.; Wegener, H.C.; Wong, D.L.F. WHO - Global Foodborne Infections Network Country Databank – A resource to link human and non-human sources of *Salmonella*. In: Proceeding of the 12th Symposium of the International Society for Veterinary Epidemiology and Economics; 10/08/2009–14/08/2009; Durban, South Africa. 2009.

[7] Tischler, A.D.; McKinney, J. Contrasting persistence strategies in *Salmonella* and *Mycobacterium*. Current Opinion in Microbiology. 2010;**13**:93–99. doi:10.1016/j.mib.2009. 12. 007

[8] Maciel, B.M.; Argôlo Filho, R.C.; Freitas, E.S.; Kruschewsky, F.F.; Santos, B.F.; Rocha, G.D.; Wetler R.M; Martins, L.A.F. Sorotipos exóticos de *Salmonella* encontrados em cães assintomáticos no município de Ilhéus/BA – Brasil (Occurrence of exotic Salmonella serovar in asymptomatic dogs in Ilhéus city / BA-Brazil). Brazilian Journal of Veterinary Research and Animal Science. 2004;**41**:247–253. doi:10.1590/S1413-95962004000400005

[9] Pasmans, F.; Blahak, S.; Martel, A.; Pantchev, N. Introducing reptiles into captive collection: the role of veterinarian. The Veterinary Journal. 2008;**175**:53–68. doi:10.1016/j.tvjl.2006.12.009

[10] Maciel, B.M.; Argôlo Filho, R.C.; Nogueira, S.S.C.; Dias, J.C.T.; Rezende, R.P. High prevalence of *Salmonella* in tegu lizards (*Tupinambis merianae*), and susceptibility of the serotypes toantibiotics. Zoonoses and Public Health. 2010;**57**:e26–e32. doi:10.1111/j.1863-2378.2009.01283.x

[11] Mastroeni, P. Mechanisms of immunity to *Salmonella* infection. In: Mastroeni P. and Maskell D, editors. *Salmonella* Infections – Clinical, Immunological and Molecular Aspects. Cambridge: Cambridge University Press; 2006. pp. 207–254. doi:10.1017/CBO9780511525360.009

[12] Kaiser, P.; Rothwell, L.; Galyov, E.E.; Barrow, P.A.; Burnside, J.; Wigley, P. Differential cytokine expression in avian cells in response to invasion by *Salmonella typhimurium*, *Salmonella enteritidis* and *Salmonella gallinarum*. Micro-biology. 2000;**146**:3217–3226.

[13] Hensel, M. Pathogenicity island and virulence of *Salmonella enterica*. In: Mastroeni P. and Maskell D, editors. *Salmonella* Infections – Clinical, Immunological and Molecular Aspects. Cambridge: Cambridge University Press; 2006. pp. 146–172. doi:10.1017/CBO9780511525360.007

[14] Schmidt, H.; Hensel, M. Pathogenicity island in bacterial pathogenesis. Clinical Microbiology Reviews. 2004;**17:**14–56. doi:10.1128/CMR.17.1.14-56.2004

[15] Jacobsen, A.; Hendriksen, R.S.; Aaresturp, F.M.; Ussery, D.W.; Friis, C. The *Salmonella enterica* Pan-genome. Microbial Ecology. 2011;**62:**487–504. doi:10.1007/s00248-011-9880-1

[16] Hensel, M. Evolution of Pathogenicity island of *Salmonella enterica*. International Journal of Medical Microbiology. 2004;**294**:95–102. doi:10.1016/j.ijmm.2004.06.025

[17] Galán, J.E. Molecular genetic bases of *Salmonella* entry into host cells. Molecular Microbiology. 1996;**20:**267–272. doi:10.1111/j.1365-2958.1996.tb02615.x

[18] Zhou, D.; Galán, J. *Salmonella* entry into host cells: the work in concert of type III secreted effector proteins. Microbes and Infection. 2002;**3:**1293–1298. doi:10.1016/S1286-4579(01)01489-7

[19] Ochman, H.F.; Soncini C.; Solomon, F.; Groisman, E.A. Identification of a pathogenicity island for *Salmonella* survival in host cells. Proceedings of the National Academy of Sciences of the United States of America. 1996;**93:**7800–7804. doi:10.1073/pnas.93.15.7800

[20] Hensel, M. *Salmonella* pathogenicity island 2. Molecular Microbiology. 2000;**36**:1015–1023. doi:10.1046/j.1365-2958.2000.01935.x

[21] Groisman E.A.; Ochman, H. Pathogenicity island: bacterial evolution in quantum leaps. Cell. 1996;**87:**791–794. doi:10.1016/S0092-8674(00)81985-6

[22] Ochman, H.; Groisman, E.A. Distribution of pathogenicity island in *Salmonella* spp. Infection and Immunity. 1996;**64:**5410–541.

[23] Santos, R.L.; Zhang, S.; Tsolis, R.M.; Kingsley, R.A.; Adams, L.G.; Bäumler, A.J. Animal models of *Salmonella* infections: enteritis versus typhoid fever. Microbes and Infection. 2001;**3:**1335–1344. doi:10.1016/S1286-4579(01)01495-2

[24] Lee, V.T.; Schneewind, O. Type III secretion machines and the pathogenesis of enteric infections caused by *Yersinia* and *Salmonella* spp. Immunological Reviews. 1999;168:241–255. doi:10.1111/j.1600-065X.1999.tb01296.x

[25] Mastroeni, P.; Sheppard, M. *Salmonella* infections in the mouse model: host resistance factors and in vivo dynamics of bacterial spread and distribution in the tissues. Microbes and Infection. 2004;**6:**398–405. doi:10.1016/j.micinf.2003.12.009

[26] Cornelis, G.R.; Van Gijsegen, F. Assembly and function of type III secretory system. Annual Review of Microbiology. 2000;**54:**735–774. doi:10.1146/annurev.micro.54.1.735

[27] Norris, F.A.; Wilson, M.P.; Wallis, T.S.; Galyov, E.E.; Majerus, P.W. SopB, a protein required for virulence of *Salmonella dublin*, is an inositol phosphate phosphatase. Proceedings of the National Academy of Sciences of the United States of America. 1998;**95:**14057–14059. doi:10.1073/pnas.95.24.14057

[28] Harrdt, W.D.; Chen, L.M.; Schuebel, K.E.; Bustelo, X.R.; Galán, J.E. *S. typhimurium* encodes an activator of Rho GTPases that induces membrane ruffling and nuclear responses in host cells. Cell. 1998;**93:**815–826. doi:10.1016/S0092-8674(00)81442-7

[29] Haraga, A.; Ohlson, M.B.; Miller, S.I. *Salmonella* interplay with cells. Nature Reviews Microbiology. 2008;**6:**53–66. doi:10.1038/nrmicro1788

[30] Fu, Y.; Galán, J.E. A *Salmonella* protein antagonizes Rac-1 and Cdc42 to mediate host-cell recovery after bacterial invasion. Nature. 1999;**401:**293–297. doi:10.1038/45829

[31] Monack, D.M.; Hersh, D.; Ghori, N.; Bouley, D.; Zychlinsky, A.; Falkow, S. *Salmonella* exploits caspase-1 to colonize Peyer's patches in a murine typhoid model. The Journal of Experimental Medicine. 2000;**192:**249–258. doi:10.1084/jem.192.2.249

[32] Zhang, S.; Adams, L.G.; Nunes, J.; Khare, S.; Tsolis, R.M.;Bäumler, A.J. Secreted effector proteins of Salmonella *enterica* serotype typhimurium elicit host specific chemokine profiles in animal models of typhoid fever and enterocolitis. Infection and Immunity. 2003;**71:**4795–4803. doi:10.1128/IAI.71.8.4795-4803.2003

[33] Galán, J.E.; Zhou, D. Striking a balance: modulation of the actin cytoskeleton by *Salmonella*. Proceedings of the National Academy of Sciences of the United States of America. 2000;**97:**8754–8761. doi:10.1073/pnas.97.16.8754

[34] Johansson, C.; Sundquist, M.; Wick, M.J. Interactions between *Salmonella* and dendritic cells: what happens along the way? In: Mastroeni P. and Maskell D, editors. *Salmonella* Infections – Clinical, Immunological and Molecular Aspects. Cambridge: Cambridge University Press; 2006. pp. 279–298. doi:10.1017/CBO9780511525360.011

[35] Vazquez-Torres, A.; Xu, Y.; Jones-Carson, J.; Holden, D.W.; Lucia, S.M.; Dinauer, M.C.; Mastroeni, P.; Fang, F.C. *Salmonella* pathogenicity island 2-dependent evasion of the phagocyte NADPH oxidase. Science. 2000;**287:**1655–1658. doi:10.1126/science.287.5458.1655

[36] Chakravortty, D.; Hansen-Wester, I.; Hensel, M. *Salmonella* pathogenicity island 2 mediates protection of intracellular Salmonella from reactive nitrogen intermediates. The Journal of Experimental Medicine. 2002;**195:**1155–1166. doi:10.1084/jem.20011547

[37] Plant, J.; Glynn, A.A. Locating *Salmonella* resistance gene on mouse chromosome 1. Clinical and Experimental Immunology. 1979;**37:**1–6.

[38] Skamene, E.; Schurr, E.; Gros, P. Infection genomics: Nramp1 as a major determinant of natural resistance to intracellular infections. Annual Review of Medicine. 1998;**49:**275–87. doi:10.1146/annurev.med.49.1.275

[39] McCollister, B.D.; Vazquez-Torres, A. Interactions of *S. enterica* with phagocytic cells. In: Mastroeni P. and Maskell D, editors. *Salmonella* Infections – Clinical, Immunological and Molecular Aspects. Cambridge: Cambridge University Press; 2006. pp. 255–278. doi:10.1017/CBO9780511525360.010

[40] Vidal, S.M.; Malo, D.; Vogan, K.; Skamene, E.; Gros, P. Natural resistance to infection with intracellular parasites. isolation of a candidate for Bcg. Cell. 1993;**73:**469–485. doi:10.1016/0092-8674(93)90135-D

[41] Monack, D.M.; Bouley, D.M.; Falkow, S. *Salmonella typhimurium* persists within macrophages in the mesenteric lymph nodes of chronically infected Nramp1$^{+/+}$ mice and can be reactivated by IFNγ neutralization. The Journal of Experimental Medicine. 2004;**199**:231–241. doi:10.1084/jem.20031319

[42] Vidal, S.; Tremblay, M.L.; Govoni, G.; Gauthier, S.; Sebastiani, G.; Malo, D.; Skamene, E.; Olivier, M.; Jothy, S.; Gros, P. The Ity/Lsh/Bcg locus: natural resistance to infection with intracellular parasites is abrogated by disruption of the Nramp1 gene. The Journal of Experimental Medicine. 1995;**182:**655–666. doi:10.1084/jem.182.3.655

[43] Maciel, B.M.; Sriranganathan, N.; Romano, C.C.; Santos, T.F.; Dias, J.C.T.; Gross, E.; Rezende, R.P. Infection cycle of *Salmonella enterica* serovar Enteritidis in latent carrier mice. Canadian Journal of Microbiology. 2012;**58**:1389–1395. doi:10.1139/cjm-2012-0375

[44] Ivanek, R.; Österberg, J.; Gautman, R.; Lewerin, S.S. *Salmonella* fecal shedding and immune responses are dose- and serotype- dependent in pigs. PLoS One. 2012;**7:**e34660. doi:10.1371/journal.pone.0034660

[45] Wigley, P.; Berchieri, Jr, A.; Page, K.L.; Smith, A.L.; Barrow, P.A. *Salmonella enterica* serovar Pullorum persists in splenic macrophages and in the reproductive tract during persistent, disease-free carriage in chickens. Infection and Immunity. 2001;**69:**7873–7879. doi:10.1128/IAI.69.12.7873-7879.2001

[46] De Buck, J.; Pasmans, F.; Van Immerseel, F.; Haesebrouck, F.; Ducatelle, R. Tubular glands of the isthmus are the predominant colonization site of *Salmonella* Enteritidis in the upper oviduct of laying hens. Poultry Science. 2004;**83:**352–358. doi:10.1093/ps/83.3.352

[47] Schröter, M.; Speicher, A.; Hofmann, J.; Roggentin, P. Analysis of the transmission of *Salmonella* spp. through generations of pet snakes. Environmental Microbiology. 2006;**8:**556–559. doi:10.1111/j.1462-2920.2005.00934.x

[48] Collins, F.M. Immunity to enteric infection in mice. Infection and Immunity. 1970;**1:**243–250.

[49] Collins, F.M. Salmonellosis in orally infected specific pathogen-free C57Bl mice. Infection and Immunity. 1972;**5:**191–198.

[50] Carter, P.; Collins, F. The route of enteric infection in normal mice. The Journal of Experimental Medicine. 1974;**139**:189–1203. doi:10.1084/jem.139.5.1189

[51] Deng, S.X.; Cheng, A.C.; Wang, M.S.; Cao, P. Gastrointestinal tract distribution of *Salmonella* enteritidis in orally infected mice with a species-specific fluorescent quantitative polymerase chain reaction. World Journal of Gastroenterology. 2007;**13:**6568–6574. doi:10.3748/wjg.13.6568

[52] Sadeyen, J.R.; Trotereau, J.; Velge, P.; Marly, J.; Beaumont, C.; Barrow, P.A.; Bumstead, N.; Lalmanach, A.C. *Salmonella* carrier state in chicken: comparison of expression of immune response genes between susceptible and resistant animals. Microbes and Infection. 2004;**6:**1278–1286. doi:10.1016/j.micinf.2004.07.005

[53] Bohnhoff, M.; Miller, C.P.; Martin, W.R. Resistance of the mouse intestinal tract to experimental Salmonella infection. I. Factors which interfere with the initiation of infection by oral inoculation. The Journal of Experimental Medicine. 1964;**120:**805–816. doi:10.1084/jem.120.5.805

[54] Round, J.L.; Mazmanian, S.K. The gut microbiota shapes intestinal immune responses during health and disease. Nature Review Immunology. 2009;**9**:313–323. doi:10.1038/nri2515

[55] Stecher, B.; Robbiani, R.; Walker, A.W.; Westendorf, A.M.; Barthel, M.; Kremer, M.; Chaffron, S.; Macpherson, A.J.; Buer, J.; Parkhill, J.; Dougan, G.; Von Mering, C.; Hardt, W.D. *Salmonella enterica* serovar typhimurium exploits in-flammation to compete with the intestinal microbiota. PLoS Biology. 2007;**5:**2177–2189. doi:10.1371/journal.pbio.0050244

[56] Barman, M.; Unold, D.; Shifley, K.; Amir, E.; Hung, K.; Bos, N.; Salzman, N. Enteric salmonellosis disrupts the microbial ecology of the murine gastrointestinal tract. Infection and Immunity. 2008;**76:**907–915. doi:10.1128/IAI.01432-07

[57] Santos, R.L.; Raffatellu, M.; Bevins, C.L.; Adams, L.G.; Tükel, Ç.; Tsolis, R.M.; Bäumler, J. Life in the inflamed intestine, *Salmonella* style. Trends in Microbiology. 2009;**17:**498–506. doi:10.1016/j.tim.2009.08.008

[58] Maciel, B.M.; Marques, E.L.S.; Dias, J.C.T.; Santos, T.F.; Brendel, M.; Rezende, R.P. Denaturing gradient gel electrophoresis analysis of 16S ribosomal DNA to monitor changes in mouse gut bacterial communities during *Salmonella enterica* serovar Enteritidis latent infection. Genetic and Molecular Research. 2013;**12:**2611–2617. doi:10.4238/2013.March.13.10

[59] Nauciel, C.; Espinasse-Maes, F. Role of gamma interferon and tumor necrosis factor alpha in resistance to Salmonella typhimurium infection. Infection and Immunity. 1992;**60:**450–454.

[60] Bao, S.; Beagley, K.W.; France, M.P.; Shen, J.; Husband, A.J. Interferon-γ plays a critical role in intestinal immunity against Salmonella typhimurium infection. Immunology. 2000;**99:**464–472. doi:10.1046/j.1365-2567.2000.00955.x

[61] Price, J.D.; Simpfender, K.R.; Mantena, R.R.; Holden, J.; Heath, W.R.; Van Rooijen, N.; Strugnell, R.A.; Wijburg, L.C. Gamma interferon-independent effects in interleukin-12 on immunity to *Salmonella enterica* serovar Typhimurium. Infection and Immunity. 2007;**75:**5753–5762. doi:10.1128/IAI.00971-07

[62] Nix, R.; Altschuler, S.; Henson, P.M.; Detweiler, C.S. Hemophagocytic macrophages harbor *Salmonella enterica* during persistent infection. PLoS Pathogens. 2007;**3**(12):e193. doi:10.1371/journal.ppat.0030193

[63] Ficht, T.A. Intracellular survival of Brucella: defining the link with persistence. Veterinary Microbiology. 2003;**92:**213–223. doi:10.1016/S0378-1135(02)00367-X

[64] Goldman, D.S.; Wagner, M.J. Enzyme systems in the mycobacteria. XIII. Glycine dehydrogenase and the glyoxylic acid cycle. Biochimica et Biophysica Acta. 1962;**65:**297–306. doi:10.1016/0006-3002(62)91048-X

[65] Hong, P.C.; Tsolis, R.M.; Ficht, T.A. Identification of genes required for chronic persistence of Brucella abortus in mice. Infection and Immunity. 2000;**68:**4102–4107. doi:10.1128/IAI.68.7.4102-4107.2000

[66] McKinney, J.D.K.; Honer zu Bentrup, K.; Mu-oz-Elías, E.J.; Miczak, A.; Chen, B.; Chan, W.T.; Swenson, D.; Sacchettini, J.C.; Jacobs, W.R Jr.; Russell, D.G. Persistence of *Mycobacterium tuberculosis* in macrophages and mice requires the glyoxylate shunt enzyme isocitrate lyase. Nature. 2000;**406:**735–738. doi:10.1038/35021074

[67] Wayne, L.G.; Lin, K.Y. Glyoxylate metabolism and adaptation of *Mycobacterium tuberculosis* to survival under anaerobic conditions. Infection and Immunity. 1982;**37**:1042–1049.

[68] Scott, D.A.; Hickerson, S.M.; Vickers, T.J.; Beverley, S.M. The role of the mitochondrial glycine cleavage complex in the metabolism and virulence of the protozoan parasite *Leishmania major*. Journal of Biological Chemistry. 2008;283:155–165. doi:10.1074/jbc.M7080 14200

Chapter 4

Salmonella Fimbriae: What is the Clue to Their Hairdo?

Karine Dufresne and France Daigle

Additional information is available at the end of the chapter

http://dx.doi.org/10.5772/67189

Abstract

Fimbriae are important virulence factors for *Salmonella* pathogenesis. They mediate adhesion to host cells (including plants), food, stainless steel and much more. The fimbrial systems are organised in gene clusters of four to fifteen genes that code for structural, assembly and regulatory proteins. There are three kinds of fimbriae depending on their mode of assembly. The chaperone/usher (CU) fimbriae use a dedicated chaperone and usher protein to coordinate the subunit biogenesis on the cell surface. The curli fimbriae are assembled by nucleation/precipitation pathway. The type IV fimbria assembly requires a transmembrane apparatus and ATP to energise the reaction. Several fimbriae are conserved among *Salmonella* serovars, while some are present in a limited set or only specific serovars. Expression and regulation of fimbrial genes are not well understood, and most *Salmonella* fimbriae are poorly expressed during in vitro culture, which further complicates research concerning their regulation and role during infection. However, *Salmonella fim* gene cluster, coding for type-1 fimbriae, was widely studied and presents its own set of regulators. Investigating fimbrial distribution, expression and regulation will further elucidate their roles in bacterial pathogenesis and host specificity. Furthermore, fimbriae are important for developing efficient diagnostic tests and antimicrobial strategies against *Salmonella*.

Keywords: fimbriae, adhesion, chaperone/usher, curli, type IV fimbria, fimbriome, *fim*

1. Introduction

Multiple virulence factors are implicated in *Salmonella* pathogenesis. These factors include type 3 secretion systems (T3SS) encoded in *Salmonella* Pathogenicity Islands (SPI)-1 and SPI-2, other SPIs, flagella, capsule, plasmids and adhesion systems [1, 2]. Among those factors, fimbriae represent a major player in pathogenesis and a source of diversity for *Salmonella* serovars. Fimbriae are the most common adhesion systems and are differentially expressed and found in a specific pattern among each serovar [3, 4].

Historically, the first observation of fimbriae was described in 1901 in *Bacillus anthracis* by Hinterberger and Reitman which hypothesised that the filaments were implicated in nutrients acquisition [5]. Then, in 1949, Anderson suggested that the filaments were artefacts due to sample preparation for electron microscopy [6]. However, many other studies contradicted Anderson and confirmed the presence of non-flagellar appendages on the bacterial surface. In 1950, Houwink and Van Iterson observed the appendages and described them as shorter and more rigid filaments than the flagella from *Escherichia coli* and suggested that the fibres were implicated in attachment to surface [7]. The name fimbria (Latin word for fibres) was suggested in 1955 by Duguid et al. to describe the filamentous structures [7, 8]. The term fimbria is preferable to use to describe non-flagellar filaments than pili, which is used to designate structures implicated in conjugation [9, 10]. In 1966, Duguid et al. classified fimbriae in seven types (types 1–6 and F) according to the morphology and haemagglutination patterns. However, another classification, based on serology, better predicted genetic relatedness of fimbrial antigens. Nowadays, fimbriae are designated by the mode of assembly of the fibril [8].

A specific fimbrial gene cluster (FGC) encodes for the structural, assembly and sometime regulatory proteins required for the production of the filamentous adhesive appendage on the bacterial surface. FGCs are usually composed of four to fifteen genes [10, 11]. An average of 12 FGCs by strains was observed in *S. enterica*. Despite that all *Salmonella* genome harbours multiple FGCs, very few are characterised so far. Most fimbriae are poorly expressed under laboratory conditions, and the functional redundancy complicates their studies [10]. However, fimbriae are implicated during infection and in a variety of other roles, like biofilm formation, seroconversion, haemagglutination, cellular invasion and macrophage interactions [2, 7, 12–16]. In mice model, S. Typhimurium fimbriae demonstrate a role in intestinal cells attachment, caecum colonisation and persistence in gut [17–19]. Moreover, fimbriae are important determinants of host adaptation by *Salmonella* [20].

In this chapter, an overview of *Salmonella* fimbriae is presented. First, the three pathways for fimbrial biogenesis (CU, precipitation/nucleation, type IV fimbriae) are described. Second, the distribution of fimbrial genes among *Salmonella* subspecies and serovars is presented. Third, the regulation of fimbrial genes is described and *fim* FGC regulation is detailed. Finally, the use of fimbriae as diagnostic and therapeutic tools is discussed.

2. Fimbrial biogenesis pathways

Three pathways for fimbrial assembly exist in *Salmonella*, the chaperone/usher (CU), the nucleation/precipitation and the type IV pathway [21]. Fimbriae of the CU pathway employ dedicated chaperones and ushers for the fimbrial assembly. The nucleation/precipitation pathway forms an aggregative fibre by precipitation of the subunits in the presence of the nucleator in the extracellular environment. Finally, the type IV fimbrial pathway uses complex machinery for the fimbriae formation and needs ATP to drive the reaction of assembly. Furthermore, the type IV fimbriae can retract and reverse its assembly [21].

The three pathways produce quite different fimbriae. CU fimbriae have the classic fimbrial shape with the repetition of major subunits emerging from the usher inserted in the outer membrane. The major subunits can be accompanied by minor subunits and/or adhesins [8]. The fimbriae produced by the nucleation/precipitation pathway have an aggregated shape, due to the precipitation of major subunits together. This kind of fimbriae is highly stable and hardly depolymerised [22]. The type IV fimbriae anchor in the inner membrane and are prolonged by the repetition of the major subunit (pilin) through the periplasm and the outer membrane reaching the extracellular medium [23]. Here, the three fimbrial assembly mechanisms will be detailed.

2.1. Chaperone/usher pathway

The CU fimbriae represent the largest and most diversified class of adhesion systems [24, 25]. Multiple CU fimbriae are present in *Salmonella* suggesting a functional redundancy [23, 26]. The assembly is characterised by an interaction between the subunits, a periplasmic chaperone and an outer membrane usher in order to form a mature fibre (**Figure 1**) [27]. Each fimbria produced by this pathway has its own unique and specific chaperone and usher [11]. Usher sequence is a good discrimination tool and is used to subdivide the CU fimbriae into six phylogenetic clades (α, κ, π, σ, γ, β) [10, 26].

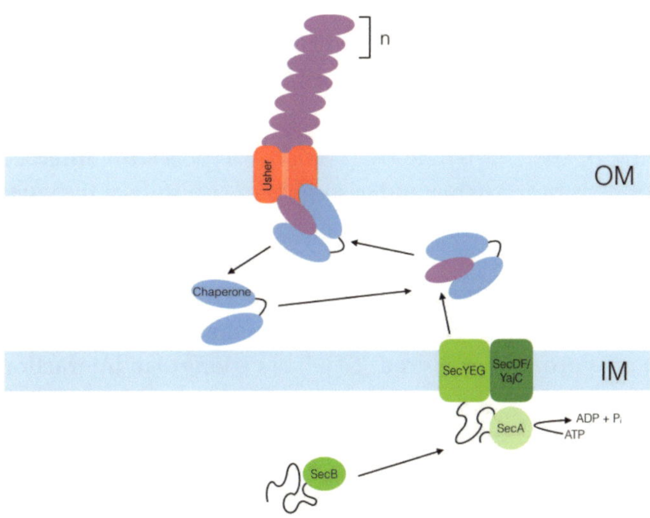

Figure 1. Chaperone/usher pathway. The subunit proteins are synthesised in the cytoplasm and translocated through the periplasm via SecYEG implying also SecDF/YajC inner membrane proteins. When the signal peptide is cleaved from the subunit, the chaperone protein complements the missing strand of the subunit in a process called donor strand complementation. The energy from the folding of the subunit is preserved by the chaperone. The chaperone drives the subunit to the usher and exchanges the donor strand. The subunit is then translocated by the usher to the extracellular medium and added to other subunits to form the fibril. IM = inner membrane; OM = outer membrane.

The biogenesis of the CU fimbriae begins with the production of the subunits in the cytoplasm and their export through the inner membrane by the general secretory pathway (GSP) [23, 27, 28]. It consists in a post-translational translocation implying the SecYEG complex and SecDF/YajC proteins. When the pre-protein is produced, it can be targeted directly to the accessory factor SecA or transported to SecA by the general chaperone SecB. Then, SecA catalyses the hydrolysis of ATP to energise the translocation through SecYEG. Use of ATP, in combination with proton-motive force, triggers the transport of the pre-protein to the periplasm. During the translocation across the inner membrane, the N-terminal signal peptide is cleaved by periplasmic peptidases [27, 29]. To prevent early folding of the subunits, the fimbrial chaperone instantly forms a complex with the translocated subunit in the periplasm [30].

Fimbrial chaperone shares conserved structural features with the general periplasmic chaperones [30]. They are formed of two β-sheet domains oriented to produce an L-shaped molecule and together form a β-barrel. Each domain has an immunoglobulin-like fold and is composed of seven primary β-strands [30–32]. Hydrophobic residues are alternated in the seven strands, facing the internal part of the barrel. These residues form the hydrophobic core of the domain that is implicated in the binding of the subunit. The fimbrial chaperones have an extended loop that lies at the extremity of one arm of the L-shaped molecule. This loop contains a conserved motif that is involved in the complex formation between the chaperone and subunits [30]. The subunit and the chaperone have a similar structure, but the subunit is missing the seventh β-strand of the C-terminal extremity [28]. The chaperone transfers the missing β-strand to the subunit to complete its structure: this mechanism is called the donor strand complementation [25]. The chaperone preserves the folding energy of the subunit to drive the last steps of the assembly due to lack of energy source (ATP) in the periplasmic space [33]. The chaperone also prevents premature fimbrial formation in the periplasm and primes the assembly through the usher [30, 34].

Then, the uncapping of the chaperone by the usher exposes the interactive surface of the subunit to the outer membrane usher and assembly of subunits at the surface can occur [33]. The transfer of the subunit from the chaperone to the usher happens very rapidly in vivo. In the absence of the usher in vitro, only a slow and inefficient assembly was observed. This suggests that the uncapping of the chaperone is important for the efficiency of mature fimbriae assembly [28, 30]. An interaction between the usher and the subunit and also between the usher and the chaperone is required [31]. This triangular interaction is important for the usher to discriminate subunit-loaded from unloaded chaperone [33]. Fimbrial usher forms a ring in the outer membrane with a transient twin-pore of 2–3 nm diameter to allow passage of subunits to the extracellular environment [35]. The usher catalyses fimbrial polymerisation by involving donor strand exchange where the N-terminal sequence of the subunit is replaced by a short sequence of the last subunit in the polymerised fibril with a zip-in-zip-out mechanism [33]. This step is triggered in part by the chaperone required for the strand exchange between the new subunit and the forming fimbria. The quaternary structure of the subunit is achieved when the protein passes through the pore. The final morphology and structure (rigid or flexible), the length (1–3 μm) and width (2–10 nm) of the fibre of the CU fimbriae depend on the subunits composition and the interactions between subunits [10, 33].

2.2. Nucleation/precipitation pathway

Curli fimbriae were initially discovered in *Escherichia coli* and are very conserved among the *Enterobacteriaceae* family, compared to any other types of FGC. The amyloid fibrils are particularly known for their role in biofilm formation and its recognition by the immune system [36]. The FGC for curli is named *csg* (curli subunit gene) for *E. coli* and *agf* (thin aggregative fimbriae) for *Salmonella*, but the term *csg* is now commonly used for *Salmonella*. Curli formation depends on two divergent operons, *csgBAC* and *csgDEFG*. The *csgBAC* genes encode for CsgA, the major subunit, CsgB, the nucleator, and CsgC, an oxidoreductase of unknown function. The *csgDEFG* genes encode for the transcription regulator of the operon (CsgD) and for the assembly proteins located in the periplasm (CsgE) or in the outer membrane (CsgG and CsgF) [37].

The curli assembly mechanism is characterised by the exportation of the subunits and their precipitation to each other in the presence of a nucleator that fixes the fibril on the bacterial surface. Exportation of curli proteins also uses the GSP to pass through the inner membrane to the periplasm. Then, the CsgA and CsgB proteins are secreted by the lipoprotein CsgG. CsgG is composed of nine anticodon-binding domain-like units that form a 36-stranded β-barrel complex that is inserted in the outer membrane. CsgG forms a pore in the outer membrane that permits the passage of the subunits and the nucleator. CsgG is accompanied by the accessory proteins CsgE and CsgF. CsgE is a specificity factor that forms a nonameric adaptor that binds to CsgG and closes the periplasmic space. The presence of CsgE optimises the uptake of CsgA by CsgG and translocation of CsgA [38]. CsgF helps the nucleation activity of CsgB. It was suggested that CsgF has a role in specific localisation and/or chaperoning of the nucleator, so CsgB will reach its full activity. Moreover, CsgF depends on CsgG and CsgE for its stability [39].

Once at the bacterial surface, the nucleator polymerises the subunits together into thin aggregative fimbriae (fibrils). This process happens only in the extracellular environment and requires the presence of the nucleator CsgB to polymerise CsgA into a filament. CsgA proteins fold into an insoluble cross β-sheet molecules [26]. CsgB anchors the curli fimbriae on the surface of the bacterial cell (**Figure 2**). In *E. coli*, it was observed that CsgB, in addition to its role of nucleator, is also part of the fimbriae with the CsgA subunits. A structurally different fibril made of CsgB subunits can be formed in the absence of CsgA [40]. CsgA and CsgB share 30% of sequence identity and have the same predicted length [37]. In *E. coli*, interbacterial complementation between a nucleator mutant and a subunit mutant is possible. However, in *Salmonella*, this complementation cannot happen, suggesting that the curli fimbriae are different in their nucleation process. However, the interbacterial complementation was observed in *Salmonella* when a lipopolysaccharide O-antigen mutant was used [41]. The nucleation/precipitation pathway is still poorly understood, and research is actually performed on the different aspects of the curli fimbrial formation.

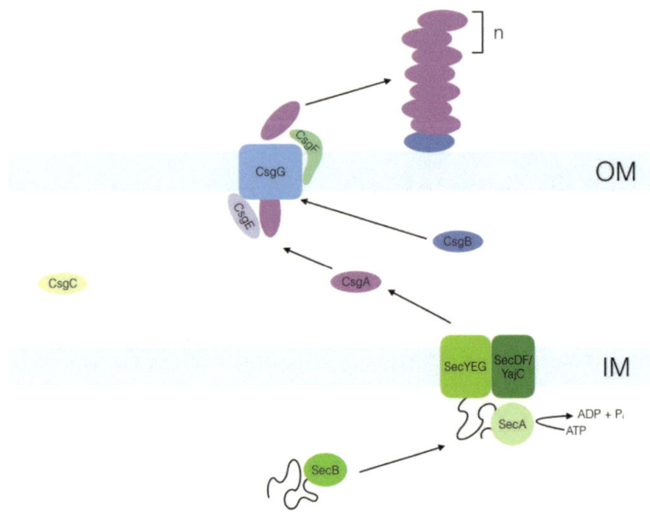

Figure 2. Nucleation/precipitation pathway. The subunit CsgA is synthesised in the cytoplasm and translocated by the GSP. CsgA passes through the periplasm and is translocated in the extracellular medium by CsgG, helped by CsgE. The nucleator CsgB is also translocated by CsgG and supported by CsgF for its stability on the bacterial surface. When CsgA is in the presence of the nucleator in the extracellular environment, the subunits precipitate in an aggregated fibril. CsgC is an oxidoreductase, but its specific role is still undiscovered. IM, inner membrane; OM, outer membrane.

2.3. Type IV fimbriae

Type IV fimbriae are usually from 1 to 5 μm long and are composed of repeated subunits of a single pilin. Type IV fimbria is subdivided into two groups based on homology of the major subunits: type IVa and type IVb fimbriae [26]. The difference between the two types is in the length of the peptide sequence and the mature major pilin sequence. Specific mechanism of assembly of type IVb fimbriae from *Salmonella* has not been characterised yet [42].

Type IV fimbriae pathway has the most complex machinery. They form an apparatus, composed of various proteins, that goes through the inner and outer membranes allowing the anchor of the fibre and energy accessibility for fimbrial assembly. The gene cluster also encodes numerous proteins with diverse functions, as the fibril is not only assembled but also disassembled. Type IV fimbriae are frequently compared to the type II secretion system (T2SS) which possesses similar structure and mechanism of assembly. Type IV fimbriae are implicated in adherence and twitching motility [11].

Type IV fimbriae are present in a variety of organisms including human pathogens such as *Neisseria gonorrhoeae*, *Neisseria meningitidis*, *Pseudomonas aeruginosa* and *Vibrio cholerae*. For *Salmonella*, they are found in *S. bongori*, *S. enterica* serovars Heidelberg, Paratyphi B and Typhi [42]. *S. bongori* type IV fimbria is encoded by the *sbe* operon that remains uncharacterised and is located on a plasmid, as well as in *S.* Paratyphi B, while the type IVb gene cluster is located on the chromosome of *S.* Heidelberg and *S.* Typhi [26].

For *S.* Typhi, the PilS subunits are produced in the cytoplasm and translocated to the periplasm by the GSP. In the periplasm, the N-terminal sequence of PilS is cleaved by PilU, a prepilin peptidase [23]. The mature pilins are then anchored to the inner membrane on platform proteins and linked together into a fibril (**Figure 3**) [26, 43]. The N-terminal domain of the mature subunits is highly hydrophobic, which permits the PilS proteins to group into a helical structure [22, 42]. The pilins are added one by one, but at three sites simultaneously, each corresponding to a strand to form a three-helix bundle [44]. An ATPase inserted in the inner membrane supplies the energy required for the assembly of the type IV fimbriae. The secretin proteins are inserted in the outer membrane and form a channel that permits the passage of the intact pilus through the bacterial surface [26]. These proteins form complexes that are then assembled in a cage-like final structure [44]. Other proteins are also involved in the assembly/disassembly mechanisms, such as another ATPase dedicated for the disassembly of the fimbriae, lipoproteins of the secretin complex (pilotins), inner membrane proteins or gene products involved in peptidoglycan remodelling to permit the passage of the fibril through the periplasm [22, 44, 45]. This assembly pathway is less understood and requires further investigations [44].

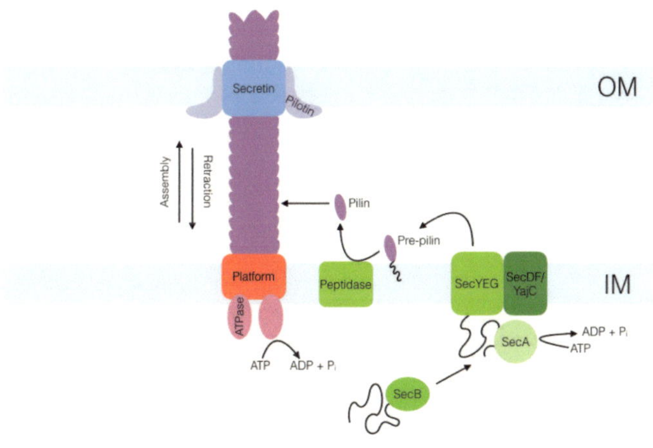

Figure 3. Type IV pathway. The pre-pilins are transported and translocated through the inner membrane (IM) to the periplasm by GSP. A peptidase cleaves the signal peptide of the pre-pilin, and the pilin can be assembled on the platform proteins. An ATPase triggers the reaction. The pilins form a three-helix structure that passes through the outer membrane (OM) by a secretin supported by pilotin. The type IV fimbriae can also retract depending on the environmental conditions.

3. *Salmonella* fimbriome

Each fimbrial pathway described above is present in *Salmonella* creating a great element of genetic diversity. CU fimbriae are the most common fimbriae detected in the *Salmonella* genome. Curli (*csg*) is found in all *Salmonella* genome, whereas only a few serovars have the type IV fimbriae. There are 38 unique FGCs identified so far in 111 sequenced genomes from 34 different serovars (**Table 1**) [46, 47]. Each serovar has its own repertoire of FGCs, but there are seven FGCs that are highly conserved in most *Salmonella* strains forming the core of *Salmonella* FGCs. Most of the FGCs are sporadic or found only in a few strains constituting the signature of each serovar.

Fimbriae	CU clade	Prevalence	Distribution	Fimbriae	CU clade	Prevalence	Distribution
bcf	γ1	Core	Absent in IV	*sdj*	γ4	Sporadic	IIIb *diarizonae*
csg	curli	Core	All *Salmonella*	*sdk/sfi*	π	Sporadic	IIIb, VI
fim	γ1	Core	Absent in *bongori*	*sdl*	π	Sporadic	IIIb *diarizonae*
lpf	γ1	Conserved	Absent in ID	*sef*	γ3	Sporadic	IB, D (pseudo)
mrk	γ4	Sporadic	Only in Montevideo	*sib*	β	Sporadic	VI *indica*
pef	κ	Sporadic	Only in IA, IC and *bongori*	*fae/skf*	κ	Sporadic	IB, IE
peg	γ4	Conserved	IB, IC, IIIa, VI, *bongori*	*ssf*	γ4	Sporadic	II *salamae*
peh	γ4	Sporadic	Only in Montevideo	*sta*	γ4	Sporadic	ID
pil		Sporadic	Type IV; ID, IE, *bongori*	*stb*	γ4	Core	I, II, IIIb;
saf	γ3	Conserved	ssp. I	*stc*	γ4	Conserved	IA, IB, ID
sba	γ4	Sporadic	*bongori*	*std*	π	Core	II, IIIa, missing in Gallinarum
sbb/sbf	π	Sporadic	*bongori*	*ste*	π	Conserved	Missing in IA, IE
sbc/spf	κ	Sporadic	IV, VI, *bongori*	*stf*	π	Conserved	Missing in ID, IE
sbs	β	Sporadic	II *salamae*	*stg*	γ1	Sporadic	ID, bongori
sdc/sas	σ	Sporadic	IIIa *arizonae*	*sth*	γ1	Core	Missing IIIa and IIIb
sdd/smf	γ1	Sporadic	IE, II, IIIa, IV	*sti*	γ1	Conserved	Missing in ID
sde	γ3	Sporadic	Tennessee (IE)	*stj*	β	Sporadic	IA, IE
sdh	γ4	Sporadic	IE	*stk*	γ4	Sporadic	IE
sdi/sdf	γ4	Sporadic	IIIb *diarizonae*	*tcf*	α	Sporadic	IC, ID, IE

Table 1. *Salmonella* fimbriome.

Each *Salmonella* strain contains 5–14 different CU fimbriae with an average of 12 fimbriae in *S. enterica*. Representatives from all the six phylogenetic clades are present in *Salmonella* (**Table 2**) [26]. The γ-fimbriae constitute the largest clade with 22 FGCs and include the highly conserved FGCs (*bcf, fim* and *sth*) that belong to the clade γ-1. The most diverse clade is γ-4, with the conserved *stb* and *stc* or *peg* (*stc-peg*) and many of the new sporadic FGCs, while the α clade (for alternate CU), also known as class 5 fimbriae, has one FGC, *tcf*, which is found in several serovars. The σ clade also had only one FGC representative, *sdc*, that was only found in *S. enterica* subspecies IIIa (*arizonae*).

The distribution of the 38 FGCs gave a signature for each species, subspecies and serovars (**Table 3**). Seven FGCs, curli and the CU *fim, bcf, sth, stb, stc-peg* and *std*, represent the conserved (core) fimbriae of *Salmonella* (positive in more than 90% of strains). The *fim* fimbriae were found in all *S. enterica* strains, only missing in *S. bongori*. The *bcf* cluster was only missing in *S. enterica* ssp. IV (*houtenae*), and the *sth* cluster was only missing in *S. enterica* ssp. IIIa and IIIb. The *stb* cluster was present in *S. enterica* ssp. I, II, IIIb and the *std* cluster was not detected in *S. enterica* serovar Gallinarum, ssp. II, IIIA and *S. bongori*. The FGC *stc* and *peg* had probably emerged from a common ancestor: they belong to the same clade (γ-4) and are inserted at the same position in the genome (between *thiM* and *mrp*); their distribution is mutually exclusive; and either one is present in the majority of *Salmonella* strains.

CU clade	**Fimbriae**
α	*tcf*
β	*sbs, sib, stj*
γ1	*bcf, fim, lpf, sdd/smf, stg, sth, sti*
γ3	*saf, sde, sef*
γ4	*mrk, peg, peh, sba, sdh, sdi, sdj, ssf, sta, stb, stc, stk*
κ	*fae/skf, pef, sbc/spf*
π	*sbb/sbf, sdk, sdl, std, ste, stf*
σ	*sdc/sas*

Table 2. *Salmonella* fimbrial type.

Most cases of salmonellosis in humans are caused by *S. enterica* ssp. I, and many of the sequenced serovars were from ssp. I. Thus, 27 out of the 38 FGCs are found in ssp. I. The ssp. I was divided into five classes using previous phylogenetic analysis [46, 47] (**Table 3**). The class IA contains broad host range serovars involved in gastroenteritis, mainly serovar Typhimurium. The class IB is formed by serovars Dublin, Enteritidis, Pullorum and Gallinarum, all sharing similar O-antigens and FGCs. The class IC contains serovars Choleraesuis and Paratyphi C and class ID contains the human-specific serovars Typhi and Paratyphi A. A separate branch of class IA, including serovars Heidelberg, Virchow and Hadar, that had the highest number of FGCs, as well as serovars Montevideo, Schwarzengrund, Welterveden, Javiana, Kentucky and Tennessee, was commonly isolated in association with edible plants and constitutes the class IE.

In addition to the seven core FGCs, five highly conserved FGCs (*saf, ste, stf, sti* and *lpf*) were associated with *S. enterica* ssp. I (**Table 3**). The *sti, lpf* and *stf* clusters are missing in human-specific serovars (class ID). The *ste* cluster is missing in class IA serovars and in some of the class IE serovars. Thus, *S. enterica* ssp. I harbours the core FGCs (*fim, bcf, sth, stb, stc-peg* and *std*), the conserved FGCs (*saf, ste, stf, sti* and *lpf*) and some sporadic FGCs unique to each serovar. Many FGCs of *Salmonella* are sporadic and form the unique repertoire in each serovar.

Despite the presence of many FGCs, extensive gene degradation was observed in most of the host-restricted and warm-blooded host-adapted serovars, mainly Gallinarum, Choleraesuis,

Paratyphi A and Typhi. Genome degradation of FGCs may correspond to the loss of genes rendered unnecessary by niche specialisation or by selective pressure in order to diminish antigen presentation at the bacterial surface during systemic disease. Intriguingly, most of FGCs were intact in Paratyphi B.

There are 11 FGCs that are not in ssp. I, with only *sbc* and *sdk* that are shared by more than one serovars. The low numbers of FGCs might be specific for cold-blooded animals' colonisation. A conserved signature specific for each subspecies was observed. As more diverse strains will be sequenced, new FGCs probably be discovered.

	Subspecies	Core	Conserved		Accessory	Absent
Salmonella enterica	I. *enterica*	*bcf, csg, fim, sth, stb, std stc-peg*	*sti,, saf, ste, stf, lpf*	A	*pef, stj*	*ste*
				B	*fae, sef*	
				C	*pef, tcf,*	
				D	*sef, sta, stg, tcf, pil*	*sti, lpf, stf*
				E	*fae, mrk, peh, sdd, sde, sdh, stj, stk, pil*	*lpf, ste, stf*
	VI. *indica*				*sbc, sdk, sib*	*stb*
	II. *salamae*				*sdd, ssf, sbs*	*std*
	IV. *houtenae*				*sbc, sdd*	*bcf, stb*
	IIIb. *diarizonae*				*sdi, sdj, sdk, sdl*	*sth*
	IIIa. *arizonae*				*sdc, sdd*	*sth, stb, std*
Salmonella bongori			*lpf*		*sba, sbb, sbc, sbe, stg(sbd)*	*fim, stb, std*

Table 3. Fimbrial distribution.

4. Fimbrial regulation

Salmonella fimbriae are usually not expressed constitutively and rarely expressed under laboratory condition, except for Fim fimbriae, a type-1 fimbria [3]. Fimbriae are important during infection [19, 48, 49], suggesting that their expression is tightly regulated. Little is known about the regulation mechanisms that promote fimbrial expression. In general, fimbrial expression is positively or negatively regulated at the genetic level. Some regulators are unique to a specific fimbriae, like the regulation of curli by CsgD, while others are global, like Dam, H-NS and Lrp (leucine-responsive regulatory protein) [50]. These mechanisms include regulatory proteins, DNA methylation, cyclic di-GMP and small RNAs [50]. In *Salmonella,* a regulation network exists between the virulence factors. Here, we present the regulation of fimbrial genes including the interaction with motility and invasion. Then, we propose an example of regulation of the *fim* FGC expression in *S.* Typhimurium, the most characterised fimbriae of *Salmonella.*

4.1. General regulation of fimbrial genes

Genes implicated in different aspects of virulence including motility, adhesion, invasion of host cells and intestinal persistence are all regulated during infection. It was proposed that there is a temporal hierarchy between the T3SS of SPI-1 (invasion), flagellar and fimbrial genes, where SPI-1 is first activated, followed by flagellar genes and then type-1 fimbrial genes (*fim*). The crosstalk between these systems seems to be critical for bacterial pathogenesis [51]. Each element of virulence is related to a large regulation network that is not completely understood. DNA adenine methylation (Dam) regulates many virulence genes in *Salmonella* [52]: it is required for SPI-1 and *pef* expression, but it also represses many genes, including the *std, csg* and flagellar genes [52–54]. It was also shown that fimbrial FGCs are repressed by the Rcs phosphorelay, a sensor of outer membrane stress [55]. Another example of regulation interaction between motility and fimbrial expression was observed by a deletion of *ydiV* in *S.* Typhimurium that results in the derepression of curli fimbriae (*csgAB*), causing an increase in swimming motility and a decrease in swarming [56].

Crosstalk regulation also occurs between the capsule and the type IVb fimbriae in *S.* Typhi. Both virulence factors are encoded on SPI-7 and facilitate invasion of monocytes, suggesting a regulation overlapped. However, the exact regulation elements that act on those two systems are unknown [57].

One of the post-transcriptional regulation mechanisms uses the binding of small RNAs and the Hfq chaperone. In an *hfq* mutant strain, the expression of fimbrial gene *sefA* was activated when most of the other fimbrial subunit genes were repressed in *S.* Enteritidis. Overall, the *hfq* deletion decreased adherence compared to wild-type strain. Thus, Hfq seems to regulate fimbrial expression of most fimbrial genes from *S.* Enteritidis [58]. There is probably more sRNAs regulation of fimbrial gene expression awaiting to be discovered.

Phase variation is a transcriptional mechanism that controls the switch between fimbriated (ON) and afimbriated (OFF) cells within a bacterial population. In *Salmonella,* expression of *lpf* and *pef* was shown to be controlled by phase variation. The regulators of this mechanism are various and depend on the FGCs concerned [54, 59].

The secondary messenger cyclic-di-GMP controls virulence and biofilm formation in *Salmonella* [60]. In *Salmonella,* curli expression was activated by AdrA, a GGDEF-domain protein that increases intracellular level of cyclic-di-GMP [61]. Fimbrial production regulated by the cyclic-di-GMP level was also observed in other species such as *Klebsiella pneumonia, E. coli* and *P. aeruginosa* [62].

In spite of all those known elements of regulation, how *Salmonella* passes from being afimbriated in vitro to a fimbriated form in vivo is still unknown.

4.2. Regulation of *fim* in *S.* Typhimurium

The *fim* FGC codes for six genes (*fimAICDHF*). This cluster is the most studied and one of the most conserved fimbriae of *Salmonella enterica* and was mainly characterised in *S.* Typhimurium. These fimbriae have a binding specificity for mannose residues [63]. The fim fimbria of *Salmonella* is not homologue with its homonym from *E. coli,* except for sharing some morphological and mechanistic features [64, 65]. Regulation and amino acid sequences of fimbrial proteins are divergent between the two species. The transition from afimbriated to fimbriated stage occurs for *fim*, but there is no inversion of the promoter region as observed for *E. coli* phase variation [66]. For *S.* Typhimurium, the major subunit FimA is accompanied by two other subunits, FimI and FimF, and by the adhesin, FimH. The *fimC* and *fimD* genes encode respectively the chaperone and the usher [67]. Ancillary genes, *fimZYW*, and a rare arginine transfer RNA (tRNA) *fimU* and *STM0551*, inserted between *fimY* and *fimW*, directly regulate *fim* expression [62].

Ancillary genes *fimZYW* regulate the expression of *fimA* [50, 68–70]. FimZ, a sensor DNA-binding protein, is the principal positive regulator of *fimA* [71]. FimY upregulates *fimZ* expression by binding to the *fimZ* promoter. FimY and FimZ then form a complex that activates the *fimA* promoter [63, 69]; *fimY* is itself regulated by the arginine tRNA *fimU* [72]. Lrp is another regulator that binds and activates the *fimZ* promoter, probably by antagonising the binding of the global repressor protein H-NS to this promoter region [67, 70, 73]. H-NS has a high affinity for AT-rich DNA region, and *fimZ* gene has an unusual AT-rich sequence [73].

At the opposite, FimW repressed directly *fimA* expression and indirectly by lowering FimZ availability by its degradation caused by FimW binding [74]. It is also suggested that STM0551, an EAL domain protein, is a negative regulator of *fim* expression by lowering the c-di-GMP level [62].

FimZ is also used as a regulator relay by two-component system for expression of *hilA*, the principal regulator of SPI-1 (invasion). The two-component system PhoBR induces *fimZ* expression, and PhoPQ activates *hilE*, one of the negative regulators of *hilA*, by a FimYZ-dependant manner. FimZ also downregulates *flhDC*, genes implicated in flagella expression [75]. Flagellar gene *fliZ* also represses *fimZ* on a post-transcriptional manner, reinforcing the fact that there is an alternated expression of flagella (motility) and fimbriae (adhesion) [51] and confirming a regulation network between SPI-1 (invasion) and fimbrial expression [76]. Thus, a combination of factors directly implicated in fimbrial genes regulation can also impact on other virulence systems of *Salmonella* (**Figure 4**).

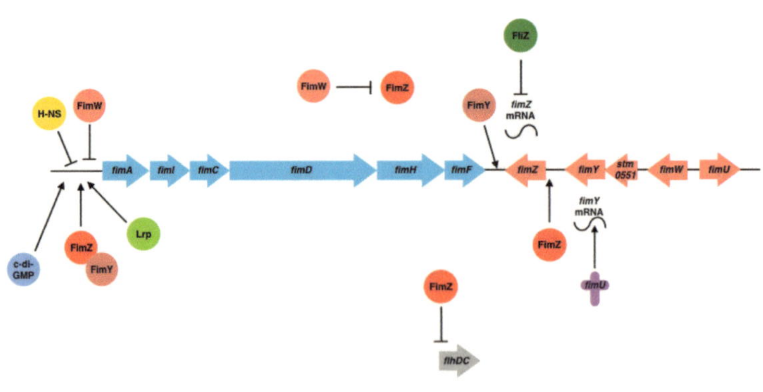

Figure 4. *fim* regulation. The fim FGC is activated and inhibited by diverse regulators. FimZ, accompanied by FimY, is the principal activator of *fimA*. Lrp and c-di-GMP also activate *fimA* at the promoter level. H-NS and FimW inhibit *fimA* expression by linking its promoter. FimW also reduces *fimA* expression by linking FimZ and decreases the availability of this activator. The gene *fimZ* is activated by FimZ itself and by FimY, but is repressed by FliZ in a post-transcriptional manner. The tRNA *fimU* regulates fimY. FimZ downregulates *flhCD*, genes implicated in flagellar expression.

5. Fimbriae as a tool

Salmonella infections are a major concern for public and animal health. Some serovars are host specific, while others are broad-spectrum pathogens and can be transmitted from food-borne animals to humans. On the other hand, animals can develop health problems and will not be suitable for consumption. To prevent those issues, it is critical to develop ways to detect *Salmonella* and protect potential hosts against infection. The importance of fimbriae for detection of *Salmonella* by molecular techniques and for vaccine development is presented in this section [77].

5.1. *Salmonella* detection using fimbrial genes

Salmonella-specific tests were performed since the end of the 1980s and mainly targeted surface antigens. Those tests include agglutination tests and ELISA (enzyme-linked immunosorbent assays) [77–79]. In 1993, Doran et al. presented a DNA-based test that targets *csgA* (*agfA*), offering a faster and more precise test for genus identification [80]. Then, in early 2000s, PCR (polymerisation chain reaction) tests using fimbrial genes, like *sef* or *csgA* (*agfA*), in combination with other virulence genes were developed to differentiate *Salmonella* strains from each other [81]. Different PCR tests (multiplex, nested and direct PCR) were elaborated for detection of *Salmonella*. Several of those tests integrated detection of fimbrial genes (i.e. *staA*, *fimW*) to discriminate between serovars [81–83]. Recently, a loop-mediated isothermal amplification (LAMP) assay was developed to detect *Salmonella* by targeting *bcfD*, a gene that belongs to the core of FGC. In isothermal conditions, the reaction occurs in an hour permitting rapid detection of *Salmonella* [84].

Salmonella-specific tests evolved from detecting antigens, which can be long and expensive to perform, to detecting specific genes in less than an hour by sensitive methods. Fimbrial genes are tools of choice for detection of *Salmonella*. The presence of conserved fimbrial genes allows the discrimination between *Salmonella* and non-*Salmonella* species. On the other hand, the presence of a specific pattern of fimbrial genes enables the discrimination between serovars.

5.2. Vaccines development

As surface structures, fimbriae constitute antigens of choice for the development of vaccines against *Salmonella* [85]. Fimbriae are difficult to study because they are poorly expressed under laboratory conditions and are redundant. The most interesting fimbriae are the ones expressed during infection. Targeting those fimbriae will confer higher chances to be recognised by the immune system in key moments of infection.

More than 20 fimbrial antigens were detected in typhoid fever patient's blood by transcriptomic analysis: SteD, StaACD, BcfDE, SafBC, TcfBCD, StbBC, FimAIDH, StdBC, StgACD and SthA [86]. Antibodies against immunogenic fimbrial proteins TcfB, StbD and CsgEFG were identified in the blood of typhoid fever patients [12]. Immunoreactive antibodies against SthDA and BcfA were found in lymphocytes supernatant (ALS) of patients with typhoid fever [87].

SefA, a protein from the SEF14 fimbriae of *S*. Enteritidis, was used as an antigen associated with liposomes for oral immunisation of chickens [88]. The immunisation of chickens by fimbrial antigens was efficient for IgG and IgA responses and reduced *Salmonella* colonisation. Four weeks after immunisation, the bacterial excretion from the intestinal tract was significantly reduced [88]. The liposome-associated immunisation was also performed with fimbrial antigen from SEF21 and resulted in a similar efficiency [89]. SefD, another antigen from SEF14, was also used to vaccinate animals in a bacterin preparation, a vaccine prepared from inactivated bacteria. This vaccine was efficient to reduce the presence of *Salmonella* from the spleens of hens [90].

As factors implicated in the first stages of infection, fimbriae are an interesting target for vaccine development [91]. Fimbrial antigens are important for the development of new anti-*Salmonella* therapies [85, 86]. However, a better understanding of their expression pattern in vivo is needed to optimise the therapeutic effects of fimbrial-targeted vaccines. Fimbrial antigens may be combined with other immunogenic proteins to increase the immune response [91].

6. Conclusion

Fimbriae are diverse proteinaceous surface structures. They diverge by their assembly mechanisms and result in different filamentous structures with roles in pathogenesis. However, their roles are not completely understood. They were first known for adherence to cells and inert surfaces, but they seem to be implicated in so much more functions during infection.

The multiplicity of adhesion systems is also an enigma. Most of the *Salmonella* serovars possess 12 fimbrial gene clusters. Some fimbriae are specific to certain serovars and may play a role in these bacteria that do not need to be fulfilled in other serovars. At the opposite, there is a core of fimbrial genes that are present in most of the serovars. Fimbriae are one of the keys to understand *Salmonella* pathogenesis. The specific pattern of each serovar, with further investigations on the sporadic fimbriae, may also bring insights into our understanding of *Salmonella* pathogenesis.

Regulation of fimbrial genes is a complex network that is tightly related to invasion and motility. Virulence factors are finely regulated, and a temporal expression hierarchy allows the success of *Salmonella* infection. General regulators are already known to regulate fimbrial genes such as stress sensor Rcs relay or the Hfq factor. Phase variation from a fimbriated to afimbriated status occurs in *Salmonella*. However, this phenomenon is not from a promoter inversion of the Fim cluster, but from the regulation by ancillary genes related to *fim* gene cluster. These ancillary genes are themselves precisely regulated by a variety of regulators known for their role in other bacterial processes.

The actual understanding of fimbrial expression opens a new area on human health prevention. Some conserved fimbrial genes, in combination with other virulence genes, are precious markers for *Salmonella* detection. These tools could permit a faster diagnostic for human patients, but also a rapid detection of contaminated food or infected animals. Fimbrial proteins can serve as good immunogens in vaccine preparation against *Salmonella* infection.

A better understanding of fimbrial expression, production and regulation processes becomes important for prevention of *Salmonella* infection. It will also enlighten the importance of fimbriae in other human pathogens, as fimbrial systems are part of virulence factors in many bacteria.

Author details

Karine Dufresne and France Daigle*

*Address all correspondence to: france.daigle@umontreal.ca

Department of Microbiology, Infectiology and Immunology, Université de Montréal, Montréal, Canada

References

[1] Daigle F. Typhi genes expressed during infection or involved in pathogenesis. J Infect Dev Ctries. 2008;2(6):431–7.

[2] Sabbagh SC, Forest CG, Lepage C, Leclerc JM, Daigle F. So similar, yet so different: uncovering distinctive features in the genomes of *Salmonella enterica* serovars Typhimurium and Typhi. FEMS Microbiol Lett. 2010;305(1):1–13.

[3] Humphries AD, Raffatellu M, Winter S, Weening EH, Kingsley RA, Droleskey R, et al. The use of flow cytometry to detect expression of subunits encoded by 11 *Salmonella enterica* serotype Typhimurium fimbrial operons. Mol Microbiol. 2003;48(5):1357–76.

[4] Townsend SM, Kramer NE, Edwards R, Baker S, Hamlin N, Simmonds M, et al. *Salmonella enterica* serovar Typhi possesses a unique repertoire of fimbrial gene sequences. Infect Immun. 2001;69(5):2894–901.

[5] Houwink AL, van IW. Electron microscopical observations on bacterial cytology; a study on flagellation. Biochim Biophys Acta. 1950;5(1):10–44.

[6] Anderson TF. On the mechanism of adsorption of bacteriophages on host cells. In: Miles AA, Pirie, N. W., editor. The nature of the bacterial surface. Oxford: Oxford University Press; 1949. p. 76–95.

[7] Duguid JP, Smith IW, Dempster G, Edmunds PN. Non-flagellar filamentous appendages (fimbriae) and haemagglutinating activity in *Bacterium coli*. J Pathol Bacteriol. 1955;70(2):335–48.

[8] Thanassi DG, Nuccio SP, Shu Kin So S, Baumler AJ. Fimbriae: Classification and Biochemistry. EcoSal Plus. 2007;2(2):1–27.

[9] Ottow JC. Ecology, physiology, and genetics of fimbriae and pili. Annu Rev Microbiol. 1975;29:79–108.

[10] Nuccio SP, Baumler AJ. Evolution of the chaperone/usher assembly pathway: fimbrial classification goes Greek. Microbiol Mol Biol Rev. 2007;71(4):551–75.

[11] Mol O, Oudega B. Molecular and structural aspects of fimbriae biosynthesis and assembly in *Escherichia coli*. FEMS Microbiol Rev. 1996;19(1):25–52.

[12] Harris JB, Baresch-Bernal A, Rollins SM, Alam A, LaRocque RC, Bikowski M, et al. Identification of in vivo-induced bacterial protein antigens during human infection with *Salmonella enterica* serovar Typhi. Infect Immun. 2006;74(9):5161–8.

[13] Boddicker JD, Ledeboer NA, Jagnow J, Jones BD, Clegg S. Differential binding to and biofilm formation on, HEp-2 cells by *Salmonella enterica* serovar Typhimurium is dependent upon allelic variation in the *fimH* gene of the *fim* gene cluster. Mol Microbiol. 2002;45(5):1255–65.

[14] Edwards RA, Schifferli DM, Maloy SR. A role for *Salmonella* fimbriae in intraperitoneal infections. Proc Natl Acad Sci U S A. 2000;97(3):1258–62.

[15] Althouse C, Patterson S, Fedorka-Cray P, Isaacson RE. Type 1 fimbriae of *Salmonella enterica* serovar Typhimurium bind to enterocytes and contribute to colonization of swine in vivo. Infect Immun. 2003;71(11):6446–52.

[16] Sabbagh SC, Lepage C, McClelland M, Daigle F. Selection of *Salmonella enterica* serovar Typhi genes involved during interaction with human macrophages by screening of a transposon mutant library. PLoS One. 2012;7(5):e36643.

[17] Chessa D, Winter MG, Jakomin M, Baumler AJ. *Salmonella enterica* serotype Typhimurium Std fimbriae bind terminal alpha(1,2)fucose residues in the cecal mucosa. Mol Microbiol. 2009;71(4):864–75.

[18] Humphries A, Deridder S, Baumler AJ. *Salmonella enterica* serotype Typhimurium fimbrial proteins serve as antigens during infection of mice. Infect Immun. 2005;73(9):5329–38.

[19] Weening EH, Barker JD, Laarakker MC, Humphries AD, Tsolis RM, Baumler AJ. The *Salmonella enterica* serotype Typhimurium *lpf, bcf, stb, stc, std,* and *sth* fimbrial operons are required for intestinal persistence in mice. Infect Immun. 2005;73(6):3358–66.

[20] Yue M, Han X, De Masi L, Zhu C, Ma X, Zhang J, et al. Allelic variation contributes to bacterial host specificity. Nat Commun. 2015;6:8754.

[21] Fronzes R, Remaut H, Waksman G. Architectures and biogenesis of non-flagellar protein appendages in Gram-negative bacteria. EMBO J. 2008;27(17):2271–80.

[22] Smyth CJ, Marron MB, Twohig JM, Smith SG. Fimbrial adhesins: similarities and variations in structure and biogenesis. FEMS Immunol Med Microbiol. 1996;16(2):127–39.

[23] Wagner C, Hensel M. Adhesive mechanisms of *Salmonella enterica*. Adv Exp Med Biol. 2011;715:17–34.

[24] Soto GE, Hultgren SJ. Bacterial adhesins: common themes and variations in architecture and assembly. J Bacteriol. 1999;181(4):1059–71.

[25] Sauer FG, Barnhart M, Choudhury D, Knight SD, Waksman G, Hultgren SJ. Chaperone-assisted pilus assembly and bacterial attachment. Curr Opin Struct Biol. 2000;10(5):548–56.

[26] Porwollik S. *Salmonella*: from genome to function. Norfolk, UK: Caister Academic Press; 2011. xii, 300, A1 p.

[27] Gerlach RG, Hensel M. Protein secretion systems and adhesins: the molecular armory of Gram-negative pathogens. Int J Med Microbiol. 2007;297(6):401–15.

[28] Thanassi DG, Saulino ET, Hultgren SJ. The chaperone/usher pathway: a major terminal branch of the general secretory pathway. Curr Opin Microbiol. 1998;1(2):223–31.

[29] Dufresne K, Paradis-Bleau C. Biology and assembly of the bacterial envelope. Adv Exp Med Biol. 2015;883:41–76.

[30] Sauer FG, Remaut H, Hultgren SJ, Waksman G. Fiber assembly by the chaperone-usher pathway. Biochim Biophys Acta. 2004;1694(1–3):259–67.

[31] Barnhart MM, Sauer FG, Pinkner JS, Hultgren SJ. Chaperone-subunit-usher interactions required for donor strand exchange during bacterial pilus assembly. J Bacteriol. 2003;185(9):2723–30.

[32] Saulino ET, Bullitt E, Hultgren SJ. Snapshots of usher-mediated protein secretion and ordered pilus assembly. Proc Natl Acad Sci USA. 2000;97(16):9240–5.

[33] Zavialov A, Zav'yalova G, Korpela T, Zav'yalov V. FGL chaperone-assembled fimbrial polyadhesins: anti-immune armament of Gram-negative bacterial pathogens. FEMS Microbiol Rev. 2007;31(4):478–514.

[34] Waksman G, Hultgren SJ. Structural biology of the chaperone-usher pathway of pilus biogenesis. Nat Rev Microbiol. 2009;7(11):765–74.

[35] Li H, Qian L, Chen Z, Thibault D, Liu G, Liu T, et al. The outer membrane usher forms a twin-pore secretion complex. J Mol Biol. 2004;344(5):1397–407.

[36] Zhan R, Han Q, Zhang C, Tian Z, Zhang J. Toll-Like receptor 2 (TLR2) and TLR9 play opposing roles in host innate immunity against *Salmonella enterica* serovar Typhimurium infection. Infect Immun. 2015;83(4):1641–9.

[37] Barnhart MM, Chapman MR. Curli biogenesis and function. Annu Rev Microbiol. 2006;60:131–47.

[38] Goyal P, Krasteva PV, Van Gerven N, Gubellini F, Van den Broeck I, Troupiotis-Tsailaki A, et al. Structural and mechanistic insights into the bacterial amyloid secretion channel CsgG. Nature. 2014;516(7530):250–3.

[39] Nenninger AA, Robinson LS, Hultgren SJ. Localized and efficient curli nucleation requires the chaperone-like amyloid assembly protein CsgF. Proc Natl Acad Sci USA. 2009;106(3):900–5.

[40] Bian Z, Normark S. Nucleator function of CsgB for the assembly of adhesive surface organelles in *Escherichia coli*. EMBO J. 1997;16(19):5827–36.

[41] White AP, Gibson DL, Collinson SK, Banser PA, Kay WW. Extracellular polysaccharides associated with thin aggregative fimbriae of *Salmonella enterica* serovar enteritidis. J Bacteriol. 2003;185(18):5398–407.

[42] Karuppiah V, Collins RF, Thistlethwaite A, Gao Y, Derrick JP. Structure and assembly of an inner membrane platform for initiation of type IV pilus biogenesis. Proc Natl Acad Sci USA. 2013;110(48):E4638–47.

[43] Takhar HK, Kemp K, Kim M, Howell PL, Burrows LL. The platform protein is essential for type IV pilus biogenesis. J Biol Chem. 2013;288(14):9721–8.

[44] Proft T, Baker EN. Pili in Gram-negative and Gram-positive bacteria—structure, assembly and their role in disease. Cell Mol Life Sci. 2009;66(4):613–35.

[45] Jain S, Moscicka KB, Bos MP, Pachulec E, Stuart MC, Keegstra W, et al. Structural characterization of outer membrane components of the type IV pili system in pathogenic *Neisseria*. PLoS One. 2011;6(1):e16624.

[46] Desai PT, Porwollik S, Long F, Cheng P, Wollam A, Bhonagiri-Palsikar V, et al. Evolutionary Genomics of *Salmonella enterica* Subspecies. MBio. 2013;4(2):e00579–12.

[47] Yue M, Rankin SC, Blanchet RT, Nulton JD, Edwards RA, Schifferli DM. Diversification of the *Salmonella* fimbriae: a model of macro- and microevolution. PLoS One. 2012;7(6):e38596.

[48] van der Velden AW, Baumler AJ, Tsolis RM, Heffron F. Multiple fimbrial adhesins are required for full virulence of *Salmonella* typhimurium in mice. Infect Immun. 1998;66(6):2803–8.

[49] Clayton DJ, Bowen AJ, Hulme SD, Buckley AM, Deacon VL, Thomson NR, et al. Analysis of the role of 13 major fimbrial subunits in colonisation of the chicken intestines by *Salmonella enterica* serovar Enteritidis reveals a role for a novel locus. BMC Microbiol. 2008;8:228.

[50] Clegg S, Wilson J, Johnson J. More than one way to control hair growth: regulatory mechanisms in enterobacteria that affect fimbriae assembled by the chaperone/usher pathway. J Bacteriol. 2011;193(9):2081–8.

[51] Saini S, Slauch JM, Aldridge PD, Rao CV. Role of cross talk in regulating the dynamic expression of the flagellar *Salmonella* pathogenicity island 1 and type 1 fimbrial genes. J Bacteriol. 2010;192(21):5767–77.

[52] Balbontin R, Rowley G, Pucciarelli MG, Lopez-Garrido J, Wormstone Y, Lucchini S, et al. DNA adenine methylation regulates virulence gene expression in *Salmonella enterica* serovar Typhimurium. J Bacteriol. 2006;188(23):8160–8.

[53] Aya Castaneda Mdel R, Sarnacki SH, Noto Llana M, Lopez Guerra AG, Giacomodonato MN, Cerquetti MC. Dam methylation is required for efficient biofilm production in *Salmonella enterica* serovar Enteritidis. Int J Food Microbiol. 2015;193:15–22.

[54] Nicholson B, Low D. DNA methylation-dependent regulation of pef expression in *Salmonella* typhimurium. Mol Microbiol. 2000;35(4):728–42.

[55] Wang Q, Zhao Y, McClelland M, Harshey RM. The RcsCDB signaling system and swarming motility in *Salmonella enterica* serovar typhimurium: dual regulation of flagellar and SPI-2 virulence genes. J Bacteriol. 2007;189(23):8447–57.

[56] Deditius JA, Felgner S, Sporing I, Kuhne C, Frahm M, Rohde M, et al. Characterization of novel factors involved in swimming and swarming motility in *Salmonella enterica* Serovar Typhimurium. PLoS One. 2015;10(8):e0135351.

[57] Lee FK, Morris C, Hackett J. The *Salmonella enterica* serovar Typhi Vi capsule and self-association pili share controls on expression. FEMS Microbiol Lett. 2006;261(1):41–6.

[58] Meng X, Meng X, Zhu C, Wang H, Wang J, Nie J, et al. The RNA chaperone Hfq regulates expression of fimbrial-related genes and virulence of *Salmonella enterica* serovar Enteritidis. FEMS Microbiol Lett. 2013;346(2):90–6.

[59] Norris TL, Kingsley RA, Bumler AJ. Expression and transcriptional control of the *Salmonella* typhimurium *lpf* fimbrial operon by phase variation. Mol Microbiol. 1998;29(1):311–20.

[60] Ahmad I, Lamprokostopoulou A, Le Guyon S, Streck E, Barthel M, Peters V, et al. Complex c-di-GMP signaling networks mediate transition between virulence properties and biofilm formation in *Salmonella enterica* serovar Typhimurium. PLoS One. 2011;6(12):e28351.

[61] Kader A, Simm R, Gerstel U, Morr M, Romling U. Hierarchical involvement of various GGDEF domain proteins in rdar morphotype development of *Salmonella enterica* serovar Typhimurium. Mol Microbiol. 2006;60(3):602–16.

[62] Wang KC, Hsu YH, Huang YN, Yeh KS. A previously uncharacterized gene *stm0551* plays a repressive role in the regulation of type 1 fimbriae in *Salmonella enterica* serotype Typhimurium. BMC Microbiol. 2012;12:111.

[63] Wang KC, Hsu YH, Huang YN, Lin JH, Yeh KS. FimY of *Salmonella enterica* serovar Typhimurium functions as a DNA-binding protein and binds the *fimZ* promoter. Microbiol Res. 2014;169(7–8):496–503.

[64] Humphries AD, Townsend SM, Kingsley RA, Nicholson TL, Tsolis RM, Baumler AJ. Role of fimbriae as antigens and intestinal colonization factors of *Salmonella* serovars. FEMS Microbiol Lett. 2001;201(2):121–5.

[65] Kisiela DI, Chattopadhyay S, Tchesnokova V, Paul S, Weissman SJ, Medenica I, et al. Evolutionary analysis points to divergent physiological roles of type 1 fimbriae in *Salmonella* and *Escherichia coli*. MBio. 2013;4(2).

[66] Clegg S, Hancox LS, Yeh KS. *Salmonella* typhimurium fimbrial phase variation and *fimA* expression. J Bacteriol. 1996;178(2):542–5.

[67] Wang KC, Hsu YH, Huang YN, Chen TH, Lin JH, Hsuan SL, et al. A low-pH medium in vitro or the environment within a macrophage decreases the transcriptional levels of *fimA*, *fimZ* and *lrp* in *Salmonella enterica* serovar Typhimurium. J Biosci. 2013;38(3):499–507.

[68] Swenson DL, Clegg S. Identification of ancillary *fim* genes affecting *fimA* expression in *Salmonella* typhimurium. J Bacteriol. 1992;174(23):7697–704.

[69] Tinker JK, Clegg S. Characterization of FimY as a coactivator of type 1 fimbrial expression in *Salmonella enterica* serovar Typhimurium. Infect Immun. 2000;68(6):3305–13.

[70] Chuang YC, Wang KC, Chen YT, Yang CH, Men SC, Fan CC, et al. Identification of the genetic determinants of *Salmonella enterica* serotype Typhimurium that may regulate the expression of the type 1 fimbriae in response to solid agar and static broth culture conditions. BMC Microbiol. 2008;8:126.

[71] Yeh KS, Tinker JK, Clegg S. FimZ binds the *Salmonella* typhimurium *fimA* promoter region and may regulate its own expression with FimY. Microbiol Immunol. 2002;46(1):1–10.

[72] Tinker JK, Clegg S. Control of FimY translation and type 1 fimbrial production by the arginine tRNA encoded by *fimU* in *Salmonella enterica* serovar Typhimurium. Mol Microbiol. 2001;40(3):757–68.

[73] McFarland KA, Lucchini S, Hinton JC, Dorman CJ. The leucine-responsive regulatory protein, Lrp, activates transcription of the *fim* operon in *Salmonella enterica* serovar typhimurium via the *fimZ* regulatory gene. J Bacteriol. 2008;190(2):602–12.

[74] Tinker JK, Hancox LS, Clegg S. FimW is a negative regulator affecting type 1 fimbrial expression in *Salmonella enterica* serovar typhimurium. J Bacteriol. 2001;183(2):435–42.

[75] Clegg S, Hughes KT. FimZ is a molecular link between sticking and swimming in *Salmonella enterica* serovar Typhimurium. J Bacteriol. 2002;184(4):1209–13.

[76] Baxter MA, Jones BD. Two-component regulators control *hilA* expression by controlling *fimZ* and *hilE* expression within *Salmonella enterica* serovar Typhimurium. Infect Immun. 2015;83(3):978–85.

[77] Thorns CJ. *Salmonella* fimbriae: novel antigens in the detection and control of *salmonella* infections. Br Vet J. 1995;151(6):643–58.

[78] Feldsine PT, Falbo-Nelson MT, Hustead DL. Polyclonal enzyme immunoassay method for detection of motile and non-motile *Salmonella* in foods: comparative study. J AOAC Int. 1993;76(3):694–7.

[79] Kerr S, Ball HJ, Mackie DP, Pollock DA, Finlay DA. Diagnostic application of monoclonal antibodies to outer membrane protein for rapid detection of *Salmonella*. J Appl Bacteriol. 1992;72(4):302–8.

[80] Doran JL, Collinson SK, Burian J, Sarlos G, Todd EC, Munro CK, et al. DNA-based diagnostic tests for *Salmonella* species targeting *agfA*, the structural gene for thin, aggregative fimbriae. J Clin Microbiol. 1993;31(9):2263–73.

[81] Craciunas C, Keul AL, Flonta M, Cristea M. DNA-based diagnostic tests for *Salmonella* strains targeting *hilA*, *agfA*, *spvC* and *sef* genes. J Environ Manage. 2012;95 Suppl:S15–8.

[82] Zhang JY, Dong LW, Ren Q, Wang XZ, Yang Y, Zhou W, et al. Simple and rapid detection of *Salmonella* by direct PCR amplification of gene *fimW*. Curr Microbiol. 2014;69(4):429–35.

[83] Pratap CB, Kumar G, Patel SK, Verma AK, Shukla VK, Kumar K, et al. Targeting of putative fimbrial gene for detection of *S*. Typhi in typhoid fever and chronic typhoid carriers by nested PCR. J Infect Dev Ctries. 2013;7(7):520–7.

[84] Zhuang L, Gong J, Li Q, Zhu C, Yu Y, Dou X, et al. Detection of *Salmonella* spp. by a loop-mediated isothermal amplification (LAMP) method targeting *bcfD* gene. Lett Appl Microbiol. 2014;59(6):658–64.

[85] Ghosh S, Chakraborty K, Nagaraja T, Basak S, Koley H, Dutta S, et al. An adhesion protein of *Salmonella enterica* serovar Typhi is required for pathogenesis and potential target for vaccine development. Proc Natl Acad Sci USA. 2011;108(8):3348–53.

[86] Sheikh A, Charles RC, Sharmeen N, Rollins SM, Harris JB, Bhuiyan MS, et al. In vivo expression of *Salmonella enterica* serotype Typhi genes in the blood of patients with typhoid fever in Bangladesh. PLoS Negl Trop Dis. 2011;5(12):e1419.

[87] Charles RC, Liang L, Khanam F, Sayeed MA, Hung C, Leung DT, et al. Immunoproteomic analysis of antibody in lymphocyte supernatant in patients with typhoid fever in Bangladesh. Clin Vaccine Immunol. 2014;21(3):280–5.

[88] Pang Y, Zhang Y, Wang H, Jin J, Piao J, Piao J, et al. Reduction of *Salmonella* enteritidis number after infections by immunization of liposome-associated recombinant SefA. Avian Dis. 2013;57(3):627–33.

[89] Pang Y, Wang H, Li Z, Piao J, Piao J, Chi Y, et al. Immune response to liposome-associated recombinant SEF21 following oral immunization in chickens. Avian Dis. 2012;56(2):347–53.

[90] Sanchez-Ingunza R, Guard J, Morales CA, Icard AH. Reduction of *Salmonella* Enteritidis in the spleens of hens by bacterins that vary in fimbrial protein SefD. Foodborne Pathog Dis. 2015;12(10):836–43.

[91] Wizemann TM, Adamou JE, Langermann S. Adhesins as targets for vaccine development. Emerg Infect Dis. 1999;5(3):395–403.

Section 2

Salmonella Detection and Antibiotic Resistance

Chapter 5

Current and Emerging Innovations for Detection of Food-Borne *Salmonella*

Wei Wu and Lingwen Zeng

Additional information is available at the end of the chapter

http://dx.doi.org/10.5772/67264

Abstract

Salmonella is one of the leading causes of food-borne illnesses worldwide, and one of the main contributors to salmonellosis is the consumption of contaminated egg, poultry, pork, beef, and milk products. Since deleterious effects of *Salmonella* on public health and the economy continue to occur, improving safety of food products by early detection of food-borne pathogens would be considered an important component for limiting exposure to *Salmonella* contamination. Therefore, there is an ongoing need to develop more advanced detection methods that can identify *Salmonella* accurately and rapidly in foods before they reach consumers. In the past three decades, there have been increasing efforts toward developing and improving rapid pathogen detection and characterization methodologies for application to food products. In this chapter, we discuss molecular methods for detection, identification, and genetic characterization of *Salmonella* in food. In addition, the advantages and disadvantages of the established and emerging rapid detection methods are addressed here. The methods with potential application to the industry are highlighted in this chapter.

Keywords: *Salmonella*, food-borne pathogens, rapid detection, molecular methods, aptamer, antibody

1. Introduction

Food-borne disease is one of the major public health problems for the food industry, especially in developing countries [1]. Failure to detect food-borne pathogens may lead to a dreadful effect. The World Health Organization (WHO) reported that in 2010 alone 1.8 million people died from diarrheal diseases, a great proportion of these cases can be attributed to contaminated food and drinking water [2]. The Centers for Disease Control and Prevention

(CDC) have estimated that 48 million cases of food-borne illnesses occur in the United States (US) annually, approximately 128,000 cases require hospitalization, and 3,000 cases result in death [3]. The CDC reported that viruses, bacteria, and parasites are major causative agents for food-borne illnesses. Among these, bacterial agents including *Salmonella*, *Listeria monocytogenes*, and *Escherichia coli* are associated with these cases, being responsible for most of the hospitalizations (63.9%) and deaths (63.7%). Especially, *Salmonella* species were considered as the leading cause for these more severe cases resulting in 35% of the hospitalizations and 28% of the deaths [4]. *Salmonella*, belonging to the family of *Enterobacteriaceae*, are Gram-negative, facultative anaerobic, and nonspore-forming bacilli. The genus *Salmonella* is consisted of two species, *enterica* and *bongori*, with six subspecies of *S. enterica*. The different serotypes are divided based on the specific surface molecules O-antigen (O-Ag) and H-antigen (H-Ag) [5]. Collectively, there are over 2500 serotypes of salmonellae capable of causing disease in humans. Most serotypes of the salmonellae could cause gastroenteritis, while a few serotypes of salmonellae would cause severe disease enteric fever, which was characterized as the onset of high fever accompanied with abdominal pain and malaise without diarrhea or vomiting [6]. Commonly, salmonellosis is self-limiting, resolving in about a week. Occasionally, however, the infection becomes systemic, a much more severe disease requiring antibiotic interventions [7]. The dose of *Salmonella* causing infection in humans indicated a wide range for the number of cells required to cause disease, ranged from 10^5 to 10^{10} cells. In contrast, enumeration of food products indicate much lower numbers of organisms, as low as ten cells, were present to cause illness [8, 9].

Most human salmonellosis cases are associated with consumption of contaminated egg, poultry, pork, beef, and milk products, which are considered one of the most important reservoirs from which *Salmonella* is passed through the food chain and ultimately transmitted to humans [10]. With increasing consumption of these food products, the number of associated salmonellosis continues to be a public health issue all around the world. It is estimated that 95% of *Salmonella* infections are due to the consumption of contaminated foodstuffs, which suggest that salmonellae may be present at low levels in food but still capable of causing a significant number of infections [11]. Yearly, in the United States, it is estimated that *Salmonella* is responsible for over a million illnesses, 19,000 hospitalizations, and almost 400 deaths. This is in part due to their marked ability to persist in a wide range of varying environmental conditions [12]. For example, *Salmonella* strains can grow in foods stored at low (2–4°C) and high (54°C) temperatures [13].

Since *Salmonella* is a major causative agent for food-associated food-borne illnesses, improving safety of poultry products by early detection of food-borne pathogens would be considered an important component for limiting exposure to *Salmonella* contamination. In order to safeguard the food supply and ensure public health, it is essential to establish rapid, reliable, and sensitive method for *Salmonella* detection. In the past two decades, there has been a thrust to develop rapid methods for identifying and detecting *Salmonella* specifically in foodstuffs [14–17]. This chapter will focus on the current culture-dependent and culture-independent methods for the rapid, accurate detection, identification, and subtyping of salmonellae in foodstuffs.

2. Methodologies for detection of *Salmonella*

2.1. Culture-dependent methods

Current testing of food samples for the presence of salmonellae can be divided into three steps: (1) detection of pathogen by plate culture, (2) identification of the isolate and its specific serovar designation, and (3) subtyping of the isolate for association with salmonellosis [18, 19]. These methods rely on traditional bacterial culture procedures that apply serial enrichments with increasing selectivity culminating in the isolation of *Salmonella* on selective differential agar plates (**Figure 1**). It always takes up to 5 days to obtain a presumptive positive result. Then traditional biochemical testing of nutrient utilization medium is needed for confirmation, another few days to complete [20]. Although innovative technologies have been applied to subtype salmonellae isolation, at least 24 h is needed for a confirmation of *Salmonella* in multiple analytes. DNA fingerprinting techniques are based on DNA size differences on an agarose gel. The digested genomic DNA of target bacteria is separated on an agarose gel and then hybridized with complementary sequences for identifying the banding pattern. A database of fingerprint species, serovar, and strain identifications is used for comparison [21–23]. The fingerprinting methods include pulsed-field gel electrophoresis (PFGE), ribotyping, and intergenic sequence (IGS) ribotyping. The use of PFGE has greatly increased the ability of track and trace back illness clusters and outbreaks. However, PFGE still requires a pure isolate and a minimum of 3 days to complete [24, 25].

Due to its sensitivity, with a limit of detection of 1 cfu, this analytical schema is considered as the "gold standard" of regulatory agencies (**Figure 1**). The disadvantages of this method are as follows. First, it is time-consuming, taking at least a week for isolation and few more days for serotyping and subtyping. The long time frame hampers its application in many food commodities, especially fresh products, before they are consumed or on hold in warehouses while awaiting test results before they spoil. Second, the operation is tedious; the amount of media and numerous plates are required for each sample. The procedures are labor-consuming and necessitate large areas of space, particularly in many sample detections. Finally, the complex ingredients in foodstuffs, such as indigenous microbiota and antimicrobials, make it notably difficult for traditional microbiological methods [11, 26–29].

2.2. Culture-independent methods

Recent advances in technology have made the detection of food-borne pathogens more rapid and convenient, while achieving improved sensitivity and specificity in comparison to conventional methods. These methods employing newer technologies are generally referred as "rapid methods," which include nucleic acid-based or antibody-based assays that are modified or improved compared to conventional methods [30–35]. These rapid detection methods can be of high value to the food industry by providing several key advantages such as speed, specificity, sensitivity, cost-efficiency, and labor efficiency.

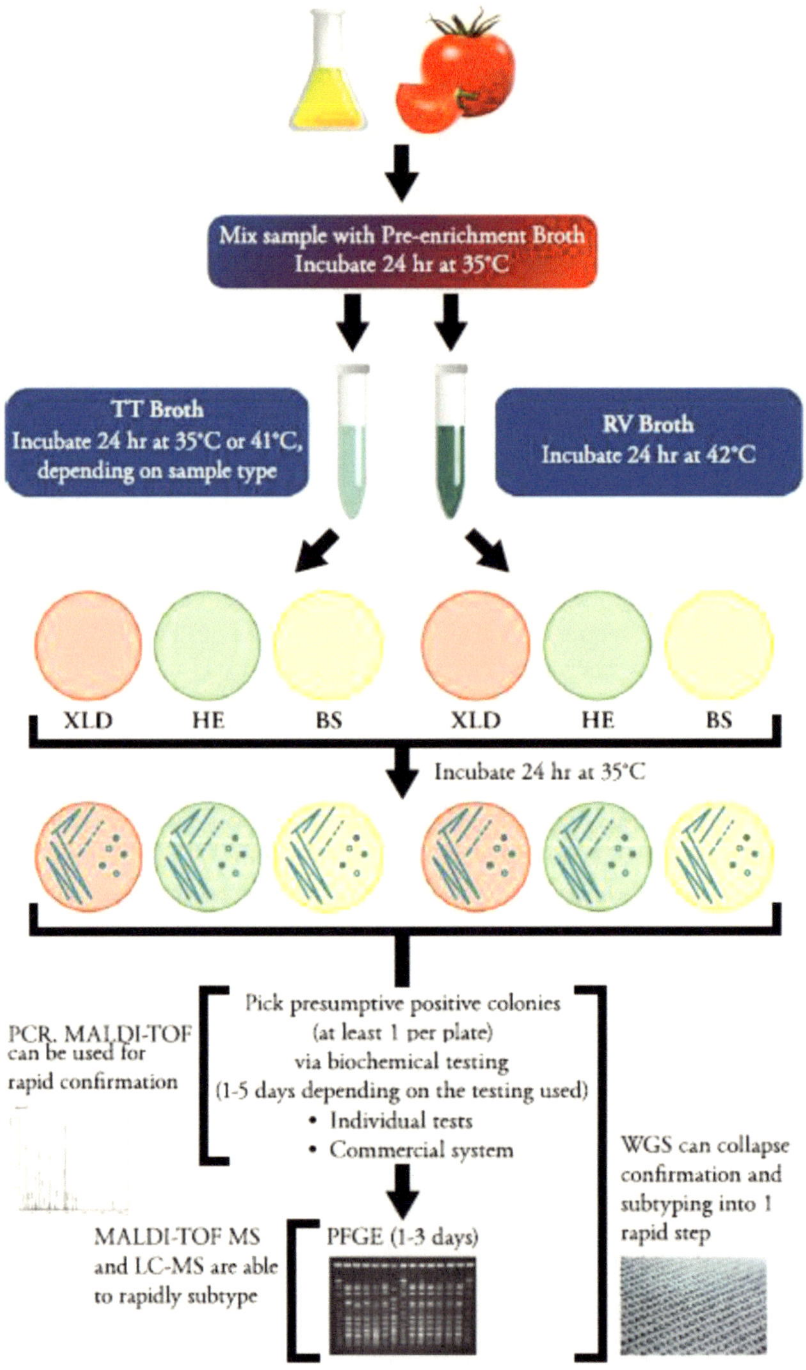

Figure 1. Overview of Bacteriological Analytical Manual (FDA-BAM) workflow for the detection, isolation, and subtyping of *Salmonella*. It takes 5 days for the detection and isolation of *Salmonella*, and a week more for subsequent confirmation and subtyping recent molecular methods, such as MS, WGS, and PCR/qPCR, may shorten the result time [36].

2.2.1. Polymerase chain reaction (PCR)

The largest advance toward faster detection of salmonellae has been in the realm of molecular biology, where polymerase chain reaction (PCR) and quantitative PCR (qPCR) are predominantly being applied as the methods of choice for the detection. Different protocols targeting different specific genes or gene regions specific to salmonellae have been published. Numerous studies have been conducted to detect and characterize *Salmonella* in poultry, poultry products, and feeds using PCR assays to target selected antibiotic resistance or virulence genes along with genus-, species-, and serotype-specific genes [16, 37–40].

Over the past years, PCR-based methods have advanced to provide high sensitivity for *Salmonella* detection and identification. Aabo et al. used PCR assay for *Salmonella* detection in minced meat and compared this method to a culture-based methodology. The sensitivity of the PCR was 89% (85 out of 96 samples), which was much higher than that of the culture method (50%, 48 out of 96 samples) [41]. Rychlik et al. established nested PCR with high sensitivity, which has a higher annealing temperature than the primers used in the first PCR, to detect *Salmonella* in chicken feces [42].

As we all know, the quality and quantity of target DNA, PCR template, are important factors during the design of a PCR assay. Although well-designed PCR primer and good PCR template can bring high specificity of the target detection, it is still not sufficient to overcome the side effects of PCR inhibitors in samples, such as denatured proteins, organic chemicals, and sucrose. Moreover, the presence of DNA and cells other than those from the targeted organism can affect the efficiency of the PCR methods. To overcome this, an enrichment step is commonly performed to enhance assay sensitivity by ensuring the detection of viable pathogens before PCR reaction. Ferretti et al. reported that PCR with a 6 h nonselective enrichment could detect various *Salmonella* serotypes in salami stuffs as low as 1 cfu in 100 ml of food homogenate [43, 44]. Myint et al. reported a PCR method for *Salmonella* detection in contaminated poultry tissue samples, and false negative results were obtained without enrichment. However, a positive rate of 90% was observed after enrichment. Generally, culture enrichment is recommended in order to distinguish live cells from dead cells before PCR [45]. Maciorowski et al. investigated different enrichment times to detect indigenous *Salmonella* in poultry dietary samples using PCR. It was found that it could not be detectable for *Salmonella* with 7 h enrichment, and the sensitivity for detection was 25 and 50% with 13 h enrichment and 24 h enrichment, respectively [46].

Improvements have also been made on the basic PCR technology as well. In particular, two primary PCR-based methods have emerged over the past several years, such as multiplex PCR and real-time quantitative PCR [47, 48]. The current status of the optimization and development of these PCR applications is summarized in the following.

Multiplex PCR is a modified PCR method that allows for multiple sequence targets to be simultaneously detected within a single reaction. This method has proven useful for the rapid identification of multiple pathogens simultaneously in a given sample. Generally, multiplex PCR amplifies the target samples using multiple primers in a reaction, which can detect and identify several target sequences in *Salmonella*. Sharma employed a multiplex fluorogenic

PCR assay for simultaneous detection of *Salmonella* and *E. coli* O157:H7, which was capable of detecting as low as 10 cfu/g in meat [49]. Similarly, Kawasaki detected multiple *Salmonella* serotypes, *L. monocytogenes*, and *E. coli* O157:H7 simultaneously in enriched meat samples using multiplex PCR [48]. Cortez et al. identified *Salmonella* from chicken abattoirs by multiplex PCR. In this paper, 29 out of 288 (~10%) samples were found to be positive for *Salmonella* spp., and 16 (~5.6%) and 7 (~2.4%) samples were characterized as *Salmonella Typhimurium* and *Salmonella enteritidis*, respectively [50]. Kim differentiated the 30 most prevalent *Salmonella* serotypes in the United States by using two five-plex PCR assays. In this study, primer pairs targeting six genetic loci from *S. Typhimurium* and four from *S. Typhi* were designed to evaluate various *Salmonella* serotypes [51]. More recently, Salemis et al. also established two five-plex assays for the detection of the most common *Salmonella* in Tunisia as well [52]. Although multiplex PCR can simultaneously detect several targets, the primary difficulties are uncommitted, in which reaction conditions are needed optimized as high amounts of DNA in the reaction mixture compared to single PCR-based assays. The complex conditions and ingredients in the reaction still increase the difficulty in discrimination between prominent PCR product sizes on traditional agarose gel electrophoresis. In practice, cross-reactivity of primer pairs and sensitivity limitations associated with the procedure make it still quite challenging to routinely use multiplex PCR for reliable simultaneous *Salmonella* serovar detection [53].

With the appearance of fluorescence technology that endows increased sensitivity (e.g., intercalating dyes such as SYBR Green or labeled probes), the limitations of conventional PCR can be overcome, such as the errors associated with end-point analyses and lack of quantification. The "real-time" aspect of real-time PCR, also referred to as qPCR, technology is linked to its ability to label and cumulatively quantify the generated PCR products at each cycle throughout the ongoing amplification process. The qPCR has been widely used to quantify *Salmonella* [54–56]. Daum screened nine foodstuffs associated with a *Salmonella* outbreak in Texas using qPCR. It was reported that only one food item was positive for *Salmonella* [57]. Wang et al. reported a qPCR method to detect *Salmonella* in raw sausage meat with detection limit of 4 cfu/g [58]. He also used this method to quantify *Salmonella* detection limits of 2.5 cfu/25 g for salmon and minced meat, 5 cfu/25 g of chicken meat, and 5 cfu/25 ml for raw milk, respectively [59]. Malorny et al. reported a duplex qPCR assay to detect *S. enteritidis* in whole chicken carcass rinses and eggs, with a detection limit of 3 cfu/50 ml of chicken carcass rinses and 3 cfu/10 ml of homogenized egg content [60]. Bohaychuk used qPCR for *Salmonella* detection in poultry cecal contents and carcasses with reported sensitivities ranging from 97 to 100% for various matrices [61]. Although qPCR is an effective tool to detect *Salmonella* with high sensitivity and specificity, it does have several limitations, which are listed in **Table 1**.

2.2.2. Enzyme-linked immunosorbent assay (ELISA)

Enzyme-linked immunosorbent assay (ELISA)-based approaches are the most prevalent antibody-based assay for pathogen detection in foods [62]. This immunological approach has been used to detect *Salmonella* in poultry production (poultry feed, feces, litter, carcass rinsing, and water samples) and has provided a better sensitivity and shorter time frame than that of culture-based methods [46]. Improvements by combination with other advanced technologies have been made to the basic ELISA method for

Salmonella detection. For example, incorporation of monoclonal antibodies can improve the sensitivity of the assay, and it can quantify *Salmonella* among poultry probiotic bacteria such as *Veillonella* [63]. In this study, the detection limit for *S. Typhimurium* was determined to be 5.5×10^4 cells/ml in pure culture. Dill combined monoclonal and polyclonal antibodies and a commercial filtering system to detect *S. Typhimurium* cells in a chicken rinsate, with detection limit of fewer than 100 *S. Typhimurium* cells [64]. As the advantages of ELISA methods for *Salmonella* detection in foods and animal feeds, they are now widely used for detection of *Salmonella* in animal-producing foods [65]. The comparison of ELISA methods with culture-based methods is performed and listed in **Table 1**.

Method	Advantages	Disadvantages
Culture-dependent methods	—Accurate	—Labor and time cost
Single and multiplex PCR	—More rapid than culture-based methods (<24 h vs. 5 ~ 7 days) —High specificity and sensitivity —Multiplex PCR (several pathogens at a time) —Labor saving —Multidetection of several *Salmonella* serotypes (5 ~ 6) in one reaction	—Costs more than culture-based methods and ELISA —Difficulty in distinguishing live and dead cells —Technically can be challenging (optimized PCR condition) —Enrichment to detect viable cells —Requires post-PCR processing of products (electrophoresis) —PCR inhibitors
qPCR	—Not influenced by nonspecific amplification; amplification can be monitored at real time —No post-PCR processing of products (gel electrophoresis) —Rapid cycling (25 min) —Confirmation of specific amplification by melting curve —Specific, sensitive, and reproducible	—Difficulty in multiplex assay —Need skilled person and support —High equipment cost —mRNA lability —Possibility of cross contamination
Antibody-based method	—More rapid than culture-based methods (2 days vs. 5 ~ 7 days) —Can be automated to reduce assay time and manual labor input —Able to handle large numbers of samples —More specific than cultural methods	—Not high sensitivity —Difficult to multidetect —False-negative results —Difficulty to differentiate damaged or stressed cells —Need to pre-enrichment —High cross-reactivity with close antigens in bacteria
Aptamer-based method	—Inexpensive, stable, and can be chemically synthesized than antibody —Time saving (2 h vs. 5 ~ 7 days of culture-based methods) —Automated to reduce manual labor input —Large numbers of sample detection at one time —Higher specificity than cultural methods	—High false-positive results —Difficulty in detecting damaged or stressed cells —Pre-enrichment for production of cell surface antigens —Possibility of cross contamination

Table 1. Advantages and disadvantages of detection methods.

2.2.3. *Aptamer-based detection assay*

Besides antibodies, other biomolecules have been investigated to selectively capture and enrich *Salmonella* from cultures, among which aptamer is the most prevalent one [66]. Aptamers are single-stranded oligonucleotides, DNA, or RNA that can fold into unique 3D structures based on their primary nucleotide sequence, rendering them capable of binding to specific ligands, like antibody interacting with an antigen [67]. Aptamers offer some advantages over antibodies in that they are relatively inexpensive to synthesize and they provide more batch-to-batch consistency [68]. However, few studies have reported their specific use in detecting *S. Typhimurium* from river water and fecal samples [66, 69]. Bacteriophages have also been explored as a means to capture *Salmonella* cells. Phages may offer some advantages over antibodies given their inherent specificity for host cells, their ease of production in bacteria versus animals or eukaryotic cell culture, and their relative stability in harsh conditions such as pH and temperature extremes [70].

Relative to culture-independent detection, researchers have focused on methods to concentrate whole cells within the sample before the pre-enrichment step. The enriched whole *Salmonella* allows for direct detection from food and environmental samples. The enrichment steps mainly rely on filtering liquids, rinsates, or mechanically disintegrated (i.e., blended or stomached) samples. Therefore, this approach has been widely used in large volumes of water, but the testing of food samples was problematic due to the food particles difficult to go through filter membranes [71]. To overcome this problem, endopeptidases have been added to apply in food samples. These degrade the small, soluble proteins and peptides so that they are unable to clog the filter and pass through with the permeate. The United States has awarded the method with grant prize. The Food and Drug Administration also recommends the method for food safety guard, (http://www.foodsafetychallenge.com), which signified its potential to greatly enhance the detection of *Salmonella* directly from foods.

2.3. Conclusion

In summary, the mentioned methods here have utility advantages for *Salmonella* detection in the food safety sector. It is important to emphasize that none of the methods will be recommended or even suited for every situation in detecting all food varieties for *Salmonella*. Application to specific food samples will be dictated by method performance. As noted previously, the performance of these methods depends on several factors, such as matrix-driven effects, general specificity and sensitivity, and their technical complexity. Meanwhile, other extrinsic factors would affect the performance, including user skill set and technical prowess, cost of the equipment, and cost per sample. Hence, the systematic validation to evaluate the methods should be considered according to its specific utility and application across the food supply.

In order to meet the current requirement of rapid detection, it is clear that several approaches have emerged including PCR-based, antibody-based, aptamer-based, and other approaches encompassing those stemming from the current genomic era. A clear character of method development direction is moving toward greater automation, cost-saving, and time-saving network integration. It is important to mention that outputs from one approach would serve to strengthen directly or tangentially other approaches. At last, it seems that a suite of tools is emerging for the food safety microbiologist, each with its specific advantages and disadvantages but all with the ability to rapidly and accurately detect *Salmonella* in certain cases and early in its contamination of the human and veterinary food supply.

Author details

Wei Wu[1] and Lingwen Zeng[2]*

*Address all correspondence to: zeng_lingwen@gibh.ac.cn

1 Institute for Translational Medicine, Qingdao University, Qingdao, China

2 Institute of Environment and Safety, Wuhan Academy of Agriculture Sciences, Wuhan, China

References

[1] Ameme DK, Abdulai M, Adjei EY, Afari EA, Nyarko KM, Asante D, Kye-Duodu G, Abbas M, Sackey S and Wurapa F. Foodborne disease outbreak in a resource-limited setting: a tale of missed opportunities and implications for response. Pan Afr Med J 2016; 23: 69.

[2] Havelaar AH, Kirk MD, Torgerson PR, Gibb HJ, Hald T, Lake RJ, Praet N, Bellinger DC, de Silva NR, Gargouri N, Speybroeck N, Cawthorne A, Mathers C, Stein C, Angulo FJ and Devleesschauwer B. World Health Organization global estimates and regional comparisons of the burden of foodborne disease in 2010. PLoS Med 2015; 12: e1001923.

[3] Talan DA and Moran GJ. Update on emerging infections: news from the Centers for Disease Control and Prevention. Surveillance for foodborne disease outbreaks – United States, 2006. Ann Emerg Med 2010; 55: 47-49.

[4] Henao OL, Scallan E, Mahon B and Hoekstra RM. Methods for monitoring trends in the incidence of foodborne diseases: foodborne diseases active surveillance network 1996–2008. Foodborne Pathog Dis 2010; 7: 1421-1426.

[5] McQuiston JR, Herrera-Leon S, Wertheim BC, Doyle J, Fields PI, Tauxe RV and Logsdon JM, Jr. Molecular phylogeny of the salmonellae: relationships among *Salmonella* species and subspecies determined from four housekeeping genes and evidence of lateral gene transfer events. J Bacteriol 2008; 190: 7060-7067.

[6] Weill FX, Tran HH, Roumagnac P, Fabre L, Minh NB, Stavnes TL, Lassen J, Bjune G, Grimont PA and Guerin PJ. Clonal reconquest of antibiotic-susceptible *Salmonella enterica* serotype Typhi in Son La Province, Vietnam. Am J Trop Med Hyg 2007; 76: 1174-1181.

[7] Kubota K, Kasuga F, Iwasaki E, Inagaki S, Sakurai Y, Komatsu M, Toyofuku H, Angulo FJ, Scallan E and Morikawa K. Estimating the burden of acute gastroenteritis and foodborne illness caused by *Campylobacter*, *Salmonella*, and *Vibrio* parahaemolyticus by using population-based telephone survey data, Miyagi Prefecture, Japan, 2005 to 2006. J Food Prot 2011; 74: 1592-1598.

[8] Tadesse G. Prevalence of human Salmonellosis in Ethiopia: a systematic review and meta-analysis. BMC Infect Dis 2014; 14: 88.

[9] Blaser MJ and Newman LS. A review of human salmonellosis: I. Infective dose. Rev Infect Dis 1982; 4: 1096-1106.

[10] Painter JA, Hoekstra RM, Ayers T, Tauxe RV, Braden CR, Angulo FJ and Griffin PM. Attribution of foodborne illnesses, hospitalizations, and deaths to food commodities by using outbreak data, United States, 1998–2008. Emerg Infect Dis 2013; 19: 407-415.

[11] Bell RL, Zheng J, Burrows E, Allard S, Wang CY, Keys CE, Melka DC, Strain E, Luo Y, Allard MW, Rideout S and Brown EW. Ecological prevalence, genetic diversity, and epidemiological aspects of *Salmonella* isolated from tomato agricultural regions of the Virginia Eastern Shore. Front Microbiol 2015; 6: 415.

[12] Scallan E, Griffin PM, Angulo FJ, Tauxe RV and Hoekstra RM. Foodborne illness acquired in the United States – unspecified agents. Emerg Infect Dis 2011; 17: 16-22.

[13] Balamurugan S and Dugan ME. Growth temperature associated protein expression and membrane fatty acid composition profiles of *Salmonella enterica* serovar *Typhimurium*. J Basic Microbiol 2010; 50: 507-518.

[14] Park SH, Aydin M, Khatiwara A, Dolan MC, Gilmore DF, Bouldin JL, Ahn S and Ricke SC. Current and emerging technologies for rapid detection and characterization of *Salmonella* in poultry and poultry products. Food Microbiol 2014; 38: 250-262.

[15] Srisawat M and Panbangred W. Efficient and specific detection of *Salmonella* in food samples using a stn-based loop-mediated isothermal amplification method. Biomed Res Int 2015; 2015: 356401.

[16] Jenikova G, Pazlarova J and Demnerova K. Detection of *Salmonella* in food samples by the combination of immunomagnetic separation and PCR assay. Int Microbiol 2000; 3: 225-229.

[17] Bolton FJ, Fritz E, Poynton S and Jensen T. Rapid enzyme-linked immunoassay for detection of *Salmonella* in food and feed products: performance testing program. J AOAC Int 2000; 83: 299-303.

[18] Belete T, Crowley E, Bird P, Gensic J and Wallace FM. A comparison of the BAX system method to the U.S. Food and Drug Administration's Bacteriological Analytical Manual and International Organization for Standardization reference methods for the detection of *Salmonella* in a variety of soy ingredients. J Food Prot 2014; 77: 1778-1783.

[19] Zhang G, Thau E, Brown EW and Hammack TS. Comparison of a novel strategy for the detection and isolation of *Salmonella* in shell eggs with the Food and Drug Administration Bacteriological Analytical Manual method. Poult Sci 2013; 92: 3266-3274.

[20] Andrews JR, Prajapati KG, Eypper E, Shrestha P, Shakya M, Pathak KR, Joshi N, Tiwari P, Risal M, Koirala S, Karkey A, Dongol S, Wen S, Smith AB, Maru D, Basnyat B, Baker S, Farrar J, Ryan ET, Hohmann E and Arjyal A. Evaluation of an electricity-free, culture-based approach for detecting typhoidal *Salmonella* bacteremia during enteric fever in a high burden, resource-limited setting. PLoS Negl Trop Dis 2013; 7: e2292.

[21] Murase T, Nagato M, Shirota K, Katoh H and Otsuki K. Pulsed-field gel electrophoresis-based subtyping of DNA degradation-sensitive *Salmonella enterica* subsp. *enterica* serovar Livingstone and serovar Cerro isolates obtained from a chicken layer farm. Vet Microbiol 2004; 99: 139-143.

[22] Fenwick SG, Duignan PJ, Nicol CM, Leyland MJ and Hunter JE. A comparison of *Salmonella* serotypes isolated from New Zealand sea lions and feral pigs on the Auckland Islands by pulsed-field gel electrophoresis. J Wildl Dis 2004; 40: 566-570.

[23] Guard J, Sanchez-Ingunza R, Morales C, Stewart T, Liljebjelke K, Van Kessel J, Ingram K, Jones D, Jackson C, Fedorka-Cray P, Frye J, Gast R and Hinton A, Jr. Comparison of dkgB-linked intergenic sequence ribotyping to DNA microarray hybridization for assigning serotype to *Salmonella enterica*. FEMS Microbiol Lett 2012; 337: 61-72.

[24] Rivoal K, Protais J, Queguiner S, Boscher E, Chidaine B, Rose V, Gautier M, Baron F, Grosset N, Ermel G and Salvat G. Use of pulsed-field gel electrophoresis to characterize the heterogeneity and clonality of *Salmonella* serotype Enteritidis, Typhimurium and Infantis isolates obtained from whole liquid eggs. Int J Food Microbiol 2009; 129: 180-186.

[25] Xi M, Zheng J, Zhao S, Brown EW and Meng J. An enhanced discriminatory pulsed-field gel electrophoresis scheme for subtyping *Salmonella* serotypes Heidelberg, Kentucky, SaintPaul, and Hadar. J Food Prot 2008; 71: 2067-2072.

[26] Singer RS, Mayer AE, Hanson TE and Isaacson RE. Do microbial interactions and cultivation media decrease the accuracy of *Salmonella* surveillance systems and outbreak investigations? J Food Prot 2009; 72: 707-713.

[27] Kim SY, Kang DH, Kim JK, Ha YG, Hwang JY, Kim T and Lee SH. Antimicrobial activity of plant extracts against *Salmonella Typhimurium*, *Escherichia coli* O157:H7, and *Listeria monocytogenes* on fresh lettuce. J Food Sci 2011; 76: M41-46.

[28] Gorski L. Selective enrichment media bias the types of *Salmonella enterica* strains isolated from mixed strain cultures and complex enrichment broths. PLoS One 2012; 7: e34722.

[29] Pettengill JB, McAvoy E, White JR, Allard M, Brown E and Ottesen A. Using metagenomic analyses to estimate the consequences of enrichment bias for pathogen detection. BMC Res Notes 2012; 5: 378.

[30] Siddique RA, Saxena M and Lakhchaura BD. PCR based rapid detection of *Salmonella* from poultry samples. Indian J Public Health 2009; 53: 226-228.

[31] McCarthy N, Reen FJ, Buckley JF, Frye JG, Boyd EF and Gilroy D. Sensitive and rapid molecular detection assays for *Salmonella enterica* serovars Typhimurium and Heidelberg. J Food Prot 2009; 72: 2350-2357.

[32] Chai Y, Li S, Horikawa S, Park MK, Vodyanoy V and Chin BA. Rapid and sensitive detection of *Salmonella Typhimurium* on eggshells by using wireless biosensors. J Food Prot 2012; 75: 631-636.

[33] Preechakasedkit P, Pinwattana K, Dungchai W, Siangproh W, Chaicumpa W, Tongtawe P and Chailapakul O. Development of a one-step immunochromatographic strip test using gold nanoparticles for the rapid detection of *Salmonella Typhi* in human serum. Biosens Bioelectron 2012; 31: 562-566.

[34] Yukawa S, Tamura Y, Tanaka K and Uchida I. Rapid detection of *Salmonella enterica* serovar Typhimurium DT104 strains by the polymerase chain reaction. Acta Vet Scand 2015; 57: 59.

[35] Sun Y, Quyen TL, Hung TQ, Chin WH, Wolff A and Bang DD. A lab-on-a-chip system with integrated sample preparation and loop-mediated isothermal amplification for rapid and quantitative detection of *Salmonella* spp. in food samples. Lab Chip 2015; 15: 1898-1904.

[36] Jacobson AP, Gill VS, Irvin KA, Wang H and Hammack TS. Evaluation of methods to prepare samples of leafy green vegetables for preenrichment with the Bacteriological Analytical Manual *Salmonella* culture method. J Food Prot 2012; 75: 400-404.

[37] Murgia M, Rubino S, Wain J, Gaind R and Paglietti B. A novel broadly applicable PCR-RFLP method for rapid identification and subtyping of H58 *Salmonella Typhi*. J Microbiol Methods 2016; 127: 219-223.

[38] Wuyts V, Mattheus W, Roosens NH, Marchal K, Bertrand S and De Keersmaecker SC. A multiplex oligonucleotide ligation-PCR as a complementary tool for subtyping of *Salmonella Typhimurium*. Appl Microbiol Biotechnol 2015; 99: 8137-8149.

[39] Ogunremi D, Kelly H, Dupras AA, Belanger S and Devenish J. Development of a new molecular subtyping tool for *Salmonella enterica* serovar Enteritidis based on single nucleotide polymorphism genotyping using PCR. J Clin Microbiol 2014; 52: 4275-4285.

[40] Baquar N, Threlfall EJ, Rowe B and Stanley J. Molecular subtyping within a single *Salmonella Typhimurium* phage type, DT204c, with a PCR-generated probe for IS200. FEMS Microbiol Lett 1993; 112: 217-221.

[41] Aabo S, Andersen JK and Olsen JE. Research note: detection of *Salmonella* in minced meat by the polymerase chain reaction method. Lett Appl Microbiol 1995; 21: 180-182.

[42] Rychlik I, van Kesteren L, Cardova L, Svestkova A, Martinkova R and Sisak F. Rapid detection of *Salmonella* in field samples by nested polymerase chain reaction. Lett Appl Microbiol 1999; 29: 269-272.

[43] Ferretti R, Mannazzu I, Cocolin L, Comi G and Clementi F. Twelve-hour PCR-based method for detection of *Salmonella* spp. in food. Appl Environ Microbiol 2001; 67: 977-978.

[44] Soumet C, Ermel G, Fach P and Colin P. Evaluation of different DNA extraction procedures for the detection of *Salmonella* from chicken products by polymerase chain reaction. Lett Appl Microbiol 1994; 19: 294-298.

[45] Myint MS, Johnson YJ, Tablante NL and Heckert RA. The effect of pre-enrichment protocol on the sensitivity and specificity of PCR for detection of naturally contaminated *Salmonella* in raw poultry compared to conventional culture. Food Microbiol 2006; 23: 599-604.

[46] Maciorowski KG, Herrera P, Jones FT, Pillai SD and Ricke SC. Cultural and immunological detection methods for *Salmonella* spp. in animal feeds – a review. Vet Res Commun 2006; 30: 127-137.

[47] Yan H, Nguyen TA, Phan TG, Okitsu S, Li Y and Ushijima H. Development of RT-multiplex PCR assay for detection of adenovirus and group A and C rotaviruses in diarrheal fecal specimens from children in China. Kansenshogaku Zasshi 2004; 78: 699-709.

[48] Kawasaki S, Horikoshi N, Okada Y, Takeshita K, Sameshima T and Kawamoto S. Multiplex PCR for simultaneous detection of *Salmonella* spp., *Listeria monocytogenes*, and *Escherichia coli* O157:H7 in meat samples. J Food Prot 2005; 68: 551-556.

[49] Sharma VK and Carlson SA. Simultaneous detection of *Salmonella* strains and *Escherichia coli* O157:H7 with fluorogenic PCR and single-enrichment-broth culture. Appl Environ Microbiol 2000; 66: 5472-5476.

[50] Cortez AL, Carvalho AC, Ikuno AA, Burger KP and Vidal-Martins AM. Identification of *Salmonella* spp. isolates from chicken abattoirs by multiplex-PCR. Res Vet Sci 2006; 81: 340-344.

[51] Kim S, Frye JG, Hu J, Fedorka-Cray PJ, Gautom R and Boyle DS. Multiplex PCR-based method for identification of common clinical serotypes of *Salmonella enterica* subsp. *enterica*. J Clin Microbiol 2006; 44: 3608-3615.

[52] Salemis NS. *Salmonella* pancolitis with acute abdomen. CT findings and review literature. Trop Gastroenterol 2010; 31: 49-51.

[53] Hyeon JY, Park C, Choi IS, Holt PS and Seo KH. Development of multiplex real-time PCR with Internal amplification control for simultaneous detection of *Salmonella* and *Cronobacter* in powdered infant formula. Int J Food Microbiol 2010; 144: 177-181.

[54] Barbau-Piednoir E, Bertrand S, Mahillon J, Roosens NH and Botteldoorn N. SYBR(R) Green qPCR *Salmonella* detection system allowing discrimination at the genus, species and subspecies levels. Appl Microbiol Biotechnol 2013; 97: 9811-9824.

[55] Sharbati S, Sharbati J, Hoeke L, Bohmer M and Einspanier R. Quantification and accurate normalisation of small RNAs through new custom RT-qPCR arrays demonstrates *Salmonella*-induced microRNAs in human monocytes. BMC Genomics 2012; 13: 23.

[56] Novinscak A, Surette C and Filion M. Quantification of *Salmonella* spp. in composted biosolids using a TaqMan qPCR assay. J Microbiol Methods 2007; 70: 119-126.

[57] Daum LT, Barnes WJ, McAvin JC, Neidert MS, Cooper LA, Huff WB, Gaul L, Riggins WS, Morris S, Salmen A and Lohman KL. Real-time PCR detection of *Salmonella* in suspect foods from a gastroenteritis outbreak in kerr county, Texas. J Clin Microbiol 2002; 40: 3050-3052.

[58] Wang L, Li Y and Mustaphai A. Rapid and simultaneous quantitation of *Escherichia coli* 0157:H7, *Salmonella,* and Shigella in ground beef by multiplex real-time PCR and immunomagnetic separation. J Food Prot 2007; 70: 1366-1372.

[59] Hein I, Flekna G, Krassnig M and Wagner M. Real-time PCR for the detection of *Salmonella* spp. in food: an alternative approach to a conventional PCR system suggested by the FOOD-PCR project. J Microbiol Methods 2006; 66: 538-547.

[60] Malorny B, Bunge C and Helmuth R. A real-time PCR for the detection of *Salmonella* Enteritidis in poultry meat and consumption eggs. J Microbiol Methods 2007; 70: 245-251.

[61] Bohaychuk VM, Gensler GE, McFall ME, King RK and Renter DG. A real-time PCR assay for the detection of *Salmonella* in a wide variety of food and food-animal matricest. J Food Prot 2007; 70: 1080-1087.

[62] Mandal TK and Parvin N. Rapid detection of bacteria by carbon quantum dots. J Biomed Nanotechnol 2011; 7: 846-848.

[63] Durant JA, Young CR, Nisbet DJ, Stanker LH and Ricke SC. Detection and quantification of poultry probiotic bacteria in mixed culture using monoclonal antibodies in an enzyme-linked immunosorbent assay. Int J Food Microbiol 1997; 38: 181-189.

[64] Dill K, Stanker LH and Young CR. Detection of *Salmonella* in poultry using a silicon chip-based biosensor. J Biochem Biophys Methods 1999; 41: 61-67.

[65] Hoorfar J. Rapid detection, characterization, and enumeration of foodborne pathogens. APMIS Suppl 2011; 133: 1-24.

[66] Jyoti A, Vajpayee P, Singh G, Patel CB, Gupta KC and Shanker R. Identification of environmental reservoirs of nontyphoidal salmonellosis: aptamer-assisted bioconcentration and subsequent detection of *Salmonella Typhimurium* by quantitative polymerase chain reaction. Environ Sci Technol 2011; 45: 8996-9002.

[67] Ozalp VC, Bayramoglu G, Erdem Z and Arica MY. Pathogen detection in complex samples by quartz crystal microbalance sensor coupled to aptamer functionalized core-shell type magnetic separation. Anal Chim Acta 2015; 853: 533-540.

[68] Bruno JG, Richarte AM, Phillips T, Savage AA, Sivils JC, Greis A and Mayo MW. Development of a fluorescent enzyme-linked DNA aptamer-magnetic bead sandwich assay and portable fluorometer for sensitive and rapid leishmania detection in sandflies. J Fluoresc 2014; 24: 267-277.

[69] Singh G, Vajpayee P, Rani N, Jyoti A, Gupta KC and Shanker R. Bio-capture of *S. Typhimurium* from surface water by aptamer for culture-free quantification. Ecotoxicol Environ Saf 2012; 78: 320-326.

[70] Laube T, Cortes P, Llagostera M, Alegret S and Pividori MI. Phagomagnetic immunoassay for the rapid detection of *Salmonella*. Appl Microbiol Biotechnol 2014; 98: 1795-1805.

[71] Vibbert HB, Ku S, Li X, Liu X, Ximenes E, Kreke T, Ladisch MR, Deering AJ and Gehring AG. Accelerating sample preparation through enzyme-assisted microfiltration of *Salmonella* in chicken extract. Biotechnol Prog 2015; 31: 1551-1562.

Chapter 6

Factors Contributing to the Emergence and Spread of Antibiotics Resistance in *Salmonella* Species

Kabiru Olusegun Akinyemi and
Samuel Oluwasegun Ajoseh

Additional information is available at the end of the chapter

http://dx.doi.org/10.5772/67701

Abstract

Salmonella, a genus of the family *Enterobacteriaceae* with over 2450 species, has been responsible for diseases ranging from non-typhoidal salmonellosis to typhoidal salmonellosis. Several groups of antibiotics such as β-lactams, aminoglycosides, tetracyclines, quinolones, cephalosporins and sulfonamides are used against *Salmonella* species. Many *Salmonella* species had developed resistance to several antibiotics over the years. Two major groups of mechanism of resistance demonstrated by this pathogen are (1) Biochemical Mechanisms; such as enzymatic inactivation, prevention of access to the target site by antibiotics and active efflux pumps. (2) Genetic mechanisms; such as mutation, horizontal gene transfer and vertical gene transfer. Some factors identified to contribute to the emergence and dissemination of antibiotic resistant-*Salmonella* include; miss-used of antibiotics, used of antibiotics in agriculture, unregulated sales of antibiotics, inappropriate prescription and dispensing practices, and poor hygiene practices (external or behavioural factors), the presence of mobile genetic elements in the organisms; plasmid DNA, transposons, integrons etc. The clinical and public health consequences, and the strategies to stem the growing tides associated with drugs resistance in Salmonella species are herein discussed. A more radical approach and commitment from the policy makers in health sector to solving problems emanating from increasing spread of resistant *Salmonella* is advocated.

Keywords: *Salmonella*, resistance, antibiotics, factors, chromosomes, plasmid

1. Introduction

Salmonella are Gram-negative, facultative anaerobes, rod-shaped bacteria and are trivially known as 'enteric bacteria' [1], with over 2587 serotypes. *Salmonella* are grouped into two basic species namely, *Salmonella enterica* and *Salmonella bongori* [2, 3]. *Salmonella* generally cause a disease termed salmonellosis, which are both typhoidal and non-typhoidal in nature. Moreover, investigation of the molecular mechanisms of *Salmonella* virulence factors have shown that pathogenic *Salmonella* species are distinguished from non-pathogenic relatives by the presence of specific pathogenicity genes, often called pathogenicity island (PIs), which contributes to both natural and acquired resistance in *Salmonella* species [4, 5]. However, the ability of *Salmonella* to cause invasive infection varies with serovars, the age of the patient and environmental factors [6].

Drug resistance among *Salmonella* serotypes has been a public health concerns at global level [7]. This could be intrinsic (natural resistance) as seen in *S. enterica* serotype typhimurium definitive phage type (DT) 104 that contains the chromosomal *Salmonella*, genomic island type 1 (SGI-1), which harbours resistance genes that confer *ACSST* phenotype (resistance to ampicillin, chloramphenicol, streptomycin, sulphonamide and tetracycline) [8, 9]. Also, the intrinsic resistance could be as a result of impermeability of bacterial cell wall to antibiotic of interest [9]. Several factors have been identified to contribute to the acquired resistance in *Salmonella*, which include: inappropriate use of antibiotic (either through over-prescription, incomplete course of treatment or inadequate dosing, etc.), use of antimicrobial agents in agriculture (either as growth promoter or for prophylaxis purposes), hospital, mutation and transferable genetic materials (plasmid, transposons and integron) [1, 9, 10]. These factors are responsible for the acquisition (emergence) and dissemination (spread) of resistance in *Salmonella* species. Various mechanisms of antimicrobial inactivation exist in *Salmonella* spp., which lead to the emergence of multi-drug resistance (MDR) strains [11, 12]. Some of these mechanisms are as follows:

(i) Enzymatic inactivation of the drug (e.g. β-lactamase)

(ii) Prevention of access to the target agent

(iii) Change or mutation in the target site

(iv) Novel penicillin binding protein (PBPs)

(v) Altered membrane permeability

(vi) Active efflux pumps

(vii) Ribosome alteration

(viii) Creation of biofilm barriers, etc.

Mobile genetic elements such as plasmids, transposons and integrons play an important role in the evolution (emergence) and dissemination (spread) of multi-drug resistance by either horizontal or vertical gene transfer [13]. The role of integrons in the acquisition and dissemination of resistance in *Salmonella* species is crucial. Integrons are DNA elements that contain collection of genes (gene cassette). Integrons are frequently associated with plasmid, transposon and are therefore easily transferable among *Salmonella* and/or between different bacteria [14].

The presence of virulence encoded plasmid DNA *spv*A, *spv*B and *spv*C in several *Salmonella* serovars had been documented and the outer membrane proteins (OMPs) of *Salmonella* typhimurium have a role in the virulence of the organism and are potent candidate for vaccine development since it is immunogenic, capable of evoking both humoral and cell-mediated immune response. These OMPs indirectly play part in intrinsic resistance and can be disseminated between or among *Salmonella* species [15, 16]. Thus, resistance acquisition or dissemination in *Salmonella* species usually involves several factors [1, 13].

2. *Salmonella* virulence and mechanisms of resistance

2.1. *Salmonella* and its virulence factors

The ability of *Salmonella* to attach itself to the host, invade and penetrate intestinal epithelial cell is determined by its virulence factor [17]. Adherence of *Salmonella* is often mediated by fimbriae and/or non-fimbrial adhesion (lipopolysaccharide) [11]. Invasion process is not merely a passive consequence of bacterial contact with epithelial cells, but instead requires the active production and transport of secreted effector proteins by a Type III secretion system (T3SS) 1 & 2 and Type 1 secretion systems, which are encoded in *Salmonella* pathogenicity island I & 2 (SPI-I & 2), respectively [17]. In addition, invasion is also induced by flagella/flagellin since *Salmonella* is a flagellated facultative anaerobe. Many invasion regulators have been described, for examples, *Hil*A [18], *Hil*C [19], InvF [20], PhoP/PhoQ, *Hil*E [21], H-NS [19] and *Inv*A genes, PhoP/PhoQ pair is also essential for the expression of genes in *Salmonella* pathogenicity island 2 (SP1-2), which encodes a second Type III secretory system. SP1-2 is required for intra-macrophage survival, which is a cell-type encountered by *Salmonella* immediately after the invasion of epithelium. PhoP/PhoQ also serves to repress SP1-1 genes, a function mediated by H*il*A [22]. PhoP/PhoQ may thus act as a genetic switch, activating traits required for macrophages survival while repressing those not needed for invasion [17].

Other factors that are involved in *Salmonella* virulence are the MgtC in *Salmonella* typhimurium. This is required for growth at low—Mg^{2+} concentrations and intra-macrophage survival. Iron acquisition (for iron deprivation survival) this is achieved by the production of two siderophores, which are enterobactin and salmochelin in response to iron deprivation. Superoxide dismutase is used to counteract the reactive oxygen produced through the activity of the phagosome NADPH oxidase (NOX_2) that are required for the killing of intracellular pathogens and enterotoxin (responsible for food-intoxication) [23]. The genes coding for the above-mentioned factors and others are conserved in *Salmonella* pathogenicity island 3 (SP1-3), and is also present in the chromosomes of other *Salmonella enterica* serovars [23]. It has been reported by several researchers [15, 24, 25], that *stn* genes coding for *Salmonella* enterotoxin) *sef* genes for *Salmonella* Enteritidis fimbriae, and *pef* genes for plasmid encoded fimbriae are widely distributed in resistant *Salmonella* strains and are responsible for *Salmonella*-associated diseases in animal and human populations globally.

2.2. Resistance mechanisms exhibited by *Salmonella* species to some antibiotics

Various mechanisms of anti-microbials inactivation have been reported by [11, 26], which invariably lead to the emergence of multidrug resistance in *Salmonella* species. These mechanisms are summarized into two broad groups, namely:

- Biochemical mechanisms and
- Genetics mechanisms.

2.2.1. Biochemical mechanisms of antibiotic resistance by Salmonella species

Enzymatic inactivation: This may result into either destruction of antimicrobial agents, such as occurs with the β-lactamases, or lead to a major modification of the antibiotic so that it does not bind to its target as it's seen with the aminoglycoside and chloramphenicol [1]. The major mechanisms of resistance to beta-lactam antibiotics among *Enterobacteriaceae* involve production of β-lactamase or extended spectrum β-lactamase (ESBLs) [1]. ESBLs have traditionally been defined as transmissible β-lactamases that can be inhibited by clavulanic acid, tazobactam or sulbactam. They are group of enzymes that break down antibiotics belonging to the penicillin and cephalosporin groups and render them ineffective [1]. ESBLs are generally encoded by mobile genes that can be exchanged between bacteria [27]. It has been noted that when ESBL strains occur, they often have co-resistance with the aminoglycosides (gentamicin), tetracycline and trimethoprim/sulphamethoxazole [27]. CTX–M ESBLs arise by plasmid acquisition of pre-existing chromosomal ESBL genes; this proved that ESBL can be plasmid mediated and thus capable of spreading to other microorganisms of either related species or genera [28].

Prevention of access to the target site: This may be by substitutions, amplifications or modification of the drug target, thereby reducing the affinity of the drug to the target. For example, in *Salmonella,* the outer membrane proteins may be altered such that antibiotics are unable to cross its cell wall [26]. Gram-negative bacteria can regulate membrane permeability by altering expression of outer membrane porin (omp) proteins that form channels for passive diffusion. Loss or reduced levels of ompF has been implicated in anti-microbial resistance in *Salmonella* over the years [29].

Active efflux pumps: This involves the expellant of multiple kinds of antibiotics out of the cytoplasm of the microorganism to the external environment [11]. Increased expression of non-specific, energy-dependent efflux systems allow bacteria to prevent the accumulation of effective concentrations of quinolones inside the cell by actively pumping out the drug. In *Escherichia coli,* the AcrAB-TolC efflux pump plays a major role in quinolone efflux and studies suggest that this may be the primary mechanism of fluoroquinolone resistance in *Salmonella* [30]. It is thoughtful that these efflux systems cause low-level resistance to quinolones that can become clinically relevant when combined with mutations in the target enzymes [31].

Reduced permeability of the antimicrobial agent: This is a common mechanism of anti-microbial resistance usually exhibited my *S. enterica.* It involves the alteration in membrane permeability, which occurs when new genetic information, change the nature of proteins in the membrane. This alteration changes a membrane transport system pores in the membrane for an anti-microbial agent not to be able to cross the membrane. This form of resistance mechanism has been discovered in *Salmonella* typhi to tetracycline, quinolones and some aminoglycosides and sulphonamide antibiotics [32, 33].

2.2.2. Genetics mechanisms of antibiotics resistance in Salmonella species

The genes coding for antibiotics resistance and virulence at times share common features of being located in the bacterial chromosome, as well as on plasmid (**Tables 1** and **2**). They are associated in gene clusters to form resistance or pathogenicity island, which are transferred by mobile genetic elements such as integrons, transposons or phage [34].

The major genetics mechanisms are as follows:

- Mutation
- Horizontal resistant gene transfer and
- Vertical resistant gene transfer.

Resistance in enteric bacteria: *Salmonella, E. coli, Shigella,* spp. etc., can be a result of gene mutation (a permanent change in the DNA of an organisms), which had been detected through several research studies globally or transfer of resistance determinant (R-determinants) between the same species or different species (Horizontal gene transfer) or by transfer of resistance genes from parental microorganism to its progeny or offspring (Vertical gene transfer) [13, 35]. Clinically, chromosomal and plasmid-mediated resistance in *Salmonella* to gentamicin and Beta-lactam antibiotics had been reported in some host animal and humans [35–37].

The role of integrons in the acquisition and dissemination of resistance in enteric bacteria such as *Salmonella* is very crucial. Integrons are genetic elements that capture and incorporate gene cassettes by using a site-specific recommendation mechanism [38]. The class 1 and class 2 integrons are known to play specific role in anti-book resistance in *Salmonella* spp., which usually contain conserved segments. For example, integron class 1 has been reported to carry *aad*A_2, *bla* and *pse*1 cassette [39, 40]. Most of these integrons are located within transposons that contribute to vertical transmission, favouring their mobilization between plasmid and

Antibiotic group	Members	Effect	Mechanism of actions
β-Lactarns	Penicillin(s), Amoxicillin Imipenem Cephalosporin (1st, 2nd, 3rd generation)	Cidal	Inhibit transpeptidation enzymes involved in cross-linking the poly saccharide chains of the bacterial cell wall peptidoglycan and also by activation of cell wall lytic enzymes (cell wall synthesis inhibition)
Aminoglycoside	Neomycin, Kanamycin, Amikacin, Tobramycin, Gentamycin and Streptomycin	Cidal	Bind to small ribosomal sub-unit (30s) and interfere with protein synthesis by directly inhibiting synthesis and causing misreading of mRNA. Thereby inhibiting protein synthesis
Tetracycline	Oxytetracycline, Chlortetracycline, Doxycycline, etc.	Static	Same as aminoglycoside
Quinolones and fluoroquinoles	Ciprofloxacin, Norfloxacin, etc.	Cidal	Inhibit DNA gyrase and topoisomerase II, thereby blocking DNA replication
Sulfonamides	Silver-sulphadiazine, Sulphamethoxazole, Sulphanilamide, Sulphisoxazole, etc.	Static	Inhibits folic acid synthesis by competing with *p*-aminobenzoic acid (PABA)

Adapted from Refs. [1, 40].

Table 1. Properties of some common antibacterial drugs commonly used against *Salmonella* species.

	Resistance genes	Resistance genes location(s)	Resistance mechanisms	Region(s)	References
Aminoglycosides	*aacC(3), aacC(3')-IIa, aacC(6'), aacC2, aadA, aadA1, aadA2, aadA12, aadB, ant(3")-Ia, aphAI, aphAI IAB, aph(3)-Ii-iv, aph(3)-IIa, strA, strB*	CH, P	Enzymatic modification and inactivation of aminoglycoside	Across the Globe	[33, 42]
β-Lactams	*ompC*, *ompF*, *bla*CMY-2, *bla*PSE-1, *bla*TEM-1, *bla*SHV-1, *bla*OXA-1, *bla*NDM-1	CH, P	β-Lactamases, ESBL, Modification of porin (*ompF*), Efflux of β-lactam(*ompC*)	Across the Globe	[33, 42, 44]
Quinolones and floro-quinolones	*GryA, GyrB, parC, parE,*	CH, P	Mutation in the Quinolones Resistance Determining Region (QRDR) *GryA, GyrB, parC, pare*	Across the Globe	[30]
Tetracycline	*tet(A), tet(B), tet(C), tet(D), tet(G)*, and *tet(H)*	P	Efflux pumps, Modification of rRNA target, Inactivation of compound	Across the Globe	[33, 42, 45]
Sulphanamides	*Sul1, sul2 sul3, dfr*	CH, P	Dihydropteroate synthase	Across the Globe	[42–44]
Phenicol eg Chloramphenicol	*floR, cmlA, cat1*	CH, P	Efflux pumps (*floR, cmlA*) and chloramphenicol acetyltransferase	Across the Globe	[42, 45]

Table 2. Antibiotic resistance genes and resistance mechanisms found in *Salmonella* species.

the bacterial chromosome by transposition events [14]. They have the ability to integrate stably into regions of other DNA, where they deliver, in a single exchange multiple new genes, particularly for drug resistance [41]. Many of the gene cassettes in resistance integrons, probably originated from super-integron (larger integron structures with hundreds of accessory genes), which encode for resistance against newer antibiotics such as cephalosporin and carbapenems [22].

2.3. Antibiotics commonly used for the treatment of salmonellosis and their mechanisms of actions

Some groups of antibiotics used in the treatment of salmonellosis globally for public health purposes as shown in **Table 1** include:

Aminoglycosides: Salmonella resistance to aminoglycosides is usually by enzymatic modification and binding to the 30S ribosomal subunit, resulting in the inhibition of protein synthesis in the organism aminoglycoside phosphotransferase confirms resistance to Kanamycin and Neomycin. Major, resistance genes include *str*A, *str*B, *aac, aad*, etc. [42, 43].

Tetracycline: Tetracycline targets the 30S ribosomal subunit of the bacteria ribosome just as aminoglycosides. Resistance mechanisms include efflux, modification of rRNA and inactivation of the compound [43]. In *Salmonella*, active efflux systems are most commonly observed and it includes *tet*A, B, C, D, G and H [43].

β-lactams: β-lactams prevent synthesis and maintenance of the peptidoglycan component of the bacteria cell wall by mimicking one of the building blocks used by enzymes to construct peptidoglycan. Most resistance to β-lactams is confirmed by β-lactamase that enzymatically cleaves the β-lactams ring and prevents it from bonding to and inactivating cell wall enzymes. Furthermore, extended spectrum β-lactamase is an important group of β-lactamases newly discovered not more than one decade ago [44]. However, other resistance mechanisms reported in major regions across the globe include efflux of the β-lactams and modification of porin (e.g. *omp*F and *omp*C) [42, 45].

Phenicols: Phenicols, e.g. chloramphenicol and related compound such as florphenicol, inhibit protein synthesis by binding to the 50S ribosome subunit. Resistance to chloramphenicol is highly prevalence in developing countries based on its cheapness and easy accessibility in the counter e.g. Nigeria [10, 44], despite its ban in developed countries, e.g. USA, based on it toxicity [43]. Most resistance mechanisms exhibited by *Enterobacteriaceae* including *Salmonella* are efflux pumps such as *flo*R and *cml*A as well as inactivating enzymes such as chloramphenicol acetyltransferase *cat*1 [46].

Sulphonamides: They are also called *folate pathway inhibitors*. These are compounds that compete for substrate of the essential folic acid pathway in bacteria at two different steps, and the sulphanilamide inhibits DHPS (dihydrofolate reductase). Sulphonamides are bacteriostatic when used alone or bactericidal when combined with trimethoprim-sulphamethoxazole [47]. Resistance to both of these antimicrobials occurs by acquisition of gene-encoding enzymes that do not bind these compounds [43], these include, the *sul* genes eg *sul*1, *sul*2 and *sul*3, which encode for insensitive DHPs enzymes, and are found in *Salmonella* globally [46].

2.4. Phenotypic and genotypic detection of resistance in *Salmonella*

Drug or antibiotic resistance is the decreased sensitivity of microbes to drug or antibiotics that are capable of causing cell death or inhibition of growth [48]. This is determined through antimicrobial sensitivity testing of *Salmonella* species (isolates) in order to determine its susceptibility or resistance to the antibiotics [49]. Resistance in *Salmonella* is encoded by genes that are present on either chromosome or extra-chromosomal DNA (plasmid) or transferable genetic materials (transposons, integrons), which is determined by genetic or molecular method [50]. The most common method is the Kirby-Bauer method [49]. Although resistance may occur due to mutation in key genetic loci in the bacterial genome, but most resistance to antimicrobial agents mediated by genes are acquired via mobile genetic elements such as plasmid and transposons [50]. The identification of resistance genotype is accomplished through detection of novel genetic materials and characterization of mutations in specific genes through polymerase chain reaction

(PCR). Several genetic methods including DNA probes, PCR and other amplification techniques are now used in varieties of clinical laboratories for identification and quantification of pathogenic organisms [51, 52].

2.5. Some identified factors for the emergence and spread of resistance in *Salmonella* species

The emergence of resistance is the natural response of microbes to the presence of antimicrobial agents [53, 54]. Several factors contribute to the increase in multi-drug resistance by *Salmonella* species, which can be grouped into two, namely:

- *Behavioural factors* (external factors): which include misuse of antibiotics, use of antibiotics in agriculture, unregulated sales of antibiotics, inappropriate prescription and dispensing practices and poor hygiene practices.
- *Genetics factors*: the mobile genetic elements, which include plasmids, transposons, integrons, etc.

2.5.1. Behavioural factors

These involve attitudinal conduct of the prescribers (Doctors), dispensers (Pharmacist), patients, agriculturists and/or government to prescription, sales, usage and regulation of antibiotics. These are elucidated as follows:

Inappropriate prescribing and dispensing: Lack of access to update information makes prescribers to prescribe less rationally [55]. Economic incentive and enticement from pharmaceutical companies further pressure the prescriber to prescribe unnecessarily or inappropriately [56]. Moreover, it is a common practice in many developing countries for antibiotics to be dispensed without a prescription. Also, over the counter sales of antibiotics is common. These practices had been attributed to weak enforcement of laws in such countries with resultant increase in acquisition of drug resistance in *Salmonella* species and high morbidity and mortality of *Salmonella*-associated diseases [10, 56].

Patients: Patient attitude contributes to the emergences of resistance through poor compliance to the prescribed course of treatment [1], especially if their symptoms are mild and resolved quickly [57]. The attitudes of self-medication in most patients has seriously contributed to the emergence of MDR in *S.* typhi to most first line drugs such as chloramphenicol, cephalosporin, streptomycin, tetracycline, ampicillin, etc. [10]. More also, poor hygiene practices of handling raw animal product and food in general with inadequate heat treatment has greatly contributed to the spread of antibiotic resistant strains from animal products and food to human [58, 59]. Furthermore, improper cooking methods; re-heating of food by food handlers in restaurants and canteens have been identified as also a major factor responsible for the spread of multidrug resistant *Salmonella* species since most of developing countries (e.g. Nigeria) population live below the average level of $1 per day meal, hence they resort to patronizing restaurants and canteens of questionable cooking standards [60, 61].

Hospitals and laboratories (*medical centres*): Majority of antimicrobials usages occur in the community, of which most intense usage occurs in hospital [64]. The strong selective pressure together with the multitude of opportunities for resistant strains of *Salmonella* to spread from patient to patient is of high increase, this then means that hospital-acquired infections (Nosocomial infection) are mainly caused by multi-drug resistant strains, as seen in *S.* typhi in the case of typhoid fever [10]. Early discharges from hospitals either through changes in practice (e.g. cost reduction in developed countries) or lack of patient's ability to pay (particularly in developing countries) contribute to the emergence and dissemination of multi-drug resistance strains of *Salmonella* species [56]. However, hospitals work based on laboratory diagnosis must of the time not relying on clinical diagnosis alone since the former is the most reliable means of diagnosing a patient. But it is in the other way in developing countries based on exclusive reliance on Widal test as a means of diagnosing typhoid fever, which can be misleading as individuals with pyrexia are assumed and erroneously diagnosed as having typhoid fever based on single Widal agglutination test [62].

Government: contributes to the emergence of resistance in *Salmonella* species and other disease causing organisms that are of public health concern in the following perspective:

(1) Weakness in legislation or its enforcement contributes to resistance by allowing the circulation in the market of substandard or counterfeit antimicrobials.

(2) Poor regulation of advertisement and promotion of drug undoubtedly increases sales, and encourages unnecessary use of antimicrobials.

(3) Lack of adequate training and certification of prescribers and dispensers may be due to poor provision or regulation by government.

(4) Poor availability of potable water.

(5) Poor diagnostic facilities of salmonellosis (typhoidal and non-typhoidal) in terms of isolation of the causative agent for quality treatment.

(6) Poor sewage disposal and waste treatment channels.

It should also be noted, that lack of information about prevalence of resistance problems or poor supply chain management or long-term facilities (poor diagnostic facilities) contribute to poor diagnosis and effective treatment of disease that are of public health concern, which result in emergence of multi-drug resistance strains that eventually result to high cost of treatment of these diseases [1, 10, 63]. Furthermore, non-availability of *S.* typhi vaccines in developing countries like Nigeria is also one of the contributing factors to the spread of resistance in *Salmonella* species [64].

Contribution of non-human uses of antimicrobials: The worldwide increase in the use of antibiotics in poultry, fishery and livestock production industries to treat and prevent infections, or as growth promoter, has greatly contributed to the increased antibiotics resistance in potential food-borne pathogens (*Salmonella, Shigella, Campylobacter*, etc.) in the past years [58, 64]. The increased use of antibiotics in agriculture has played a significant role in the emergence and spread of antibiotic resistant food-borne pathogens in human as a result of the consumption of poultry and dairy products [59]. The summary of the behavioural factors and their contribution to antibiotic resistance is shown in **Figure 1**.

2.5.2. The genetic factors

The major mechanism in the spread (dissemination of resistance genes between or among bacteria of the same species or different species is through genetic mechanism. Since resistance genes for instance in *Salmonella* have often been located within plasmid, integrons sometimes

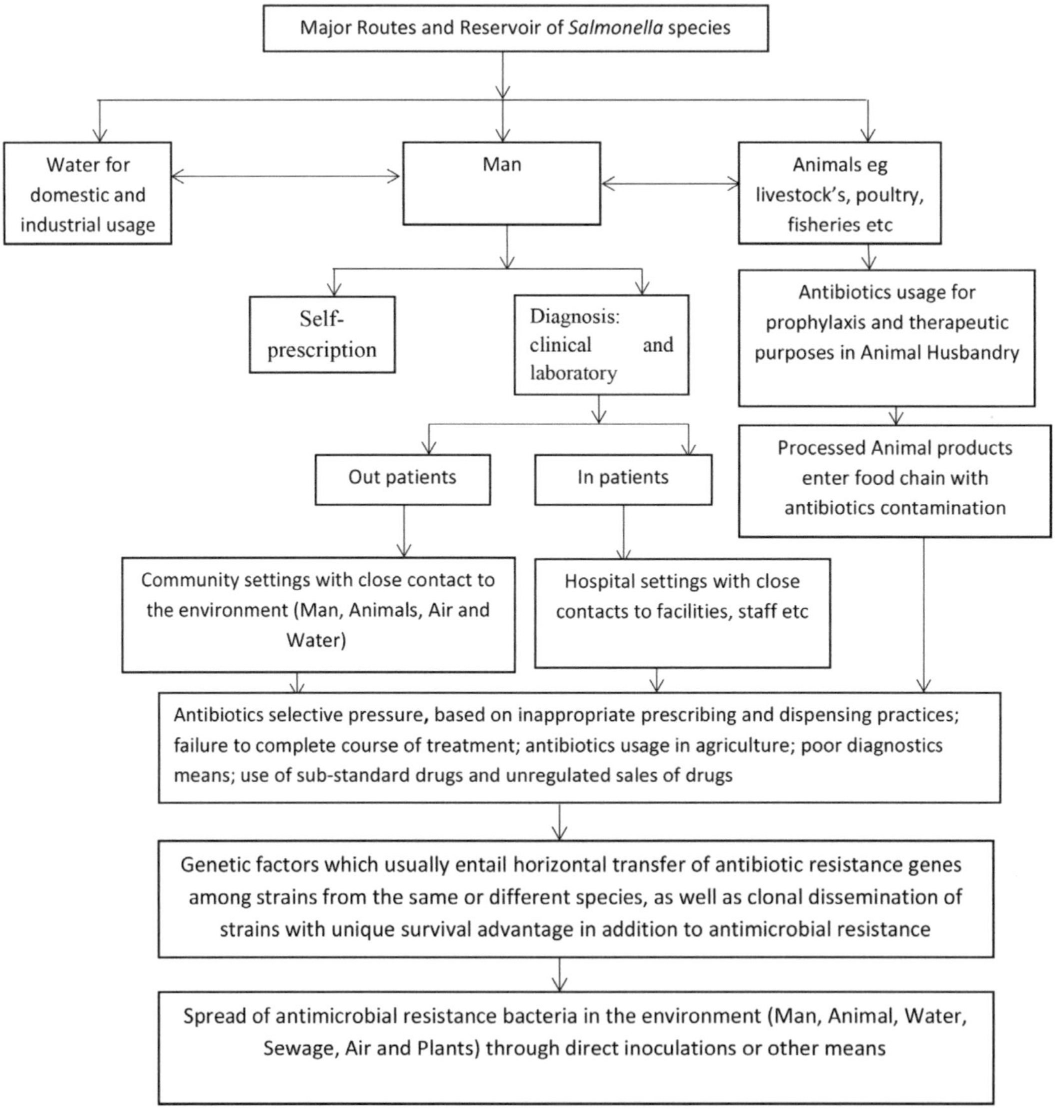

Figure 1. A flow chart showing the spread of antibiotic resistance in *Salmonella* species in both man and animal populations.

associated with transposons and also insertion sequence [1, 56, 65]. The major factors involved in the genetic mechanism of spread are the integrons, transposomes and plasmids [13].

Integrons are mobile genetic elements of specific structure that consist of two conserved segment capable of flanking through a central region in which resistance gene cassettes are inserted [36]. Also, on the 5^1-conserved segment is an *int* gene that encodes a site-specific recombinase, capable of capturing DNA, including resistance genes [66].

Transposons: These are mobile genetic elements that contain insertion sequence (0.2–6.0kb), which can move (transpose) from one site to the other site within the same or different chromosome or plasmid and thus replicate along with it [56].

Plasmid (4–400kb) are self-replicating, extra chromosomal DNA that contain genes either for resistance, virulence and other functions and are dispensable under certain conditions. Incompatibility group of plasmid DNA (Inc) HI1 are important vectors of antibiotic resistance in *S.* typhi. It was first detected from a large outbreak in 1972 in Mexico [64]. However, some larger plasmids are conjugative (R-plasmid) and are transferable between organisms, spreading along resistance genes in *S.* typhi [38]. It is should be noted that, as resistance genes move to other plasmids or chromosomes, they sometimes link with other resistance genes in resistance clusters, whose transfer can then result in spontaneous acquisition of resistance to several unrelated drugs, which eventually result to multi-drug resistance by recombination process [56].

2.6. Consequences of resistance in *Salmonella* species to public health

There are several clinical and public health consequences associated with antimicrobial drugs resistance in *Salmonella* species. These include:

(1) Failure in therapy, thereby resulting to limitation in the choice of treatment after the establishment of microbial diagnosis [67].

(2) Increased burden of illness and outbreaks in settings where patients are treated with antimicrobial drugs [67].

(3) Increased virulence of *Salmonella* species as a result of 'drug-bug combination' that poses selective pressure on the microorganism [25].

(4) Increased mortality and morbidity, thereby posing threats to public health [10, 67].

(5) Increased cost of treatments [1].

(6) Longer stay in hospital, which increases the risk of acquisition of nosocomial infections.

(7) Increased transmission of resistant *Salmonella* strains [67].

2.7. Strategies to combat resistance problems posed by *Salmonella* species

Several efforts have been adopted by several organizations, government and researchers to combat antimicrobial resistance imposed by some pathogenic organism that are of public health significant (*Salmonella* spp.) [68]. The 2006 IFT report led to the publication of the World Health Organization (WHO) list of critically important antimicrobials for human medicine and veterinary importance. This propelled the U.S Food and Drug Administration (FDA) to categorize various classes of anti-microbials as important, highly important and critically important and has since issued rules that prohibit most extra labelled use of some critically important antimicrobials such as fluoroquinolones and cephalosporin in food animal species [69].

Other efforts to address threats posed by antimicrobial resistance include: monitoring programmes for antimicrobial resistance microbes that integrates human, animals and food sampling scheme. Examples include: National Antimicrobial Resistance Monitoring System (NARMS) in the United States and the Danish Integrated Antimicrobial Resistance Monitoring Programme (DANMAP) in Denmark. These programmes in collaboration with CDC, WHO and FDA had really helped to trace the incidence of resistance particularly in foodborne pathogens (*Salmonella* and *Campylobacter*) globally, thereby embarking several strategies such as giving updated information, rules/laws, social and financial help, etc. to combat resistance threats.

Also, effort to combat resistance posed by *Salmonella* is the modification of drugs that led to the production of third – and fourth generation cephalosporins, and the use of medicinal plants also known as herbal medicine had been proven to have bactericidal effect on *S.* typhi; the causative agent of typhoid fever, also with the use of combined therapy, that is, the use of two or more different classes of antibiotics for the treatments of a particular disease e.g. Salmonellosis [1, 57].

Furthermore, the following are also needed to be done to track-down the current rise in the spread of resistant *S. enterica*: Intensive surveillance of vended foods in developing countries to reduce microbial risk associated with their consumption [60]. Public enlightenment to discourage the patronage of vended foods should be intensified as vended foods especially in Lagos is a potential vector responsible for the spread of resistant *Salmonella* species, or high level of hygiene practice should be maintained by food vendors under strict supervision and monitoring by food regulatory authorities if at all vended foods will be patronized [60].

3. Conclusion

Several factors such as misuse of antibiotics, use of antibiotics in agriculture, poor hygiene practices by hospitals and individuals, unregulated sales of antibiotics and genetic factors, such as plasmids, integron, transposons, etc., contribute to selective pressure on antibiotics and resistance gene transfer, respectively, in *Salmonella* species. This has led to the emergence and spread of resistance in this microorganism and resultant therapeutic failures. Several strategies have been adopted by governmental organizations and pharmaceutical companies in the areas of resistance monitoring, restriction in the use of antibiotics in agriculture, production of modified drugs, the use of combined therapy, future plans on the use of bioactive compounds from medicinal plants against MDR bacterial strains. There is a need to enforce regulatory laws governing procurement and sales of antibiotics in developing countries.

http://dx.doi.org/10.5772/67701

Also, good sanitation and hygiene practices as well as sensitization of people about the danger associated with indiscriminate purchase and use of antibiotics are essential to steam the growing trends of antibiotic resistance in bacterial pathogens especially *Salmonella* species.

Author details

Kabiru Olusegun Akinyemi* and Samuel Oluwasegun Ajoseh

*Address all correspondence to: akinyemiko@yahoo.com

Department of Microbiology, Faculty of Science, Lagos State University, Ojo, Lagos, Nigeria

References

[1] Bisi-Johnson, M.A., Obich-Kambizil, and Nkomo, M. (2012). A review of *Escherichia coli* and *Salmonella* species: Molecular landscape and therapeutic consideration. Tanbo district, Easters Cape Province, South Africa. *J. Med. Sci. Adv.*, **1** (1): 1–16

[2] Grimont, P.A.D. and Weill, F.X. (2007). Antigenic formulae of the *Salmonella* serovars, 9th edition. Paris: WHO Collaborating Center for Reference and Research on Salmonella at Institut Pasteur in France 150 p.

[3] Centre for disease control and prevention (2012). *Salmonella surveillance report.*

[4] Brooks, J.T., Ochieng, J.B., Kumar, L., Okoth, G., Shapiro, R.L., Well, G.J., Bird, M., Bop, C., Cheqe, W., Beatty, M.E., Chiller, T., Vulule, J.M., Mintz, E. and Slutsker, L. (2006). Surveillance for bacterial antimicrobial resistance in rural western Kenya (1997–2000). *Cin. Infect. Dis.*, **43:** 393–401.

[5] Micheal, G.B., Butage, P., Cloeckaert, A. and Schwarz, S. (2006). Genes and mutation conferring antimicrobial resistance in *Salmonella: an update. Microbes infects*, **8** (7): 1898–1914.

[6] Uzzau, S., Brown, D.J., Wallis, T., Rubino, S., Leori, G., Bernard, S., Casadesus, J., Platt, D.J. and Olsen, J.E. (2000). Host adapted serotypes of *Salmonella enterica. Epidemiol. Infect.*, **125**: 229–255.

[7] Sharma, R., Sharma, C. and Kapoor, B. (2005). Antibacteria resistance: current problems and possible solutions. *Indian J. Med. Sci.*, **5** (1): 129.

[8] Murugkar, H.V., Rahman, H. and Dutta, P.K. (2003). Distribution of virulence genes in *Salmonella* serovars isolates from man and animals. *Indian J. Med. Res.*, **117:**66–70.

[9] Meervenne, E.V., Coilliev, and Kercklif, F.M., et al. (2012). Strain specific transfer of antibiotic resistance from an environmental planning to food-borne pathogens. *J. Biomed. Biotechnol.*, **101** (11): 83–98.

[10] Akinyemi, K.O., Bamiro, B.S. and Coker, A.O. (2007). *Salmonella* in Lagos, Nigeria: incidence of plasmodium falciparum-associated with co-infection, patterns of antimicrobial resistance, and emergence of reduced susceptibility fluoroquinolones. *J. Health Popul. Nutr.*, **25**:351–358.

[11] Aleksun, M.N. and Levy, S.B. (2007). Molecular mechanism of antibacterial multidrug resistance cell. *J. Med. Microbol.*, **128**(7):1037–1050.

[12] Sundsfjord, A., Simonsen, G.S., Haldersen, B.C., Haaheim, H., Hjelmevoll, S.O., Littauer, P. and Dahl, K.H. (2000). Genetic methods for detection of antimicrobial resistance. *Apruis*, **112**(11–12): 815–837.

[13] David, M.O., Rose, K., Waini, E.N., Ghebremedhin, B., Konig, W. and Kong, B. (2010). Integron-plasmid mediated antibiotic resistance and enhance factors in clinical *Salmonella entericaserovars. African J. Pharm.*, **4** (7): 490–497.

[14] Carattoli, A. (2003). Plasmid-mediated antimicrobial resistance in *Salmonella enterica. Clin. Micrbiol.*, **5**(4): 113–122.

[15] Guiney, D.G., Frang, F.C., Krause, M. and Libby, S. (1994). Plasmid-mediated virulence genes. In non-typhoidal *Salmonella serovars. FEMS Microbiol.*, **124**: 1–9.

[16] Hamid, N. and Jain, S.K. (2008). Characterization of an outer membrane protein of *Salmonella enterica Ser.*Typhimurium that confers protection against typhoid. *Vaccine Imunol.*, **15**:1461–1495.

[17] Altier, C. (2005).Genetic and environmental control of *Salmonella* invasion. *J. Microbiol.*, **43**: 85–92.

[18] Lostrol, C.P. and Lee, C.A. (2001). The *Salmonella* pathogenecity Island–1 type III secretion system. *Microbes Infect.*, **3**(14–15): 1281–1291.

[19] Schechter, L.M., Dammuer, S.M. and Lee, C.A. (1999). Two araclxyls family members can independently conteract the effect of repressing sequences upstream of the *HIL*A promoter. *Mol. Microbial.*, **32**: 629–642.

[20] Davies, J. and Wright, G.D.(1997). Bacteria resistance to aminoglycoside antibiotics. *EUJ Pharm.*, **5**: 234–240.

[21] Baxter, M.A., Fahlen, T.F., Wilson R.L. and Jones, B.D. (2003). H*il*E interact with H*il*D and negatively regulates l*il*A transcription and expression of the *Salmonella enterica serovar* Typhimurium invasive phenotype. *Infect. Immun.*, **71**: 1292–1305.

[22] Fluit, A.C. and Schmitz, F.J. (2004). Resistance integrons and super integrons. *Clin. Microbial. Infect.*, **10**: 272–288.

[23] Retainal, P., Castillo–Ruiz, M. and Mora, G.C. (2009). Characterization of mgtc, a virulence factor of *Salmonella enterica*serovar.Typhi. *Antibiol. Agent Chemother.*, **4**(5): 5551.

[24] Akinyemi, K.O., Iwalokun, B.A., Foli, F., Oshodi, K. and Coker, A.O. (2011). Prevalence of multiple drug resistance and screening of enterotoxin (stn) gene in *Salmonella enterica*serovars from water sources in Lagos, Nigeria. *Public Health* (impact factor:1.26), **125(**2): 65–71.

[25] Sara, M., Soto, Irene, R., Rosario, M.R., Jordi,V. and Carmen, M.M. (2006). Detection of virulence determinants in clinical strains of *Salmonella enterica*serovar Enteritidis and mapping on macrorestriction profile. *J. Med. Microbiol.*, **55**: 365–373.

[26] Sivakumar,T., Avinash N., Saravanavel, D., Prablue, T., Shankar and Vijaghbaskar P. (2012). Characterization of multi drug resistance pattern of *Salmonella* species. *J. Med. Sci.*, **7**(2): 64–67.

[27] Winokur, P.L., Canton, R., Casella, J.N. and Legakis, N. (2001). Variation in the prevalence of strains expressing an extended — spectrum B-latamase phenotype and characterization of isolation from Europe, the Americas, and the Western pacific region. *Clin. Infect. Dis.*, **32**(2): 4–5103.

[28] Babic, M., Hujer, A.M. and Bonomo, P.A. (2006). What's new in antibiotic resistance? Focus on beta-lactamases. *Drug Resist. update*, **9**(3): 142–156.

[29] Thompson, P.R., Schwatzenhaver, J., Hughes, D.W., Bertillis, A.M. and Wright, G.D. (1999).The aminoglycoside phosphotransferase (3') for antibiotic recognition and resistance. *J. Biochem.*, **274**: 30697–30706.

[30] Dimitrovi, T., Dashti, A.A., Albaksami, O., Udo, E.E., Jadaon, M.M. and Albert, M.J.(2009). Ciprofloxacin resistant *Salmonella enterica* serovar Typhi from Kuwait with novel mutation in *gyr*Aand *par*C genes. *J. Clin. Microbiol.*, **47**(1): 208.

[31] Hooper, D.C. (1999). Mechanism of fluoroquinolone resistance. *Drug Resist. Update*, **2**: 38–55.

[32] Kotra, L.P., Hadad, J. and Mobashery, S. (2000). Aminoglycosides: perspectives on mechanisms of action and resistance and strategies to counter resistance. *Antimicrobs Agents Chemother.*, **44**: 3249–3256.

[33] Miller, G.H., Sabatelli, F.J. Hare, R.S, Glupczynski, Y. et al.(1997). The most frequent aminoglycoside resistance mechanisms—changes with time and geographical area: a reflection of aminoglycoside pattern. *Clin. Infect. Dis.*, **24**(1): 46–62.

[34] Villa, H. and Carattoli, A. (2005). Integron and transposons on the *Salmonella enterica*serovea Typhimurium associated with virulence plasmid. *Antimicrob. Agents Chemother*, **49**(3): 1194–1197.

[35] Cournvalin, P.(1994). Transfer of antibiotic resistance in gram-positive and gram-negative bacteria. *Antimicrob. Agents Chemother.*, **38**: 1447–1451.

[36] Hall, R.M. and Collins, C.M. (1998). Antibiotic resistance in gram-negative bacteria: the rate of gene cassettes and integrons. *Drug Resist. Updates*, **1**: 109–119.

[37] Threlfall, E.J., Ward, L.R., Skinner, J.A. and Rowe, B. (1997). Increase in multiple antibiotic resistance in non-typhoidal *Salmonella* from human. *FEMS Microbiol. Rev.*, **4**: 251–31.

[38] Cambray, G., Guerout, A.M. and Mazel, D. (2010). Integrons annel. *Rev. Genet.*, **44**: 141–166.

[39] Randall, L.P., Cooles, S.W., Osborn, M.K., Piddock, L.J.V. and Woodward, M.J. (2004). Antibiotic resistance genes, integrons and multiple antibiotic resistance in thirty-five serotypes of *Salmonella enterica* from human and animal in the UK. *J. Antimicrobial. Chemother.*, **53**: 208–216.

[40] Peter, E. D, Leverstein–van, H.M.A., Box, A.T., Verhoef, J. and Fluit, A.C. (2001). Novel genes cassette and integrons. *Anitmicrob. Agents Chemother.*, **45**: 2961–2964.

[41] Nemergut, D.R., Robeson, M.A., Kysela, R.F., Martin, A.P., Schmidt, S.K. and Knight, R. (2008). Insight and inferance about integron evolution from genomic data. *BMC Genomics*, **9**: 261–264.

[42] Glenn. M., Lindsey, R.L., Frank,J. F., Meinersmann, R. J., Englen, M.D., Fedorka-Cray, P. J., et al. (2011). Analysis of antimicrobial resistance genes detected in multidrug-resistant *Salmonella enterica* serovar Typhimurium isolated from food animals. *Microb. Drug Resist.*, **17**: 407–418.

[43] Frye, J. G., Lindsey, R. L., Meinersmann, R. J., Berrang, M. E., Jackson, C. R., Englen, M. D., et al. (2011). Related antimicrobial resistance genes detected in different bacterial species co-isolated from swine fecal samples. *Foodborne Pathog. Dis.*, **8**: 663–679.

[44] Akinyemi, K.O., Iwalokun, B.A., Alafe, O.O. Mudashiru, S.A. and Fakorede, C. (2015). $Bla_{CTX\text{-}M\text{-}1}$ group extended spectrum bête-lactamase producing *Salmonella* Typhi from hospitalized patients in Lagos, Nigeria. *Infect. Drug Resist.*, **8**: 99–106.

[45] Harriet, U. and Nandita De (2014). Mechanisms of antimicrobial resistance in *Salmonella* Typhi. *Int. J. Curr. Microbiol. Appl. Sci.*, **3**(12): 461–476.

[46] Joanne, M.W., Linda, M.S. and Christopher, J.W. (2011). Order *Enteriobacterioceae*, Prescott microbiology. Eight edn. New York: McGraw-Hill companies, Inc. pp. 536–539.

[47] Grey, D., Hamilton-miller, J.M., and Brumfilt, W. (1979). Incidence and mechanisms of resistance to trimethoprim in clinically isolated gram-negative bacteria. *Chemotherapy*, **25**: 147–156.

[48] Al-Sanouri, T.M., Paglietti, B., Haddadin, A., Murgia, M., Bacciu, D., Youssef, M. and Rubino, S. (2008). Emergence of plasmid-mediated multidrug resistance in epidemic and non-epidemic strains of *Salmonella enterica* serotype Typhi from Jordan. *J. Infect. Dev. Ctries.*, **2**: 295–301.

[49] Bauer, A.W., Kirby, W.M., Shorns, J.C. andTurch, M. (1966). Antibiotic susceptibility testing by a standard single disk method. *Am. J. Clin. Pathol.*, **45**(4): 493–496.

[50] Maria De T., Yolanda S., Emilia C., Rojo-Bezares, B., Garcia-Campello, M., Undabeitia, E. and Carmen T. (2011). Genetic characterization of the mechanisms of resistance to

amoxillin/clavulanate and third generation cephalosporium in *Salmonella enterica* from three Spanish hospitals. *Int. Microbial.*, **14**: 173–181.

[51] Anees, A., Indu, S., Fatima, K. and Anjum, P. (2015). Multi-drug resistance *Salmonella enterica* subspecies *enterica* serotype Typhi: A diagnostic and therapeutic challenge. *Int. J. Curr. Microbiol. Appl. Sci.*, Special issue-**1**: 19–25.

[52] Flamm, R.K., Phillips, K.L., Tenover, F.C. and Plorde, J.J. (1993). A survey of clinical isolates of*enterobacteriaceae* using a series of DNA probes for aminoglycoside resistance genes. *Mol. Cell Probes.*, **7**: 139–144.

[53] Gonzales, R., Steiner, J.F. and Saude, M.A. (1997). Antibiotics prescription for adults with cold upper respiration tract infections and brouchitis by ambulatory care physician. *JAMA*, **278**: 901–904.

[54] Guillemout, D., Carbon, C., Vauzethe-Kervoectran, F. et al. (1998). Inappropriateness and variability of antibiotics prescription among French office-based physicians. *J. Dis. Epidemiol.*, **51**: 61–68.

[55] Kunin, N. (1997). Antibiotic amageddon. *Clin. Infect. Dis.*, **5**: 240–241.

[56] Kim, L., Abigail, A.S., Harry, W.T. and Richard, G.W. (2002). Bacterial Resistance to antimicrobials. New York: Maree Dekker. pp. 2–490.

[57] Laubert, H.P.(1999). Don't keep taking the tablet. *Laucet*. **354**: 943–945.

[58] Apata, D.F. (2009). Antibiotic resistance in Poultry. *Int. J. Poult. Sci.*, **8**: 404–408.

[59] Ashraf, R. and Shah, N.P. (2011). Antibiotic resistance of probiotic organisms and safety of probiotic drug products. *Int. Food Res. J.*, **18**: 837–853.

[60] Akinyemi, K.O., Fashola, M.O., Habib, N. and Akinwande, E. (2013). Vended foods in Lagos, Nigeria: a potential reservoir for the spread of emerging strains of drug resistant bacteria. *Health.*, **5**(4): 675–680.

[61] David, O.M. and Oluyege, A.O. (2015). Antibiotic resistance and plasmid carriage among *Salmonella* Typhi isolated from food handlers in a Nigeria University. *Int. J. Curr. Microbiol. Appl. Sci*, **4**(3): 906–914.

[62] Akinyemi, K.O., Oyefolu, A.O., Omonigbehin E.O., Akinside, K.A. and Coker, A.O. (2000). Evaluation of blood collected from clinically diagnose typhoid fever patients in the metropolis of Lagos. *J. Niger. Infect. Contr. Assoc.*, **3**(2): 25–30.

[63] WHO (2005).World Health Organisation. Drug resistance *Salmonella*, REF 1-6. Fact sheet N^{0}139. Revised April, 2005.

[64] Zaki, K.O. and Karande, S. (2011). Multidrug resistance typhoid fever: a review. *J. Infect. Dev. Ctries.*, **5**(5): 324–337.

[65] Akinyemi, K.O., Smith, S.I., Oyefolu, A.O. and Coker A.O. (2005). Multi drug resistance in *Salmonella enterica* ser. Typhi isolated from patients with typhoid fever complications in Lagos, Nigeria. *Public Health*, **119**: 321–327.

[66] Skold, O. (2000). Sulfonamide resistance: mechanisms and trends. *Drug Resist. Updates*, **3**: 155–160.

[67] Frederic, J.A. (2011). Human health consequences of antimicrobial drug-resistant *Salmonella* and other foodborne pathogens. *Clin. Infect. Dis.*, **41**(11):1613–1620.

[68] DANMAP. (2012). Use of antimicrobial agents and occurrence of antimicrobial resistance in bacteria from food animals, food and human in Denmark. Danish integrated antimicrobial resistance monitoring and research programmes. National food inst., Technical univ. of Denmark and statens serum Institut. Available from: http//www.danmap.org

[69] FDA. (2012). National Antimicrobial Resistance Monitoring System (NARMS)— Enteric Bacteria Exercutive Report. Rockville, MD: U.S. Department of Health and Human Service, Food and Drug Admistration. 114

Chapter 7

Quinolone Resistance in Non-typhoidal *Salmonella*

Siriporn Kongsoi, Chie Nakajima and
Yasuhiko Suzuki

Additional information is available at the end of the chapter

http://dx.doi.org/10.5772/67154

Abstract

Non-typhoidal *Salmonella* is the primary foodborne zoonotic agent of salmonellosis in many countries. Non-typhoidal *Salmonella* infections are transmitted to humans primarily through consumption of contaminated foods from animal origin, whereas *S.* Typhi and Paratyphi infections are spread directly or indirectly by contact with an infected person. Quinolones exhibit potent antibacterial activity against *Salmonella* and are usually the first choice of treatment for life-threatening salmonellosis due to multidrug-resistant strains. However, by the early 1990s, quinolones have been approved for use in food-producing animals. The increased use of this group of antimicrobials in animal has led to the concomitant emergence of quinolone-resistant non-typhoidal *Salmonella* strains. However, in some countries, there are no legal provisions, which apply to veterinary drugs. This situation provides favorable conditions for spread and persistence of quinolone-resistant bacteria in food-producing animals. The objective of this chapter is to review the current regulatory controls for the use of quinolones in food-producing animals, its effect on development of quinolone resistance, and the potential impact on human and animal health. Moreover, this chapter reviews the current knowledge of quinolone resistance mechanisms and the future directions of research with particular attention to the strategies to control the emergence of quinolone-resistant *Salmonella*.

Keywords: non-typhoidal *Salmonella*, quinolones, resistance

1. Introduction

Non-typhoidal *Salmonella* refers to a group of bacteria that cause diarrheal illness in humans and domestic animals. More than 2500 different serovars of non-typhoidal *Salmonella* have been described: all serovars of *Salmonella* except for Typhi, Paratyphi A, Paratyphi B (tartrate negative), and Paratyphi C. Non-typhoidal *Salmonella* are important causes of foodborne infection because *Salmonella* have a broad host range and are strongly associated with animal and plant products. Humans are infected by consumption of food or water contaminated with *Salmonella* and direct contact transmission between infected animals and humans in a variety of ways or contaminated environment and directly between humans. The recent outbreaks show that fresh fruits and vegetables can be contaminated with non-typhoidal *Salmonella* especially sprouts, tomatoes, fruits, peanuts, and spinach [1–5]. Non-typhoidal *Salmonella* is commonly found in food products derived from the animal species such as poultry, eggs, dairy products, and contaminated pets such as cats, dogs, rodents, reptiles, or amphibians [6–9].

Non-typhoidal *Salmonella* is a leading cause of bacterial diarrhea worldwide, in contrast to typhoid fever, which remains endemic in developing countries. There are an estimated 93.8 million cases of non-typhoidal *Salmonella* gastroenteritis, resulting in approximately 155,000 deaths globally each year [10]. Gastroenteritis is the most frequent clinical symptom of non-typhoidal *Salmonella* infection. The incubation period of non-typhoidal *Salmonella* gastroenteritis is 6–72 h, usually 12–36 h after initial exposure. The classic presentation in non-typhoidal *Salmonella* gastroenteritis has self-limiting, acute gastroenteritis, watery diarrhea, abdominal pain, fever, nausea, and sometimes vomiting [11]. The gastroenteritis usually lasts 4–7 days, and most people recover with little or no treatment [12]. Non-typhoidal salmonellosis clinical presentations differ significantly by serovars such as *S.* Typhimurium and *S.* Enteritidis, have a broad host range, and can cause gastrointestinal infections with less severity than typhoidal enteric fever which affects both humans and a wide variety of animal hosts. An infection with *S.* Choleraesuis is primarily responsible for the severe systemic illness of salmonellosis in human and swine. Some serotypes such as *S.* Dublin are responsible for the systemic salmonellosis in humans and also cause death in young calves, occasionally death in mature cattle and results in decreased milk production, diarrhea, and abortion in cattle. Rates of invasive systemic salmonellosis and death are generally higher among persons with high-risk conditions, infants aged <3 months, elderly aged ≥60 years, the debilitated, immunosuppressive conditions, and malignant neoplasms.

Antimicrobial therapy can prolong the duration of excretion of non-typhoidal *Salmonella* and, therefore, is only considered for gastroenteritis patients caused by *Salmonella* species with moderate-to-severe diarrhea, high fever, or systemic infection and for gastroenteritis in people at increased risk of invasive disease (persons with high-risk conditions). Current recommendations are that fluoroquinolones (FQs) be reserved for patients with moderate-to-severe diarrhea by non-typhoidal *Salmonella* infection. Resistance among non-typhoidal *Salmonella* serovars to the first-line antibiotics such as chloramphenicol, ampicillin, trimethoprim-sulfamethoxazole, and cotrimoxazole has been present for many years, and resistance to FQs has also increased over the last decade.

The emergence of quinolone-resistant non-typhoidal *Salmonella* varies by serotype and geographic location. Therefore, the control of quinolone-resistant non-typhoidal *Salmonella* infection is difficult. There is a high need to understand the quinolone resistance mechanisms for preventing the further quinolone resistance development through the better interventional strategies that prevent spread of quinolone-resistant *Salmonella* between humans and animal reservoirs along the food chain.

http://dx.doi.org/10.5772/67154

2. Quinolone use in food-producing animals

The first quinolone was generated in the early 1960s. The first member of the quinolones is nalidixic acid (NAL), a 1,8-naphthyridine as shown in **Figure 1**, which had a good activity against Gram-negative pathogens and was used to treat urinary tract infections. However, the use of NAL was decreased due to the increasing resistance of this drug and because of the synthesis of new, broad-spectrum, and safer antimicrobials. The molecular modifications of the core quinolone structure significantly affect their antimicrobial activity, allowing the synthesis of various compounds of this drug class.

FQs (fluorinated derivatives of quinolones) were first developed since the 1980s. The presence of fluorine in position 6 of the core quinolone structure provides broad and potent antimicrobial activity against Gram-positive and Gram-negative bacteria because it significantly enhances the antibiotics' penetration into the bacterial cell membrane. Norfloxacin (NOR), launched in 1980, is a first broad-spectrum FQ which consisted of a piperazinyl ring that replaces the methyl group at position 7 (**Figure 1**) results in enhancing activity against Gram-negative bacteria [13]. Ciprofloxacin (CIP) has similar structure to NOR except the ethyl group at N-1 of CIP is replaced by a cyclopropyl group (**Figure 1**) that increasing the spectrum of action which not only active against Gram-negative bacteria but also against Gram-positive bacteria [14]. The structure of enrofloxacin (ENR) is similar to CIP but with an additional ethyl group on the piperazinyl ring (**Figure 1**).

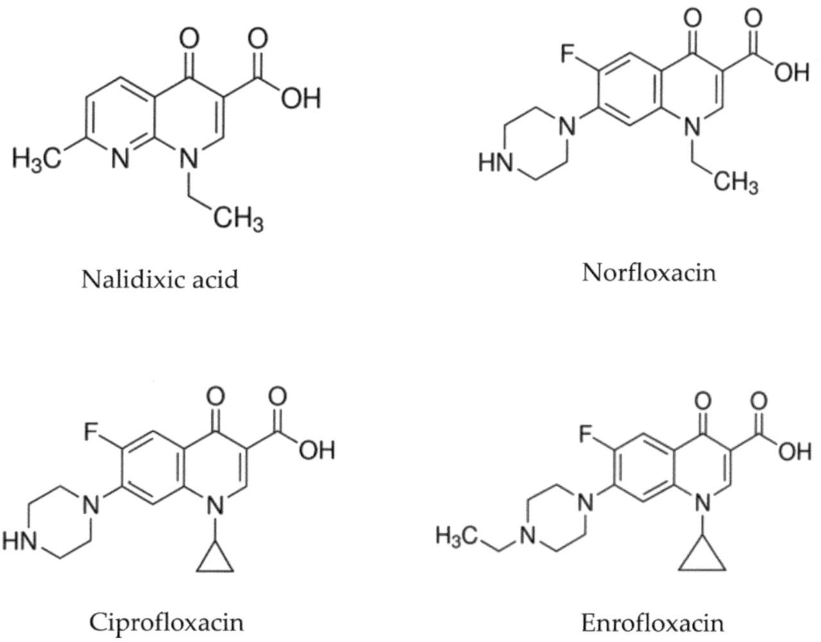

Figure 1. The structural features of four different quinolones.

All these structural modifications in the molecular molecule of quinolones improved a spectrum of drug activity, tissue penetration, long half-life in the body, lower toxicity, and greater capacity to cross bacterial cell membranes and consequently better activity against Gram-negative bacteria and Gram-positive species. Their treatment indications developed from urinary infection to applications against many other systemic diseases. The last generations of quinolones provide the activity against anaerobic bacteria.

FQs have been licensed for use in food animals at the beginning of the 1990s, and subsequently, a new FQs extensively have been authorized, and a large number of different veterinary pharmaceutical products have been launched in the market [15]. ENR exhibits good activity against most Gram-negative bacteria, including *Escherichia coli*, *Campylobacter*, *Enterobacter*, *Serratia*, *Chlamydia*, and *Mycobacterium*, and has a variable effect on *Pseudomonas*, *Enterococcus*, *Clostridium*, *Staphylococcus*, and *Streptococcus*. The efficacies of ENR treatment in food-producing animals have been reported in turkeys against *Pasteurella multocida* infections and in chickens against *E. coli* infections. Danofloxacin (DFX) and ENR are licensed for use in food-producing animals in the United States. ENR and DFX are currently approved to be good choices for therapy of bovine respiratory disease (BRD) in high-risk cattle. ENR is also currently approved for treatment of swine respiratory disease (SRD). DFX and ENR are only available as a sterile injectable solution for animal usage and should be administered under a prescription from a veterinarian. ENR is FQ antimicrobial agent frequently used in poultry production, sold by the Bayer Corporation under the trade name Baytril; however, it is also sold under the various generic names. ENR is a FQ antibiotic that is very similar to the human drug CIP. Under current legislation, if a small number of chickens present the clinical signs and symptoms, ENR can be used to treat the whole flock by adding the drug into the drinking water, even when most of the chickens are not sick. FQs can also be used to treat infections in breeding flocks, and the transmission of drug-resistant organisms may occur among chicks.

Finland and Denmark ban all the uses of FQs in poultry; however, they are used in other species of farm livestock. Australia has never approved the use of FQs in poultry and any farm animals, and consequently, resistance to FQs in zoonotic bacteria such as *Campylobacter* and *Salmonella* has a low prevalence in farm animals. The prevalence in human infected with resistant bacteria is also much lower than in many other countries. Resistant *Campylobacter* infections were low just 0% in 2003 and 2.6% in 2006; however, nearly all of these cases were returning travelers [16]. Human infections with resistant *E. coli* were also low in prevalence at 4–5% [16]. Finland does not approve the use of FQs in poultry result in no resistant *Campylobacter* from poultry productions in 2007, and the resistance in *Campylobacter* was found only 1% in 2008 and 2009. Resistant *Campylobacter* infections of Finnish patients who had not traveled abroad were found 2–3% and 61% were investigated from the patients who have traveled abroad within 2 weeks [17].

In September 2005, the U.S. Food and Drug Administration (FDA) banned the use of FQs for treating bacterial infections in U.S. poultry result from concerns about increasing in FQ resistance among *Campylobacter* isolates of poultry and humans. Although the FQs were banned in the US in 2005, the impact of the ban on resistance in human *C. jejuni* is not clear because the resistant isolates in 2013 remained at the same level as in 2005 (22%). In retail chicken,

CIP resistance in *C. coli* has decreased to 13.5% in 2010 from 29% in 2005; however, resistance in *C. jejuni* significantly increased from 15.2 to 22.5% from 2002 to 2010. It may be caused by the illegal use of FQs in the U.S. poultry industry.

3. A contribution of veterinary usage of quinolones to resistance in human non-typhoidal *Salmonella* isolates

Multidrug resistance in non-typhoidal *Salmonella* is a global problem, and these strains are linked to more severe disease outcome. Serovars Typhimurium and Newport, two of most common serotypes, are more resistant to multiple antimicrobial agents than the other serotypes [18]. Multidrug-resistant *S.* Typhimurium definitive type (DT) 104, was first detected in 1980s, emerged as a public health concern because of its global distribution in diseases among animal species such as poultry, pigs, and sheep and humans [19, 20]. The emergence and worldwide spread of multidrug-resistant *S.* Typhimurium DT104 isolates are associated with the intake of contaminated meat and meat products. Many strains of *S.* Typhimurium DT104 are generally resistant to ampicillin, chloramphenicol, streptomycin, sulphonamides, and tetracycline [21]. Moreover, new resistant strains of non-typhoidal *Salmonella* are constantly rising worldwide and resistant against ampicillin, chloramphenicol, kanamycin, streptomycin, trimethoprim, and cotrimoxazole [22–24], for example, a multidrug-resistant strains of serovars Virchow [25], Heidelberg [26], and Infantis [27, 28].

Quinolones were introduced for veterinary use in various countries, and subsequent use has been followed by the development of quinolone resistance in bacteria of food-producing animals and consequently transmits the resistant zoonotic bacteria to humans [29]. In many countries, FQs are drug of first choice for prescription in acute gastrointestinal symptoms caused by *Salmonella* infection, and resistance to this drug group has often been described, particularly to NAL [15]. In a study performed between 1996 and 2003, *Salmonella* isolates were investigated for quinolone susceptibility; the results revealed that NAL and CIP resistances were 1.6 and 7%, respectively. A significant upward trend in resistance was observed for NAL from 0.4% in 1996 to 2.3% in 2003 [30]. In Germany, an increase in the frequency of NAL-resistant *Salmonella* strains was discovered after the approval and use of ENR [31]. Concurrent increase in resistance was observed in France among *Salmonella* isolates from animals and humans, and the same clones were determined among the different hosts [32]. In the United Kingdom, also in Spain, the incidence of NAL-resistant *Salmonella* illnesses in humans was increased followed the introduction for veterinary use of FQs in 1993 [33, 34]. A study from Denmark and Taiwan described the emergence of salmonellosis caused by multidrug and quinolone-resistant *S.* Typhimurium DT104 linked to a swine herd and the subsequent spread of those isolates to humans [35–37]. In European countries, similar associations between FQ resistance development in *Salmonella* infecting humans and retail poultry products have been described. Therefore, the FQ-resistant *Salmonella* in poultry has reached alarming proportions in some countries [38]. In the United States, there was an increase in the proportion of FQ resistance development in *Salmonella* infections following the first approved use of FQs in food-producing animals in 1995 [39].

The data indicate that it would be reasonable to assume that the veterinary usage of FQs will have made a remarkable contribution to FQ resistance in human *Salmonella* infections.

4. The potential impact on human health

FQ resistance in *Salmonella* is clearly associated with FQ use in food-producing animals, and foodborne infections caused by such resistant bacteria are well investigated in human. FQ resistance in *S.* Typhimurium DT104 has been associated with increased hospitalization, more frequent and longer illness, treatment failures, and a higher risk of death [40]. Many studies also investigated that infections with multidrug-resistant *Salmonella* were associated with longer hospitalization and a higher death rate than infections with susceptible isolates [41–43]. Previous study has found a 3.15 times increased mortality when patients infected with NAL-resistant *S.* Typhimurium compared to patients infected with susceptible isolates [44]. For treatment of the infections with FQ-resistant *Salmonella,* alternative antimicrobials are the third or fourth generation cephalosporin. Nevertheless, it should be considered contraindications for treatment of uncomplicated non-typhoidal *Salmonella* infection because FQ treatment can induce prolonged excretion of *Salmonella* and increased frequency of relapses [45]. However, for patients at risk such as immunocompromised, severely infected and elderly, FQs are considered first choice drugs and effective in reducing the disease length if the treatment starts early in the infection.

5. The potential impact on animal health

FQs are highly potent antimicrobial agents rapidly absorbed after oral administration and have a long half-life and widespread distribution to most body tissues, which made them suitable for using in herd treatment of food-producing animals. FQs are effective for serious infections in food-producing animals such as systematic gastroenteritis and severe respiratory diseases and are also used to treat urinary tract, skin, and soft-tissue infections caused by Gram-negative or some Gram-positive aerobic bacteria. Moreover, they also have potential for treatment of infections caused by *Mycoplasma, Mycobacterium, Chlamydia, Ehrlichia,* and *Rickettsia.* However, documentation about authorized dosages and the effectiveness of FQs to treat all these infections in animals have not been determined on the base of the pharmacokinetic and pharmacodynamics properties. Sufficient knowledge about the selecting optimal dose and duration of FQs could help to develop appropriate dosing regimens to maximize the clinical efficacy, avoid therapeutic failure, and decrease the selection of resistance which would ensure for the benefit of animals and their future use.

However, the potential clinical disadvantage associated with FQ use was a rapid selection for resistance. Several pathogenic bacteria of food-producing animals have been investigated the increasing of resistance to FQs following the introduction of ENR [46]. If FQ resistance emerges in animal pathogenic bacteria, this may result in treatment failure and increased mortality. This is a risk for poor animal welfare conditions and will result in economical losses. Consequently, for some animal infectious diseases, antimicrobial therapeutic use will be complicated if FQs lose their efficacy. As described in a previous study, multidrug-resistant *S.* Typhimurium infections in veal calves were resistant to most conventionally used antimicrobials and also resistant to ENR resulted in a mortality exceeding 90%. FQs are also considered effective in other infections such as pneumonia, neonatal diarrhea, and mastitis caused by Gram-negative organisms in piglets and calves. However, there were insufficient data to support the animal health or welfare problems when diseases cannot be treated result from FQ resistance during treatment.

6. The current state of knowledge of quinolone resistance mechanisms

FQs are strong inhibitors of bacterial enzymes, which are necessary enzymes associated in major biological processes including DNA replication [47–49]. In prokaryotes, DNA is known as a double helix because there are two strands that intertwine around each other. However, additional complexity comes from the further twisting (supercoiling) of the double-strand structure to put the double helix under torsion stress [50]. This supercoiling process that enables the long strands of DNA is condensed into compact supercoils permitting large amounts of DNA to be packed into the cell [51].

Topoisomerase I and topoisomerase II enzymes are enzymes that regulate the overwinding or underwinding of DNA and control the level of twisting within DNA. Topoisomerase I removes the number of negative supercoils, in contrast to topoisomerase II, which introduces negative supercoils that facilitate the unwinding of the over-twisted DNA and can further change the DNA topology into an under-twisted DNA [50]. DNA gyrase and DNA topoisomerase IV are type II topoisomerase comprising 2 A subunits and 2 B subunits encoded by the *gyrA* and *gyrB* genes or 2 C subunits and 2 E subunits encoded by the *parC* and *parE* genes, respectively [52]. DNA gyrase and topoisomerase IV have distinct roles although both enzymes have homologous action to relax positively supercoiled DNA. DNA gyrase decatenates replicating DNA by introducing negative supercoils into relaxed DNA while topoisomerase IV unlinks the newly replicated daughter chromosomes during cell division [52–54].

FQs are direct inhibitors of bacterial DNA synthesis by inhibiting two enzymes, DNA gyrase and topoisomerase IV, which have important roles in DNA replication. The quinolones bind to these enzymes with DNA to form drug-enzyme-DNA complexes (known as a ternary complex) subsequently induces double-strand DNA breaks and blocks replication, therefore, results in damage to bacterial DNA and bacterial cell death [55–58]. However, the primary target enzyme, either DNA gyrase or topoisomerase IV, of FQs varies depending on the bacterial species. The preferential target of FQs in Gram-negative bacteria is DNA gyrase, whereas in Gram-positive microorganisms, topoisomerase IV is the primary target [58].

Resistance to quinolones occurs by different ways. The major mechanisms of bacterial resistance to FQs are altered target enzymes, expression of an active efflux, and altered membrane permeability.

6.1. Target-site mutation

The main mechanism of FQ resistance is due to mutation in target genes (*gyrA*, *gyrB*, *parC*, and *parE*) that encode the primary and secondary target enzymes of these drugs. The mutations in quinolone resistance-determining region (QRDR) of target genes alter the target enzyme conformation by amino acid substitutions and subsequently decrease in the drug binding affinity of the target enzyme, leading to FQ resistance [59–62].

In *Salmonella*, quinolone resistance was firstly investigated in the *gyrA* gene coding for the A subunit of gyrase. Mutations associated with FQ resistance in GyrA have been clustered between amino acids 67 and 106, termed the QRDR region. Amino acid substitutions of GyrA at Ser83 (to Phe, Tyr, or Ala) or at Asp87 (to Gly, Asn, or Tyr) are most usually identified in NAL-resistant *Salmonella* strains. Previous studies have observed that single point mutation in QRDR of *gyrA* led to reduced sensitivity to CIP in *Salmonella* isolates [63]. Similar decreasing in CIP susceptibility was also found in three amino acid mutations of *parC* at Ser67 (to Cys), Arg76 (to Cys), and Cys80 (to Arg) in *S.* Enteritidis [64, 65]. Nevertheless, less frequently, the previous study detected novel mutations inside QRDR of GyrA at codon Asp72, Asp82, and Ala119 and also outside the QRDR [66]. Moreover, in another studies, the authors found double mutations in GyrA at both Ser83 and Asp87 in *S.* Typhimurium DT204 [67] and a single mutation at Asp87 (to Tyr) in all *Salmonella* strains [68] showing high-level resistance to FQs. A *gyrB* gene mutation has also been observed in a quinolone-resistant *S.* Typhimurium at Ser463 (to Tyr) [69].

These target-site mutations show that different mutations of FQ-resistant *Salmonella* isolates can result in very different resistance levels of quinolones, and this is not the same for all strains and all resistance mutations. Therefore, amino acid substitutions in topoisomerases are inadequate to clarify the level of resistance to quinolones in *S. enterica*. Nevertheless, it remains to be investigated what the specific role of these mutations on quinolone resistance in *Salmonella*.

6.2. Transmissible quinolone-resistance mechanisms

Plasmid-mediated quinolone resistance (PMQR) genes on mobile genetic elements are able to reduce susceptibility of quinolone or FQ antimicrobials. The PMQR gene, *qnr*, encodes a pentapeptide repeat motif protein (Qnr) that protects the target enzyme DNA gyrase and topoisomerase IV by blocking the quinolone inhibition [70]. Recently, several Qnr proteins were investigated in Enterobacteriaceae (QnrA, QnrB, QnrC, QnrD, QnrS) [71, 72]. A recent study reported six variants of *qnrB* genes in *Salmonella* and *E. coli* isolates of human and animal isolates [73]. Nonetheless, the prevalence of *qnrS* genes is higher than the other *qnr* genes in *Salmonella*. A study from different European countries investigated a *qnrS* gene in 10% of the *Salmonella* isolates [73]. Moreover, *qnrS* gene has been identified in non-typhoidal *Salmonella* clinical isolate from the USA [74]. The *qnrD* gene also has been investigated in eight different *Salmonella* serovars from 13 European countries [73].

Another plasmid-encoded quinolone resistance determinant is a variant of an aminoglycoside acetyl transferase gene, *aac(6')-Ib-cr*, which is able to acetylate the amino nitrogen on the piperazinyl substituent in aminoglycoside, and FQ drug classes lead to decreased susceptibility of these drugs [75–77]. However, the variant enzyme is not able to acetylate moxifloxacin and levofloxacin due to the absence of a piperazinyl substituent at position C-7. Recently, this *aac(6')-Ib-cr* gene has been reported in *Salmonella* isolated from chickens in China [78]. Plasmid-mediated quinolone resistance determinants in *Salmonella* isolated from food-producing animals are serious public health concern. Continuous surveillance of quinolone resistance determinants at national and international levels needs for limiting the dissemination of quinolone-resistant *Salmonella* strains.

6.3. Membrane permeability

The membrane permeability and the ability of FQs to enter the bacterial cells are an important determinant of the potency of these drugs that have intracellular targets [79]. The outer-membrane proteins (OMPs) of Gram-negative bacteria consist of pore-forming outer-membrane proteins which serve as a particular barrier for the entry of hydrophilic molecules into the cell. It has been shown that CIP (hydrophilic quinolones) preferentially entry into the cells via porin pathway [80]. Down-regulation of OMPs results in reduced FQ susceptibility in FQ-resistant isolates of different species [81–84]. Very few researches have investigated on alterations of OMP expression or the role of lipopolysaccharide composition in quinolone-resistant *Salmonella* isolates [68, 85–89]. The lengthening of the O chains has been studied in quinolone-resistant *Salmonella* that could also lead to a lower level in the permeability of the outer membrane [85]. The previous studies have found the lack of OmpF porin expression result from SoxS up-regulates micF transcription in quinolone-resistant *Salmonella* strains [86–88, 90]. However, it remains unclear whether such alterations contributed to significant reduction of outer-membrane permeability and reduced susceptibility of quinolones in *Salmonella* isolates.

6.4. Efflux

Chromosomal multidrug efflux pumps are capable of actively removing FQs and a broad range of antimicrobial agents from the bacterial cell and are mostly encoded by chromosomal genes. These efflux systems consist of different classes of transporters such as the resistance nodulation division (RND) family of tripartite transporters of Gram-negative pathogens [91, 92]. These systems are mainly responsible for the intrinsic pattern of reduced susceptibility to FQs and other antimicrobial agents but are also responsible for increased resistance resulting from derepression of the transporter. Previous studies showed the evidence for the participation of active efflux in quinolone-resistant *Salmonella* isolates [85, 93]. It was concluded that the overproduction of the AcrAB-TolC efflux pump appeared prior to *gyrA* mutations in *in vitro* selected quinolone-resistant *Salmonella* mutants [85]; therefore, the AcrAB-TolC efflux system is the major mechanism that involved in quinolone resistance in *S.* Typhimurium DT104 strains. However, both target gene mutations and active efflux mediated by AcrAB-TolC are necessary to obtain high-level FQ resistance for *S.* Typhimurium DT204 strains [94]. Nevertheless, there is no direct evidence to demonstrate the role of the AcrAB-TolC efflux system in quinolone-resistant *Salmonella*; therefore, substantial work remains to be done in order to understand the role of efflux and its regulation in *Salmonella*.

6.5. The fitness costs

Mechanisms associated with high-level FQ resistance are multiple mutations in the type II topoisomerase-encoding genes and the over-expression of multidrug resistance efflux pumps. The presence of mutations in these structural or regulatory genes not only increases resistance to quinolones but also affects fitness costs such as reduced growth rates and virulence of the bacterial cell in a lack of antibiotic selective pressure [95–99]. However, maintenance of resistance can arise through the development of second-site compensatory mutations that restore fitness and virulence without loss of resistance [100].

The fitness cost of the genes responsible for quinolone resistance traits has not been fully elucidated in high-level FQ-resistant *Salmonella*. Nevertheless, results from previous studies suggest that high-level CIP resistance mechanisms in *Salmonella* lead to restrictive conditions of fitness costs and minimizing the emergence and spread of highly resistant clones in the absence of drug selection pressure [101, 102]. As demonstrated in previous study [103], high-level CIP-resistant S. Enteritidis *in vitro* derived mutants in the absence of antibiotic selective pressure result in compensatory evolution favoring a reversion back to a more sensitive phenotype associated with lesser fitness costs, rather than the compensatory mutations that would restore resistance. However, under *in vivo* conditions, a previous study has found that chromosomal mutations of S. Typhimurium that confer resistance to NAL, streptomycin, or rifampicin decrease growth rate and ability to colonize in mice rather than a reversion to the susceptible phenotype and restore virulence [104]. In contrast to the high-level FQ resistance, an intermediate level of resistance to CIP of S. Typhimurium mutants apparently favored a partial reversion to a susceptible level and a normal growth rate with successfully colonized the gut of chickens, rather than the acquisition of resistance to FQs [101].

Quinolone resistance of non-typhoidal *Salmonella* is complicated. The understanding of the various mechanisms of quinolone resistance, the fitness costs of each *Salmonella* strain, and the interplay between different quinolone resistance mechanisms has increased in recent years. Increased resistance to quinolones could be selected under a wide range of selective conditions even in the absence of quinolone selective pressure. Therefore, minimizing the emergence and spread of quinolone resistance will not be as simple as limiting the use of these drugs.

7. To decrease the emergence and spread of quinolone resistance

FQs are intensively used in animal production and have allowed better treatment of several animal infectious diseases. The risks of the overuse and misuse of FQs in food-animal production can contribute to higher levels of resistance in human *Salmonella* infections. Therefore, the FQ resistance of *Salmonella* should be taken into account and prevented as resistant bacteria or resistance genes may be transferred to humans through the food chain. Given the importance of FQ resistance as a global health concern, many researchers have reviewed the existing scientific literatures and developed guidelines to limit all compounds of FQ use, including use in food-producing animals. FQs should be banned for all preventive use and mass medication, but only used as life-saving therapeutic treatment of individual sick animals.

Priority setting of agendas for research on minimizing the emergence of FQ resistance in *Salmonella* is needed to identify missing scientific data and to specify research designs and methods to address these resistance problems in food-producing animals and human medicine. The priorities identified by the research agenda must include contributions by different experts in basic genetics and microbiology sciences, veterinary medicine, human medicine, public health organization, social sciences, economics sciences, and public policy.

Furthermore, sufficient research funding for minimizing the FQ resistance of *Salmonella* in human and food-producing animals has likely contributed to the adequate scientific evidence which necessary for informing public health decisions. Given the scale of the FQ resistance problem and the demonstrated role of FQ uses in food-producing animals in this public health crisis, adequate support for research specific to the role of food-producing animal uses of FQs in the development of resistance must be a national priority.

Urgently address complex barriers that limit the quality of data on the use of FQs in food-producing animals and human medicine. Currently, such data from human and veterinary medicine are provided on a voluntary basis, and the methods used to collect, analyze, and report are not standardized because of political, economic, and social barriers. Effective surveillance of FQ use in food-producing animals and humans is a key first step toward for estimating the full scope of FQ resistance in *Salmonella*. Despite increasingly widespread recognition that FQ use in food-producing animals is a major factor of human infections with FQ-resistant *Salmonella*, there remains a significant need for scientific evidence of the FQ use practices that affect the human health risk.

8. Conclusion

Infections in humans with quinolone-resistant *Salmonella* resulted in increased risk of hospitalization and mortality. FQs are efficient and valuable antimicrobials in some serious animal indications because FQs are the only alternative available. Therefore, if FQs lose their ability for the treatment of animal diseases, the therapeutic effect of some diseases will be complicated and may result in poor animal welfare and economical losses. Recently, it is now critical that food-producing animal use of FQs be recognized as one of the major contributors to the development of resistant *Salmonella* strains that result in life-threatening human infections and included as part of the strategy to control the public health crisis of FQ resistance.

Author details

Siriporn Kongsoi[1], Chie Nakajima[2,3] and Yasuhiko Suzuki[2,3]*

*Address all correspondence to: suzuki@czc.hokudai.ac.jp

1 Faculty of Veterinary Medicine, Kasetsart University, Nakorn Pathom, Thailand

2 Research Center for Zoonosis Control, Hokkaido University, Sapporo, Japan

3 The Global Station for Zoonosis Control, Hokkaido University, Sapporo, Japan

References

[1] Berger CN, Shaw RK, Brown DJ, Mather H, Clare S, Dougan G, et al. Interaction of *Salmonella enterica* with basil and other salad leaves. ISME J [Internet]. 2009 Feb 2 [cited 2016 Aug 7];3(2):261–5. doi:10.1038/ismej.2008.95

[2] Barton Behravesh C, Mody RK, Jungk J, Gaul L, Redd JT, Chen S, et al. 2008 outbreak of Salmonella Saintpaul infections associated with raw produce. N Engl J Med [Internet]. 2011 Mar 10 [cited 2016 Aug 7];364(10):918–27. Available from: http://www.ncbi.nlm.nih.gov/pubmed/21345092

[3] Cavallaro E, Date K, Medus C, Meyer S, Miller B, Kim C, et al. Salmonella typhimurium infections associated with peanut products. N Engl J Med [Internet]. 2011 Aug 18 [cited 2016 Aug 7];365(7):601–10. Available from: http://www.ncbi.nlm.nih.gov/pubmed/21848461

[4] Jackson BR, Griffin PM, Cole D, Walsh KA, Chai SJ. Outbreak-associated *Salmonella enterica* serotypes and food Commodities, United States, 1998–2008. Emerg Infect Dis [Internet]. 2013 Aug [cited 2016 Aug 7];19(8):1239–44. Available from: http://www.ncbi.nlm.nih.gov/pubmed/23876503

[5] Bayer C, Bernard H, Prager R, Rabsch W, Hiller P, Malorny B, et al. Surveillance and outbreak reports Rosner BM. An outbreak of Salmonella Newport associated with mung bean sprouts in Germany and the. Euro Surveill [Internet]. [cited 2016 Aug 7];19(1). Available from: www.eurosurveillance.org:pii=20665.

[6] Acheson D, Hohmann EL. Nontyphoidal Salmonellosis. Clin Infect Dis [Internet]. 2001 Jan 15 [cited 2016 Aug 7];32(2):263–9. doi:10.1086/318457

[7] Mermin J, Hutwagner L, Vugia D, Shallow S, Daily P, Bender J, et al. Reptiles, amphibians, and human Salmonella infection: a population-based, case-control study. Clin Infect Dis [Internet]. 2004 Apr 15 [cited 2016 Aug 7];38 Suppl 3:S253–61. Available from: http://www.ncbi.nlm.nih.gov/pubmed/15095197

[8] Braden CR. Salmonella enterica serotype Enteritidis and eggs: a national epidemic in the United States. Clin Infect Dis [Internet]. 2006 Aug 15 [cited 2016 Aug 7];43(4):512–7. Available from: http://www.ncbi.nlm.nih.gov/pubmed/16838242

[9] Haeusler GM, Curtis N. Non-typhoidal Salmonella in children: microbiology, epidemiology and treatment. Adv Exp Med Biol [Internet]. 2013 [cited 2016 Aug 7];764:13–26. Available from: http://www.ncbi.nlm.nih.gov/pubmed/23654054

[10] Majowicz SE, Musto J, Scallan E, Angulo FJ, Kirk M, O'Brien SJ, et al. The global burden of nontyphoidal *Salmonella gastroenteritis*. Clin Infect Dis [Internet]. 2010 Mar 15 [cited 2016 Aug 7];50(6):882–9. Available from: http://www.ncbi.nlm.nih.gov/pubmed/20158401

[11] McGovern VJ, Slavutin LJ. Pathology of *Salmonella colitis*. Am J Surg Pathol [Internet]. 1979 Dec [cited 2016 Aug 7];3(6):483–90. Available from: http://www.ncbi.nlm.nih.gov/pubmed/534385

[12] Glynn JR, Palmer SR. Incubation period, severity of disease, and infecting dose: evidence from a Salmonella outbreak. Am J Epidemiol [Internet]. 1992 Dec 1 [cited 2016 Aug 7];136(11):1369–77. Available from: http://www.ncbi.nlm.nih.gov/pubmed/1488963

[13] Andriole VT. The quinolones: past, present, and future. Clin Infect Dis [Internet]. 2005 Jul 15 [cited 2016 Aug 7];41 Suppl 2(Supplement 2):S113–9. Available from: http://www.ncbi.nlm.nih.gov/pubmed/15942877

[14] Sharma PC, Jain A, Jain S. Fluoroquinolone antibacterials: a review on chemistry, microbiology and therapeutic prospects. Acta Pol Pharm [Internet]. [cited 2016 Aug 7];-66(6):587–604. Available from: http://www.ncbi.nlm.nih.gov/pubmed/20050522

[15] Antibiotic Resistance in the European Union Associated with Therapeutic Use of Veterinary Medicines Report and Qualitative Risk Assessment by the Committee for Veterinary Medicinal Products. 1999 [cited 2016 Aug 7]; Available from: http://www.eudra.org/emea.html

[16] Cheng AC, Turnidge J, Collignon P, Looke D, Barton M, Gottlieb T. Control of Fluoroquinolone Resistance through Successful Regulation, Australia. 2012 [cited 2016 Aug 7]; Available from: doi:10.3201/eid1809.111515

[17] Rautelin H, Vierikko A, Hänninen M-L, Vaara M. Antimicrobial susceptibilities of Campylobacter strains isolated from Finnish subjects infected domestically or from those infected abroad. Antimicrob Agents Chemother [Internet]. 2003 Jan [cited 2016 Aug 7];47(1):102–5. Available from: http://www.ncbi.nlm.nih.gov/pubmed/12499176

[18] Krueger AL, Greene SA, Barzilay EJ, Henao O, Vugia D, Hanna S, et al. Clinical outcomes of nalidixic acid, ceftriaxone, and multidrug-resistant nontyphoidal Salmonella infections compared with pansusceptible infections in FoodNet sites, 2006–2008. Foodborne Pathog Dis [Internet]. 2014 May [cited 2016 Aug 7];11(5):335–41. Available from: http://www.ncbi.nlm.nih.gov/pubmed/24617446

[19] Helms M, Ethelberg S, Mølbak K, Lightfoot D, Powling J, Berghold C, et al. International Salmonella typhimurium DT104 infections, 1992–2001. Emerg Infect Dis. 2005;11:859–67.

[20] Threlfall EJ. Epidemic Salmonella typhimurium DT 104—a truly international multiresistant clone. J Antimicrob Chemother [Internet]. 2000 Jul [cited 2016 Aug 7];46(1):7–10. Available from: http://www.ncbi.nlm.nih.gov/pubmed/10882682

[21] Mather AE, Reid SWJ, Maskell DJ, Parkhill J, Fookes MC, Harris SR, et al. Distinguishable epidemics of multidrug-resistant Salmonella Typhimurium DT104 in different hosts. Science [Internet]. 2013 Sep 27 [cited 2016 Aug 7];341(6153):1514–7. Available from: http://www.ncbi.nlm.nih.gov/pubmed/24030491

[22] Gordon MA. Salmonella infections in immunocompromised adults. J Infect. 2008; 56(6):413–22.

[23] Kingsley RA, Msefula CL, Thomson NR, Kariuki S, Holt KE, Gordon MA, et al. Epidemic multiple drug resistant Salmonella Typhimurium causing invasive disease in

sub-Saharan Africa have a distinct genotype. Genome Res [Internet]. 2009 Dec [cited 2016 Aug 7];19(12):2279–87. Available from: http://www.ncbi.nlm.nih.gov/pubmed/19901036

[24] Msefula CL, Kingsley RA, Gordon MA, Molyneux E, Molyneux ME, MacLennan CA, et al. Genotypic homogeneity of multidrug resistant S. Typhimurium infecting distinct adult and childhood susceptibility groups in Blantyre, Malawi. PLoS One [Internet]. 2012 [cited 2016 Aug 7];7(7):e42085. Available from: http://www.ncbi.nlm.nih.gov/pubmed/22848711

[25] Weill F-X, Lailler R, Praud K, Kérouanton A, Fabre L, Brisabois A, et al. Emergence of extended-spectrum-beta-lactamase (CTX-M-9)-producing multiresistant strains of *Salmonella enterica* serotype Virchow in poultry and humans in France. J Clin Microbiol [Internet]. 2004 Dec [cited 2016 Aug 7];42(12):5767–73. Available from: http://www.ncbi.nlm.nih.gov/pubmed/15583311

[26] Dutil L, Irwin R, Finley R, Ng LK, Avery B, Boerlin P, et al. Ceftiofur resistance in *Salmonella enterica* serovar Heidelberg from chicken meat and humans, Canada. Emerg Infect Dis [Internet]. 2010 Jan [cited 2016 Aug 7];16(1):48–54. Available from: http://www.ncbi.nlm.nih.gov/pubmed/20031042

[27] Gal-Mor O, Valinsky L, Weinberger M, Guy S, Jaffe J, Schorr YI, et al. Multidrug-resistant *Salmonella enterica* serovar Infantis, Israel. Emerg Infect Dis [Internet]. 2010 Nov [cited 2016 Aug 7];16(11):1754–7. Available from: http://www.ncbi.nlm.nih.gov/pubmed/21029536

[28] Aviv G, Tsyba K, Steck N, Salmon-Divon M, Cornelius A, Rahav G, et al. A unique megaplasmid contributes to stress tolerance and pathogenicity of an emergent *Salmonella enterica* serovar Infantis strain. Environ Microbiol [Internet]. 2014 Apr [cited 2016 Aug 7];16(4):977–94. Available from: http://www.ncbi.nlm.nih.gov/pubmed/24320043

[29] Engberg J, Aarestrup FM, Taylor DE, Gerner-Smidt P, Nachamkin I. Quinolone and macrolide resistance in *Campylobacter jejuni* and *C. coli*: resistance mechanisms and trends in human isolates. Emerg Infect Dis [Internet]. 2001 [cited 2016 Aug 7];7(1):24–34. Available from: http://www.ncbi.nlm.nih.gov/pubmed/11266291

[30] Stevenson JE, Gay K, Barrett TJ, Medalla F, Chiller TM, Angulo FJ. Increase in nalidixic acid resistance among non-Typhi *Salmonella enterica* isolates in the United States from 1996 to 2003. Antimicrob Agents Chemother [Internet]. 2007 Jan [cited 2016 Aug 7];51(1):195–7. Available from: http://www.ncbi.nlm.nih.gov/pubmed/17088493

[31] Malorny B, Schroeter A, Helmuth R. Incidence of quinolone resistance over the period 1986 to 1998 in veterinary Salmonella isolates from Germany. Antimicrob Agents Chemother [Internet]. 1999 Sep [cited 2016 Aug 7];43(9):2278–82. Available from: http://www.ncbi.nlm.nih.gov/pubmed/10471579

[32] Heurtin-Le Corre C, Donnio PY, Perrin M, Travert MF, Avril JL. Increasing incidence and comparison of nalidixic acid-resistant *Salmonella enterica* subsp. enterica serotype typhimurium isolates from humans and animals. J Clin Microbiol [Internet].

1999 Jan [cited 2016 Aug 7];37(1):266–9. Available from: http://www.ncbi.nlm.nih.gov/pubmed/9854111

[33] Marimón JM, Gomáriz M, Zigorraga C, Cilla G, Pérez-Trallero E. Increasing prevalence of quinolone resistance in human nontyphoid *Salmonella enterica* isolates obtained in Spain from 1981 to 2003. Antimicrob Agents Chemother [Internet]. 2004 Oct [cited 2016 Aug 7];48(10):3789–93. Available from: http://www.ncbi.nlm.nih.gov/pubmed/15388435

[34] Threlfall EJ, Ward LR, Skinner JA, Rowe B. Increase in multiple antibiotic resistance in nontyphoidal salmonellas from humans in England and Wales: a comparison of data for 1994 and 1996. Microb Drug Resist [Internet]. 1997 [cited 2016 Aug 7];3(3):263–6. Available from: http://www.ncbi.nlm.nih.gov/pubmed/9270996

[35] Su LH, Chiu CH, Kuo AJ, Chia JH, Sun CF, Leu HS, et al. Secular trends in incidence and antimicrobial resistance among clinical isolates of Salmonella at a university hospital in Taiwan, 1983–1999. Epidemiol Infect [Internet]. 2001 Oct [cited 2016 Aug 7];127(2):207–13. Available from: http://www.ncbi.nlm.nih.gov/pubmed/11693497

[36] Chiu C-H, Wu T-L, Su L-H, Chu C, Chia J-H, Kuo A-J, et al. The emergence in Taiwan of fluoroquinolone resistance in *Salmonella enterica* serotype choleraesuis. N Engl J Med [Internet]. 2002 Feb 7 [cited 2016 Aug 7];346(6):413–9. Available from: http://www.ncbi.nlm.nih.gov/pubmed/11832529

[37] Hsueh P-R, Teng L-J, Tseng S-P, Chang C-F, Wan J-H, Yan J-J, et al. Ciprofloxacin-resistant *Salmonella enterica* Typhimurium and Choleraesuis from pigs to humans, Taiwan. Emerg Infect Dis [Internet]. 2004 Jan [cited 2016 Aug 7];10(1):60–8. Available from: http://www.ncbi.nlm.nih.gov/pubmed/15078598

[38] European Union summary report on antimicrobial resistance in zoonotic and indicator bacteria from animals and food in the European Union in 2009. EFSA J [Internet]. 2011 Jul [cited 2016 Aug 7];9(7):2154. doi:10.2903/j.efsa.2011.2154

[39] Geneva. Food and Agriculture Organization of the United Nations World Health Organization World Organization for Animal Health Joint FAO/OIE/WHO Expert Workshop on Non-Human Antimicrobial Usage and Antimicrobial Resistance: Scientific assessment. 2003.

[40] Andorra A. The WHO Regional Office for Europe Tackling antibiotic resistance from a food safety perspective in Europe.

[41] Lee LA, Puhr ND, Maloney EK, Bean NH, Tauxe R V. Increase in antimicrobial-resistant Salmonella infections in the United States, 1989–1990. J Infect Dis [Internet]. 1994 Jul [cited 2016 Aug 7];170(1):128–34. Available from: http://www.ncbi.nlm.nih.gov/pubmed/8014487

[42] Holmberg SD, Solomon SL, Blake PA. Health and economic impacts of antimicrobial resistance. Rev Infect Dis [Internet]. [cited 2016 Aug 7];9(6):1065–78. Available from: http://www.ncbi.nlm.nih.gov/pubmed/3321356

[43] Martin LJ, Fyfe M, Doré K, Buxton JA, Pollari F, Henry B, et al. Increased burden of illness associated with antimicrobial-resistant *Salmonella enterica* serotype typhimurium infections. J Infect Dis [Internet]. 2004 Feb 1 [cited 2016 Aug 7];189(3):377–84. Available from: http://www.ncbi.nlm.nih.gov/pubmed/14745694

[44] Helms M, Simonsen J, Molbak K. Quinolone resistance is associated with increased risk of invasive illness or death during infection with Salmonella serotype Typhimurium. J Infect Dis [Internet]. 2004 Nov 1 [cited 2016 Aug 7];190(9):1652–4. Available from: http://www.ncbi.nlm.nih.gov/pubmed/15478071

[45] Sirinavin S, Garner P. Antibiotics for treating salmonella gut infections. Cochrane database Syst Rev [Internet]. 2000 [cited 2016 Aug 7];(2):CD001167. Available from: http://www.ncbi.nlm.nih.gov/pubmed/10796610

[46] Aarestrup FM, Jensen NE, Jorsal SE, Nielsen TK. Emergence of resistance to fluoroquinolones among bacteria causing infections in food animals in Denmark. Vet Rec [Internet]. 2000 Jan 15 [cited 2016 Aug 7];146(3):76–8. Available from: http://www.ncbi.nlm.nih.gov/pubmed/10674696

[47] Hooper DC. Mechanisms of action of antimicrobials: focus on fluoroquinolones. Clin Infect Dis [Internet]. 2001 Mar 15 [cited 2016 Aug 7];32(Supplement 1):S9–15. doi:10.1086/319370

[48] Drlica K. Bacterial topoisomerases and the control of DNA supercoiling. Trends Genet [Internet]. 1990 Dec [cited 2016 Aug 7];6(12):433–7. Available from: http://www.ncbi.nlm.nih.gov/pubmed/1965069

[49] Pruss GJ, Franco RJ, Chevalier SG, Manes SH, Drlica K. Effects of DNA gyrase inhibitors in *Escherichia coli* topoisomerase I mutants. J Bacteriol [Internet]. 1986 Oct [cited 2016 Aug 7];168(1):276–82. Available from: http://www.ncbi.nlm.nih.gov/pubmed/3019999

[50] Baranello L, Levens D, Gupta A, Kouzine F. The importance of being supercoiled: How DNA mechanics regulate dynamic processes. Biochim Biophys Acta Gene Regul Mech. 2012;1819(7):632–8.

[51] Webber MA, Ricci V, Whitehead R, Patel M, Fookes M, Ivens A, et al. Clinically relevant mutant DNA gyrase alters supercoiling, changes the transcriptome, and confers multidrug resistance. MBio [Internet]. 2013 Jul 23 [cited 2016 Aug 7];4(4):e00273–13. doi:10.1128/mBio.00273-13

[52] Corbett KD, Schoeffler AJ, Thomsen ND, Berger JM. The Structural basis for substrate specificity in DNA topoisomerase IV. J Mol Biol. 2005;351(3):545–61.

[53] Arnoldi E, Pan X-S, Fisher LM. Functional determinants of gate-DNA selection and cleavage by bacterial type II topoisomerases. Nucleic Acids Res [Internet]. 2013 Nov [cited 2016 Aug 7];41(20):9411–23. Available from: http://www.ncbi.nlm.nih.gov/pubmed/23939623

[54] Drlica K. Mechanism of fluoroquinolone action. Curr Opin Microbiol. 1999;2(5):504–8.

[55] Drlica K, Malik M, Kerns RJ, Zhao X. Quinolone-mediated bacterial death. Antimicrob Agents Chemother [Internet]. 2008 Feb 1 [cited 2016 Aug 7];52(2):385–92. doi:10.1128/AAC.01617-06

[56] Drlica K, Zhao X. DNA gyrase, topoisomerase IV, and the 4-quinolones. Microbiol Mol Biol Rev [Internet]. 1997 Sep [cited 2016 Aug 7];61(3):377–92. Available from: http://www.ncbi.nlm.nih.gov/pubmed/9293187

[57] Zhao X, Xu C, Domagala J, Drlica K. DNA topoisomerase targets of the fluoroquinolones: a strategy for avoiding bacterial resistance. Proc Natl Acad Sci USA [Internet]. 1997 Dec 9 [cited 2016 Aug 7];94(25):13991–6. Available from: http://www.ncbi.nlm.nih.gov/pubmed/9391140

[58] Hooper DC. Mechanisms of fluoroquinolone resistance. Drug Resist Updat [Internet]. 1999 Feb [cited 2016 Aug 7];2(1):38–55. Available from: http://linkinghub.elsevier.com/retrieve/pii/S1368764698900681

[59] Yoshida H, Bogaki M, Nakamura M, Nakamura S. Quinolone resistance-determining region in the DNA gyrase gyrA gene of *Escherichia coli*. Antimicrob Agents Chemother [Internet]. 1990 Jun 1 [cited 2016 Aug 7];34(6):1271–2. doi:10.1128/AAC.34.6.1271

[60] Yoshida H, Bogaki M, Nakamura M, Yamanaka LM, Nakamura S. Quinolone resistance-determining region in the DNA gyrase gyrB gene of *Escherichia coli*. Antimicrob Agents Chemother [Internet]. 1991 Aug 1 [cited 2016 Aug 7];35(8):1647–50. doi:10.1128/AAC.35.8.1647

[61] Hooper DC. Mechanisms of action and resistance of older and newer fluoroquinolones. Clin Infect Dis [Internet]. 2000 Aug 1 [cited 2016 Aug 7];31(Supplement 2):S24–8. doi:10.1086/314056

[62] Piddock LJV. Mechanisms of fluoroquinolone resistance: an update 1994–1998. Drugs [Internet]. 1999 [cited 2016 Aug 7];58(Supplement 2):11–8. Available from: http://link.springer.com/10.2165/00003495-199958002-00003

[63] Hirose K, Hashimoto A, Tamura K, Kawamura Y, Ezaki T, Sagara H, et al. DNA sequence analysis of DNA gyrase and DNA topoisomerase IV quinolone resistance-determining regions of *Salmonella enterica* Serovar Typhi and Serovar Paratyphi A. Antimicrob Agents Chemother [Internet]. 2002 Oct 1 [cited 2016 Aug 7];46(10):3249–52. doi:10.1128/AAC.46.10.3249-3252.2002

[64] Choi SH, Woo JH, Lee JE, Park SJ, Choo EJ, Kwak YG, et al. Increasing incidence of quinolone resistance in human non-typhoid *Salmonella enterica* isolates in Korea and mechanisms involved in quinolone resistance. 2005;56(6):1111–4.

[65] Wu W, Wang H, Lu J, Wu J, Chen M, Xu Y, et al. Genetic diversity of *Salmonella enterica* serovar Typhi and Paratyphi in Shenzhen, China from 2002 through 2007. BMC Microbiol [Internet]. 2010 [cited 2016 Aug 7];10(1):32. Available from: http://bmcmicrobiol.biomedcentral.com/articles/10.1186/1471-2180-10-32

[66] Eaves DJ, Liebana E, Woodward MJ, Piddock LJV. Detection of gyrA mutations in quinolone-resistant *Salmonella enterica* by denaturing high-performance liquid chromatography. J Clin Microbiol [Internet]. 2002 Nov 1 [cited 2016 Aug 7];40(11):4121–5. doi:10.1128/JCM.40.11.4121-4125.2002

[67] Guerra B, Malorny B, Schroeter A, Helmuth R. Multiple resistance mechanisms in fluoroquinolone-resistant Salmonella isolates from Germany. Antimicrob Agents Chemother [Internet]. 2003 Jun 1 [cited 2016 Aug 7];47(6):2059–2059. doi:10.1128/AAC.47.6.2059.2003

[68] O'Regan E, Quinn T, Pages J-M, McCusker M, Piddock L, Fanning S. Multiple regulatory pathways associated with high-level ciprofloxacin and multidrug resistance in *Salmonella enterica* Serovar Enteritidis: involvement of ramA and other global regulators. Antimicrob Agents Chemother [Internet]. 2009 Mar 1 [cited 2016 Aug 7];53(3):1080–7. doi:10.1128/AAC.01005-08

[69] Gensberg K, Jin YF, Piddock LJ. A novel gyrB mutation in a fluoroquinolone-resistant clinical isolate of Salmonella typhimurium. FEMS Microbiol Lett [Internet]. 1995 Oct 1 [cited 2016 Aug 7];132(1–2):57–60. Available from: http://www.ncbi.nlm.nih.gov/pubmed/7590165

[70] Xiong X, Bromley EHC, Oelschlaeger P, Woolfson DN, Spencer J. Structural insights into quinolone antibiotic resistance mediated by pentapeptide repeat proteins: conserved surface loops direct the activity of a Qnr protein from a gram-negative bacterium. Nucleic Acids Res [Internet]. 2011 May [cited 2016 Aug 7];39(9):3917–27. Available from: http://www.ncbi.nlm.nih.gov/pubmed/21227918

[71] Jacoby G, Cattoir V, Hooper D, Martinez-Martinez L, Nordmann P, Pascual A, et al. qnr Gene Nomenclature. Antimicrob Agents Chemother [Internet]. 2008 Jul 1 [cited 2016 Aug 7];52(7):2297–9. doi:10.1128/AAC.00147-08

[72] Baquirin MHC, Barlow M. Evolution and recombination of the Plasmidic qnr Alleles. J Mol Evol [Internet]. 2008 Jul 1 [cited 2016 Aug 7];67(1):103–10. Available from: http://link.springer.com/10.1007/s00239-008-9131-3

[73] Veldman K, Cavaco LM, Mevius D, Battisti A, Franco A, Botteldoorn N, et al. International collaborative study on the occurrence of plasmid-mediated quinolone resistance in *Salmonella enterica* and *Escherichia coli* isolated from animals, humans, food and the environment in 13 European countries. J Antimicrob Chemother [Internet]. 2011 Jun [cited 2016 Aug 7];66(6):1278–86. Available from: http://www.ncbi.nlm.nih.gov/pubmed/21393198

[74] Gay K, Robicsek A, Strahilevitz J, Park CH, Jacoby G, Barrett TJ, et al. Plasmid-mediated quinolone resistance in non-Typhi serotypes of *Salmonella enterica*. Clin Infect Dis [Internet]. 2006 Aug 1 [cited 2016 Aug 7];43(3):297–304. Available from: http://www.ncbi.nlm.nih.gov/pubmed/16804843

[75] Vetting MW, Park CH, Hegde SS, Jacoby GA, Hooper DC, Blanchard JS. Mechanistic and structural analysis of aminoglycoside *N*-Acetyltransferase AAC(6')-Ib and its bifunctional, fluoroquinolone-active AAC(6')-Ib-cr Variant[†‡]. Biochemistry [Internet]. 2008 Sep 16 [cited 2016 Aug 7];47(37):9825–35. doi:10.1021/bi800664x

[76] Martínez-Martínez L, Pascual A, Jacoby GA, Goldstein F, Acar J, Threlfall E, et al. Quinolone resistance from a transferable plasmid. Lancet (London, England) [Internet]. 1998 Mar 14 [cited 2016 Aug 7];351(9105):797–9. Available from: http://www.ncbi.nlm.nih.gov/pubmed/9519952

[77] Robicsek A, Jacoby GA, Hooper DC, Ball P, Paton J, Reeves D, et al. The worldwide emergence of plasmid-mediated quinolone resistance. Lancet Infect Dis [Internet]. 2006 Oct [cited 2016 Aug 7];6(10):629–40. Available from: http://www.ncbi.nlm.nih.gov/pubmed/17008172

[78] Du X-D, Li D-X, Hu G-Z, Wang Y, Shang Y-H, Wu C-M, et al. Tn1548-associated armA is co-located with qnrB2, aac(6')-Ib-cr and blaCTX-M-3 on an IncFII plasmid in a *Salmonella enterica* subsp. enterica serovar Paratyphi B strain isolated from chickens in China. J Antimicrob Chemother [Internet]. 2012 Jan [cited 2016 Aug 7];67(1):246–8. Available from: http://www.ncbi.nlm.nih.gov/pubmed/21965429

[79] Hirai K, Aoyama H, Suzue S, Irikura T, Iyobe S, Mitsuhashi S. Isolation and characterization of norfloxacin-resistant mutants of *Escherichia coli* K-12. Antimicrob Agents Chemother [Internet]. 1986 Aug 1 [cited 2016 Aug 7];30(2):248–53. doi:10.1128/AAC.30.2.248

[80] Chapman JS, Georgopapadakou NH. Routes of quinolone permeation in *Escherichia coli*. Antimicrob Agents Chemother [Internet]. 1988 Apr [cited 2016 Aug 7];32(4):438–42. Available from: http://www.ncbi.nlm.nih.gov/pubmed/3132091

[81] Chenia HY, Pillay B, Pillay D. Analysis of the mechanisms of fluoroquinolone resistance in urinary tract pathogens. J Antimicrob Chemother [Internet]. 2006 Dec [cited 2016 Aug 7];58(6):1274–8. Available from: http://www.ncbi.nlm.nih.gov/pubmed/17040923

[82] Zeth K, Kozjak-Pavlovic V, Faulstich M, Fraunholz M, Hurwitz R, Kepp O, et al. Structure and function of the PorB porin from disseminating *Neisseria gonorrhoeae*. Biochem J [Internet]. 2013 Feb 1 [cited 2016 Aug 7];449(3):631–42. Available from: http://www.ncbi.nlm.nih.gov/pubmed/23095086

[83] Everett MJ, Jin YF, Ricci V, Piddock LJ. Contributions of individual mechanisms to fluoroquinolone resistance in 36 *Escherichia coli* strains isolated from humans and animals. Antimicrob Agents Chemother [Internet]. 1996 Oct [cited 2016 Aug 7];40(10):2380–6. Available from: http://www.ncbi.nlm.nih.gov/pubmed/8891148

[84] Danilchanka O, Pavlenok M, Niederweis M. Role of porins for uptake of antibiotics by *Mycobacterium smegmatis*. Antimicrob Agents Chemother [Internet]. 2008 Sep [cited 2016 Aug 7];52(9):3127–34. Available from: http://www.ncbi.nlm.nih.gov/pubmed/18559650

[85] Giraud E, Cloeckaert A, Kerboeuf D, Chaslus-Dancla E. Evidence for active efflux as the primary mechanism of resistance to ciprofloxacin in *Salmonella enterica* serovar typhimurium. Antimicrob Agents Chemother [Internet]. 2000 May [cited 2016 Aug 7];44(5):1223–8. Available from: http://www.ncbi.nlm.nih.gov/pubmed/10770755

[86] Griggs DJ, Hall MC, Jin YF, Piddock LJ. Quinolone resistance in veterinary isolates of Salmonella. J Antimicrob Chemother [Internet]. 1994 Jun [cited 2016 Aug 7];33(6):1173–89. Available from: http://www.ncbi.nlm.nih.gov/pubmed/7928811

[87] Piddock LJ, Griggs DJ, Hall MC, Jin YF. Ciprofloxacin resistance in clinical isolates of Salmonella typhimurium obtained from two patients. Antimicrob Agents Chemother [Internet]. 1993 Apr 1 [cited 2016 Aug 7];37(4):662–6. doi:10.1128/AAC.37.4.662

[88] Piddock LJ, Ricci V, McLaren I, Griggs DJ. Role of mutation in the gyrA and parC genes of nalidixic-acid-resistant salmonella serotypes isolated from animals in the United Kingdom. J Antimicrob Chemother [Internet]. 1998 Jun [cited 2016 Aug 7];41(6):635–41. Available from: http://www.ncbi.nlm.nih.gov/pubmed/9687102

[89] Davin-Regli A, Bolla JM, James CE, Lavigne JP, Chevalier J, Garnotel E, et al. Membrane permeability and regulation of drug "influx and efflux" in enterobacterial pathogens. 2008;9:750–9.

[90] Pomposiello PJ, Demple B. Identification of SoxS-regulated genes in *Salmonella enterica* serovar typhimurium. J Bacteriol [Internet]. 2000 Jan [cited 2016 Aug 7];182(1):23–9. Available from: http://www.ncbi.nlm.nih.gov/pubmed/10613858

[91] Kaatz GW, Seo SM. Inducible NorA-mediated multidrug resistance in *Staphylococcus aureus*. Antimicrob Agents Chemother [Internet]. 1995 Dec 1 [cited 2016 Aug 7];39(12):2650–5. doi:10.1128/AAC.39.12.2650

[92] Piddock LJ V. Multidrug-resistance efflux pumps—not just for resistance. Nat Rev Microbiol [Internet]. 2006 Aug [cited 2016 Aug 7];4(8):629–36. Available from: http://www.ncbi.nlm.nih.gov/pubmed/16845433

[93] Piddock LJ, White DG, Gensberg K, Pumbwe L, Griggs DJ. Evidence for an efflux pump mediating multiple antibiotic resistance in *Salmonella enterica* serovar Typhimurium. Antimicrob Agents Chemother [Internet]. 2000 Nov [cited 2016 Aug 7];44(11):3118–21. Available from: http://www.ncbi.nlm.nih.gov/pubmed/11036033

[94] Baucheron S, Imberechts H, Chaslus-Dancla E, Cloeckaert A. The AcrB multidrug transporter plays a major role in high-level fluoroquinolone resistance in *Salmonella enterica* serovar typhimurium phage type DT204. Microb Drug Resist [Internet]. 2002 [cited 2016 Aug 7];8(4):281–9. Available from: http://www.ncbi.nlm.nih.gov/pubmed/12523625

[95] Alonso A, Morales G, Escalante R, Campanario E, Sastre L, Martinez JL. Overexpression of the multidrug efflux pump SmeDEF impairs *Stenotrophomonas maltophilia* physiology. J Antimicrob Chemother [Internet]. 2004 Feb 12 [cited 2016 Aug 7];53(3):432–4. doi:10.1093/jac/dkh074

[96] Bagel S, Hüllen V, Wiedemann B, Heisig P. Impact of gyrA and parC mutations on quinolone resistance, doubling time, and supercoiling degree of *Escherichia coli*. Antimicrob Agents Chemother [Internet]. 1999 Apr [cited 2016 Aug 7];43(4):868–75. Available from: http://www.ncbi.nlm.nih.gov/pubmed/10103193

[97] Kugelberg E, Löfmark S, Wretlind B, Andersson DI. Reduction of the fitness burden of quinolone resistance in *Pseudomonas aeruginosa*. J Antimicrob Chemother [Internet]. 2005 Jan [cited 2016 Aug 7];55(1):22–30. Available from: http://www.ncbi.nlm.nih.gov/pubmed/15574475

[98] Sánchez P, Linares JF, Ruiz-Díez B, Campanario E, Navas A, Baquero F, et al. Fitness of in vitro selected *Pseudomonas aeruginosa* nalB and nfxB multidrug resistant mutants. J Antimicrob Chemother [Internet]. 2002 Nov [cited 2016 Aug 7];50(5):657–64. Available from: http://www.ncbi.nlm.nih.gov/pubmed/12407121

[99] Zhang Q, Sahin O, McDermott PF, Payot S. Fitness of antimicrobial-resistant Campylobacter and Salmonella. Microbes Infect. 2006;8(7):1972–8.

[100] Andersson DI. The biological cost of mutational antibiotic resistance: any practical conclusions? Curr Opin Microbiol. 2006;9(5):461–5.

[101] Giraud E, Cloeckaert A, Baucheron S, Mouline C, Chaslus-Dancla E. Fitness cost of fluoroquinolone resistance in *Salmonella enterica* serovar Typhimurium. J Med Microbiol [Internet]. 2003 Aug 1 [cited 2016 Aug 7];52(8):697–703. Available from: http://jmm.microbiologyresearch.org/content/journal/jmm/10.1099/jmm.0.05178-0

[102] Wang Y-P, Li L, Shen J-Z, Yang F-J, Wu Y-N. Quinolone-resistance in Salmonella is associated with decreased mRNA expression of virulence genes invA and avrA, growth and intracellular invasion and survival. Vet Microbiol. 2009;133(4):328–34.

[103] O'Regan E, Quinn T, Frye JG, Pages J-M, Porwollik S, Fedorka-Cray PJ, et al. Fitness costs and stability of a high-level ciprofloxacin resistance phenotype in *Salmonella enterica* Serotype Enteritidis: reduced infectivity associated with decreased expression of Salmonella Pathogenicity Island 1 Genes. Antimicrob Agents Chemother [Internet]. 2010 Jan 1 [cited 2016 Aug 7];54(1):367–74. doi:10.1128/AAC.00801-09

[104] Björkman J, Hughes D, Andersson DI. Virulence of antibiotic-resistant Salmonella typhimurium. Proc Natl Acad Sci USA [Internet]. 1998 Mar 31 [cited 2016 Aug 7];95(7):3949–53. Available from: http://www.ncbi.nlm.nih.gov/pubmed/9520473

Chapter 8

Salmonella in Wastewater: Identification, Antibiotic Resistance and the Impact on the Marine Environment

Abdellah El Boulani, Rachida Mimouni,
Hasna Mannas, Fatima Hamadi and
Nouredine Chaouqy

Additional information is available at the end of the chapter

http://dx.doi.org/10.5772/67298

Abstract

Many coastal cities around the world discharge their wastewaters into the marine environment. These wastewaters contain a high variety of pathogenic microorganisms that would have a role in the contamination of this ecosystem and may have potential risks for public health and environment. Using an environmental approach, we investigate the presence of *Salmonella* in wastewater treatment plants and its presence after the treatment in its receiving marine environment. In this environmental approach, we provide information about the inefficiency of wastewater treatment to remove *Salmonella*, especially that wastewater is considered as a good tank of high diversity of *Salmonella* serotypes. The identified *Salmonella* serotypes in the receiving marine environment almost coincide with those identified in wastewater. This characterization of *Salmonella* strains from wastewater and marine environment involves the direct impact of municipal wastewater discharges on this environment. Antibiotic susceptibility tests reveal generally the presence of multiresistant *Salmonella* strains in wastewater, which usually end up in the marine environment and may have a significant risk on the public health.

Keywords: antibiotic susceptibility, marine environment, *Salmonella*, Wastewater, wastewater treatment

1. Introduction

Many major coastal cities around the world discharge their wastewaters into the marine environment. Wastewater may consist of a combination of domestic, industrial and agricultural effluent. Generally, wastewater treatment plants (WWTPs) are mostly designed to effectively remove fecal bacteria, some chemical pollutants but are not provided to eliminate pathogenic microorganisms [1, 2]. Furthermore, most of these treatment systems remain imperfect and continue to reject varied concentrations of enteric bacteria in the environment [1–5].

Pathogenic bacteria become normally more harmful to environment and humans when they acquire resistance to antibiotics. Moreover, many studies [5–7] confirmed the detection of antibiotic concentrations in wastewater that treatment systems generally fail to eliminate. Therefore, when there is a contact between bacteria and antibiotics traces, the wastewater could be an ideal environment to the exchange of genetic material between bacteria and consequently the acquisition of antibiotic resistance [5, 6, 8, 9].

The *Salmonella* genus is one of the pathogen bacteria that could be conveyed to the environmental waters through sewage pollution. Therefore, the determination of the presence of *Salmonella*, its levels and its antibiotic resistance at the same time in wastewaters and environmental waters are crucial and are required to assess the related health risks.

Previous works [1, 9–13] have studied the presence of *Salmonella* in wastewater but they stay insufficient to provide enough information on the diversity and the antibiotic resistance profiles of *Salmonella*. This makes transmission of *Salmonella* via wastewater, its impact on the environment and the origin of contamination poorly understood. In Morocco, *Salmonella* in wastewater is rarely discussed and its bibliography is very scarce. In this context, we are currently leading the first study about *Salmonella* in the southern region of Morocco. This work is focusing on the identification, serotyping and antibiotic susceptibility of *Salmonella* strains isolated from Agadir wastewater treatment plant.

The aim of this chapter is first to provide qualitative information on the capacity of wastewater treatment process to eliminate *Salmonella* considered among the most pathogenic bacteria easily transmissible in water. The second aim is to present the most *Salmonella* serotypes isolated from wastewater and marine environment and the possible impact of wastewater discharges on marine environment.

2. WWTPs removal efficiency of *Salmonella*

Wastewater treatment plants know a growing pressure which leads to the evacuation of untreated or insufficiently treated effluents into the environment. Thus, the efficient removal of pathogenic bacteria in wastewater is a crucial task because wastewater discharges can significantly increase the contamination of surface water and lead to water and seafood-borne infections. Generally, an optimal wastewater treatment process can attain 90–99% of reduction of microbial load [2, 14, 15]. However, in some cases, the reduction level decreases are mostly due to a nonrespective operating mode or due to bad or inadequate plant maintenance.

Several studies have shown the presence of *Salmonella* in wastewater before and after treatment even if treatment processes are different [1, 9, 10, 13]. This could be explained by the fact that WWTPs are mostly designed just to reduce microbial load but are not conceived specifically to completely eliminate the pathogenic bacteria.

An activated sludge treatment process remains unable to totally remove *Salmonella* [9, 12]. Koivunen et al. have also shown that activated sludge process coupled with phosphorus precipitation followed by a secondary settling or coupled with denitrification-nitrification fails to remove *Salmonella* from municipal wastewater [1].

Until now, no study has been conducted on the elimination of *Salmonella* by infiltration percolation treatment process through sand. However, a current study conducted by our research team (unpublished data) showed the inefficiency of this treatment system to remove *Salmonella*. Thus, treated wastewater still contains *Salmonella* which continues to be detected at the treatment plant exit.

To get an efficient reduction or a total removal of *Salmonella*, a tertiary wastewater treatment is needed. Indeed, Koivunen et al. show that tertiary treatment by rapid sand contact filter allows a very good efficiency to remove *Salmonella*. Consequently, *Salmonella* was not found in wastewaters after tertiary filtration [1]. Furthermore, a current study conducted by our team showed that tertiary treatment by UV irradiation applied just on a portion of the secondary treated effluents (which are intended for the irrigation of golf courses) allows total elimination of *Salmonella* (unpublished data).

3. Microbiological risks associated with *Salmonella* in wastewater

Wastewater is known to be a common vehicle for the transport and transmission of *Salmonella* serovars and is able to pollute environment and infect humans. Indeed, several outbreaks and contaminations have been related to *Salmonella* in wastewater through irrigation of crops [16–18], infiltration and transport in soil to groundwater [19–21] or to its discharge into the marine environment [22, 23]. In this last case, although some pathogens are naturally present in the aquatic environment, *Salmonella* may be introduced through animal or human fecal and sewage pollution [24].

The risk of contamination linked to *Salmonella* is enhanced by its ability to survive longer in the environment. Indeed, contamination of groundwater, environmental water and soil by *Salmonella* is due to its ability to survive very long time in these environments [25]. Furthermore, contaminations related to *Salmonella* in seawater and seafood are increased by the capacity of *Salmonella* to survive in relatively high salt conditions [26]. Thus, the persistence of wastewater discharges in coastal waters may increase the load of *Salmonella* in marine environment, and therefore increase the higher incidence of seawater and seafood-borne infections.

4. Identification methods of *Salmonella*

Various methods have been developed for the subtyping of *Salmonella*. Each of them has its advantages and drawbacks in terms of cost, speed, robustness, and sensitivity [27]. The choice of identification techniques of bacteria is generally done according to the objectives of identifying and the available means. Biochemical techniques are usually used to isolate and identify only species. For further characterization, determination of the origins and the relationships between different isolates, many other accurate methods are needed.

Conventional serotyping using somatic and flagellar *Salmonella* antisera is the most frequently used reference method for serotyping *Salmonella* isolated from wastewater [1, 9, 28, 29]. This method is based on the direct agglutination technique blade, involving *Salmonella* strains with different antisera to identify variants of the somatic O and flagellar H antigens. Serotyping is generally performed according to the antigenic formulae of Kauffmann-White-Le Minor scheme [30]. The main limitation of this technique is that not all O serotypes are included in Polyvalent O antisera which *Salmonella* species should agglutinate with [31]. A combination between conventional serotyping and the ribosomal spacer-heteroduplex polymorphism (RS-HP) methods was also used to characterize *Salmonella* strains from wastewater [13]. This technique based on the PCR amplification of the intergenic spacer region between the 16S and 23S rRNA genes can produce amplicon profiles allowing the discrimination of species at both serotype and intraserotype levels [13].

PFGE allows a high discrimination and it is usually used for outbreak investigations and it is also widely used for characterizing epidemic *Salmonella* strains. The capacity of PFGE to differentiate strains of bacterial pathogens makes it a standard method used to assess the epidemic spread of infectious diseases and to trace *Salmonella* outbreaks. However, even if it is reproducible and discriminatory, some strains of *Salmonella* cannot be typed by PFGE [27]. Recently, matrix-assisted laser desorption/ionization time of light mass spectrometry (MALDI-TOF MS) has been used for the identification of *Salmonella*. It is also utilized to discriminate *Salmonella Typhi* from other *Salmonella* serovars [32]. Despite its rapidity and simplicity, the preparation of MALDI-TOF requires more modifications and improvements to available protocols before being adopted as an autonomous method [32]. Other molecular methods developed as alternatives to conventional serotyping (MLST, MLVA, SNP, and molecular typing with composite microarrays) seem successful. However, these methods do not provide exactly similar results like those obtained by the current reference method which is agglutination serotyping [27].

5. *Salmonella* serotypes isolated from wastewater

As reported, wastewater is an ideal tank of *Salmonella* strains. Furthermore, identified *Salmonella* showed generally high variability of serotypes. The major serotypes isolated in wastewater from different countries are presented in **Table 1**.

Data concerning *Salmonella* serotyping (**Table 1**) show high heterogeneity of serotypes isolated from wastewater. This high diversity can be explained by the variety of the origin of effluents carrying these *Salmonella* strains. The most frequent serotypes identified in France wastewater were Newport, Saintpaul, and Brandenburg [13]. Indeed, Serotypes Mbandaka, Virchow, Hadar, Indiana, Infantis, Saintpaul, and Senftenberg are commonly isolated from poultry farms. Also, Typhimurium and Indiana serotypes are generally isolated in human pathology and can derive from healthy carriers [13]. Espigares et al. have also explained this diversity by the variety of the origin of *Salmonella* which may be of human or animal origin [9]. *Salmonella* Agona, Saintpaul, Virchow, and Corvallis are the most frequent serotypes identified in Finnish wastewater [1]. According to Koivunen et al., this diversity may be reported to the size of the population suggesting, therefore, that larger populations produce larger spectra of serovars [1]. However, despite these explanations, the origin of this diversity remains unknown. The large variability in serovars identified in USA wastewater indicates multiple sources of the isolates. This variability may be due to fecal shedding in clinical salmonellosis or to animal agriculture [33]. Our current study (not shown data) concerning isolated *Salmonella* from wastewater in Agadir, a coastal city in Morocco, show high variability of serotypes. Thus, among 52 *Salmonella* strains we identified 18 different serotypes. *Salmonella Muenster* was the major serotype which showed a high incidence with 14 isolates followed by *Salmonella Infantis*, *Salmonella Senftenberg*, *Salmonella Montevideo*, and *Salmonella Kentucky* as the most frequent serotypes identified. This high diversity of serotypes in Agadir wastewater can be explained by its various origins including domestic and industrial effluents especially those coming from poultry slaughterhouse and fish processing plants very widespread in the city.

Country	**France**	**Spain**	**Finland**	**Morocco**	**Mexico**	**USA**
Serotypes	Agona	Anatum	Agona	Anatum	Typhimurium	Agona
	Bardo	Enteritidis	Corvallis	Give	Vejle	Banana
	Brandenburg	Hadar	Blockley	Newport	Corvallis	Montevideo
	Derby	London	Enteritidis	Senftenberg	Nchanga	Derby
	Hadar	Newport	Hadar	Typhimurium	Nitra	Edinburg
	Indiana	Typhimurium	Infantis		Stanleyville	Hadar
	Infantis		Lexington			Havana
	Manhattan		Mbandaka			Infantis
	Newport		Muenster			Saintpaul
	Saintpaul		Panama			Senftenberg
	Senftenberg		Saintpaul			Typhimurium
	Typhimurium		Typhimurium			Newport
	Virchow		Virchow			Thompson
References	[13]	[9]	[1]	[28]	[29]	[33]

Table 1. *Salmonella* serotypes isolated from wastewater.

6. *Salmonella* serotypes isolated from a wastewater receiving marine environment

In coastal cities, the marine environment is usually the final end of treated and untreated sewage. **Table 2** shows some studies throughout the world carried in this regard.

Country	France	Spain	Mexico	Morocco	USA
	Cerro	Anatum	Stanley	Altona	Adelaide
	Newport	Enteritidis	Galiema	Anatum	Agona
	Typhimurium	Goldcoast	Bulovka	Corvallis	Arizona
Serotypes	Virchow	Hadar	Othmarschen	Hadar	Bardo
		London	Tonev	Senftenberg	Hartford
		Newport	Subaru	Typhimurium	Newport
		Typhimurium	Typhimurium	Kentucky	Poona
			Vejle	London	Reading
			Winnipeg	Mbandaka	Typhimurium
				Muenster	
				Oakland	
				Blockley	
				Labadi	
References	[13]	[34]	[29]	[35, 36, 38]	[47]

Table 2. *Salmonella* serotypes isolated from marine environment.

As reported in wastewater, data from marine environment also reveal a large diversity of *Salmonella* serotypes. However, the origin of these serovars remains little known. Following to data in **Tables 1** and **2**, it appears that the most serotypes found in wastewater are also isolated in the surrounding marine environment. Furthermore, studies from France [13] and Mexico [29] showed that Newport and Typhimurium were respectively the major *Salmonella* serotypes isolated in wastewater. These serotypes were also the same major serotypes isolated from marine environment [13, 29]. Serovar Typhimurium has been shown to be the most common serovar isolated from marine environment in different parts of the world [13, 29, 34–36]. It was suggested previously that this serotype shows an excellent adaptation to the marine water stress after passing through wastewater [37]. In Agadir, study conducted by our team [38] in marine environment has identified *S. Muenster* as the major serotype (13 strains among 46 isolates). This high occurrence of serotype Muenster coincides with its high incidence in Agadir wastewater. Therefore, these findings reveal that wastewater discharges into the marine environment could be the main source of contamination and the principal origin of *Salmonella* strains found in this environment.

7. Antimicrobial resistance of *Salmonella* isolated from wastewater

Urban wastewater treatment plants (UWTPs) are suspected to be among the main anthropogenic sources for antibiotics, antibiotic resistant genes (ARGs) and antibiotic resistant bacteria (ARB) spread into the environment [14, 39, 40]. The presence of antibiotics in effluents is generally due to incomplete metabolism in humans or because of the mismanagement of unused antibiotics [4, 41].

Generally, bacteria in wastewater are in permanent contact with various elements including antibiotics and other chemical products. Furthermore, antibiotic resistance was positively correlated with the occurrence of antibiotic residues. In addition, a relationship between antibiotic residues, bacterial community structure and antibiotic resistance was demonstrated [42]. Therefore, the elimination of these antibiotics from wastewater is a major concern. Sorption and hydrolysis could be a degradation pathway that may lead to the removal of antibiotics in wastewater [39]. However, in previous reports, it has been demonstrated that UV radiation is not effective to remove antibiotics [43]. This indicates that photolysis is not an important mechanism for degradation of these compounds in wastewater. A combination of physico-chemical and biological treatment and the optimization of their operating conditions might prove an effective removal increase of persistent antibiotic residues in wastewater [39].

According to previous studies [6, 44, 45], ARB have been detected widely in wastewater samples and comparatively to surface water, higher proportion of ARB was reported in raw and treated wastewater than in surface water [4, 40]. It has also been reported that *Salmonella* strains show a high proportion among other multidrug resistant bacteria [46]. According to these studies, conditions in wastewater treatment plants (WWTPs) seem to be favorable for the proliferation of ARB.

Antibiotic resistance (ABR) of *Salmonella* isolated from wastewater has been discussed in some studies. A wide variety of antibiotic resistance patterns of *Salmonella* serotypes have been found in USA wastewater [33]. Indeed, 86% of 647 *Salmonella* isolates were susceptible, 4% were monoresistant and 10% were multiresistant. *Salmonella* serovars multiresistant to at least four antibiotics were *Salmonella Braenderup*, Derby, Edinburg, Hadar, Saintpaul, Typhimurium, Uganda and Virchow. A resistance to the third generation of cephalosporins considered as one of the first drugs of choice to treat human salmonellosis has also been reported [33]. From Finnish wastewater [1], among 197 isolates, 44% of the *Salmonella* strains were resistant to antimicrobial agents, almost 20% were multiresistant. The most multiresistant serotype was *Salmonella Saintpaul* (to 6 antibiotics). Moreover, 32% of strains were resistant to nalidixic acid which can indicates the reduction of sensitivity to ciprofloxacin considered as the selected drug in severe infections [1]. The most resistant serotype isolated in wastewater from Spain was *Salmonella Hadar* with a pattern of multiresistance to six antibiotics [9]. In Morocco, among 42 strains isolated from wastewater, 19 (45.2%) were resistant at least to two antibiotics. The most multiresistant serotype was *S. Typhimurium* followed by *S. Hadar* and *S. Senftenberg*. *S. Typhimurium* was resistant to ampicillin, chloramphenicol, streptomycin, sulfametoxazole/trimetoprim, and tetracycline. Serovars Give, Newport and Anatum were susceptible to all used antibiotics [28]. Antibiotic susceptibility test (ATS) of *Salmonella* serotypes from Agadir wastewater treatment plant carried out by our team showed that among 52 isolates 23% of strains were multiresistant. ATS was carried out by the disk diffusion method, with a panel of 32 antimicrobial drugs (Bio-Rad) and interpreted according to the EUCAST clinical guidelines (http://www.eucast.org/clinical_breakpoints/). Multiresistant serovars were Chester, Kentucky, and Typhimurium. The most multiresistant serotype identified in this study was Typhimurium with a pattern of multiresistance to 18 antibiotics.

All these data showed that wastewater is a tank of a wide variety of *Salmonella enterica* serovars and ABR patterns. Other data showed that multiresistant bacteria have been detected extensively in wastewater samples which pass through WWTPs and arrive to the receiving environment [14, 40, 44]. Consequently, this problem is of great concern for the wastewater management of coastal cities because multiresistant bacteria have become a significant public health problem. The caused infection is much more difficult to be treated because the panel of effective antibiotics will be reduced.

8. Conclusions

- Conventional wastewater treatment without efficient tertiary treatment, like filtration or disinfection by UV, is generally insufficient and consequently constitutes a risk for public health.
- Wastewater is an ideal tank of high diversity of *Salmonella* serotypes and ABR patterns which usually end up in the marine environment in coastal cities.
- The presence of the same major *Salmonella* serovars simultaneously in sewage and in the marine environment confirms that the principal source of contamination of marine environment by *Salmonella* is wastewater discharges.
- Improvement in the efficiency of treating antibiotics residues in WWTPs is the first line of defense against the potential ecological impacts of these chemicals in the environment.
- On the one hand, wastewater treatment must adopt effective methods for treatment, and on the other hand, there should be a rigorous approach for surveillance and monitoring effluents before and after treatment and discharge into the environment.

Acknowledgements

We wish to thank the Institute Pasteur (IP) of Paris, France for help. We are grateful to the Laboratory of Microbiology, National Health Security Food Office (ONSSA) Agadir, Morocco for their excellent technical assistance. We thank also AGROTECH Agadir for their cooperation.

Author details

Abdellah El Boulani[1], Rachida Mimouni[1*], Hasna Mannas[1], Fatima Hamadi[1] and Nouredine Chaouqy[2]

*Address all correspondence to: r_mimouni@yahoo.fr

1 Faculty of Sciences, Laboratory of Microbial Biotechnology & Plant Protection, University Ibn Zohr, Agadir, Morocco

2 Laboratory of Microbiology, National Health Security Food Office (ONSSA), Agadir, Morocco

References

[1] Koivunen J, Siitonen A, Heinonen-Tanski H. Elimination of enteric bacteria in biological–chemical wastewater treatment and tertiary filtration units.*Water Research*. 2003;**37**: 690–698. DOI : 10.1016/S0043-1354(02)00305-6

[2] Mannas H. Phenotypic and molecular characterization of microorganisms of sanitary interest isolated from marine environments polluted by urban and industrial liquid discharges. Thesis, University of Ibn Zohr, Agadir, Morocco. 2016.

[3] Naidoo S, Olaniran AO. Treated wastewater effluent as a source of microbial pollution of surface water resources. *International Journal of Environmental Research and Public Health*. 2013;**11**: 249–270. DOI: 10.3390/ijerph110100249

[4] Bouki C, Venieri D, Diamadopoulos E. Detection and fate of antibiotic resistant bacteria in wastewater treatment plants: a review. *Ecotoxicology and Environmental Safety*. 2013;**91**: 1–9. DOI: 10.1016/j.ecoenv.2013.01.016

[5] Huang J-J, Hu H-Y, Lu S-Q, Li Y, Tang F, Lu Y, Wei B. Monitoring and evaluation of antibiotic-resistant bacteria at a municipal wastewater treatment plant in China. *Environment International*. 2012;**42**: 31–36. DOI: 10.1016/j.envint.2011.03.001

[6] Michael I, Rizzo L, McArdell C, Manaia C, Merlin C, Schwartz T, Dagot C, Fatta-Kassinos D. Urban wastewater treatment plants as hotspots for the release of antibiotics in the environment: a review. *Water Research*. 2013;**47**: 957–995. DOI: 10.1016/j.watres.2012.11.027

[7] Hartig C, Storm T, Jekel M. Detection and identification of sulphonamide drugs in municipal waste water by liquid chromatography coupled with electrospray ionisation tandem mass spectrometry. *Journal of Chromatography A*. 1999;**854**: 163–173. DOI: 10.1016/S0021-9673(99)00378-7

[8] Vaz-Moreira I, Nunes OC, Manaia CM. Bacterial diversity and antibiotic resistance in water habitats: searching the links with the human microbiome. *FEMS Microbiology Reviews*. 2014;**38**: 761–778. DOI: 10.1111/1574-6976.12062

[9] Espigares E, Bueno A, Espigares M, Gálvez R. Isolation of Salmonella serotypes in wastewater and effluent: effect of treatment and potential risk. *International Journal of Hygiene and Environmental Health*. 2006;**209**: 103–107. DOI: 10.1016/j.ijheh.2005.08.006

[10] Ben Salem I, Ouardani I, Hassine M, Aouni M. Bacteriological and physico-chemical assessment of wastewater in different region of Tunisia: impact on human health. *BMC Research Notes*. 2011;**4**: 1. DOI: 10.1186/1756-0500-4-144

[11] Levantesi C, La Mantia R, Masciopinto C, Böckelmann U, Ayuso-Gabella MN, Salgot M, Tandoi V, Van Houtte E, Wintgens T, Grohmann E. Quantification of pathogenic microorganisms and microbial indicators in three wastewater reclamation and managed aquifer recharge facilities in Europe. *Science of the Total Environment*. 2010;**408**: 4923–4930. DOI: 10.1016/j.scitotenv.2010.07.042

[12] Howard I, Espigares E, Lardelli P, Martin J, Espigares M. Evaluation of microbiological and physicochemical indicators for wastewater treatment. *Environmental Toxicology*. 2004;**19**: 241–249. DOI: 10.1002/tox.20016

[13] Baudart J, Lemarchand K, Brisabois A, Lebaron P. Diversity of Salmonella strains isolated from the aquatic environment as determined by serotyping and amplification of the ribosomal DNA spacer regions. *Applied and Environmental Microbiology*. 2000;**66**: 1544–1552. DOI: 10.1128/AEM.66.4.1544-1552.2000

[14] Kümmerer K. Antibiotics in the aquatic environment–a review–part II. *Chemosphere*. 2009;**75**: 435–441. DOI: 10.1016/j.chemosphere.2008.12.006

[15] Kayser R, Boll R, Muller H. Quantitative determinations of the elimination of salmonellae by biological treatment of wastewater. *Zentralblatt fuer Bacteriologie, Mikrobiologie und Hygiene, Serie B*. 1987; **184**: 195–205 (In German).

[16] Melloul AA, Hassani L. Salmonella infection in children from the wastewater-spreading zone of Marrakesh city (Morocco). *Journal of Applied Microbiology*. 1999;**87**: 536–539. DOI: 10.1046/j.1365-2672.1999.00847.x

[17] Melloul AA, Hassani L, Rafouk L. Salmonella contamination of vegetables irrigated with untreated wastewater. *World Journal of Microbiology and Biotechnology*. 2001;**17**: 207–209. DOI: 10.1023/A:1016686501953

[18] Heaton J, Jones K. Microbial contamination of fruit and vegetables and the behaviour of enteropathogens in the phyllosphere: a review. *Journal of Applied Microbiology*. 2008;**104**: 613–626. DOI: 10.1111/j.1365-2672.2007.03587.x

[19] Graun G. A Summary of waterborne illness transmitted through contaminated groundwater. *Journal of Environmental Health*. 1985; **48**: 122–127.

[20] Matthess G, Pekdeger A. Survival and transport of pathogenic bacteria and viruses in groundwater. 1985; (ed. C. H. Ward, W. Giger, and P. L. McCarty), Groundwater quality, Wiley, New York, 472–482.

[21] El Heloui M, Mimouni R, Hamadi F. Impact of treated wastewater on groundwater quality in the region of Tiznit (Morocco). *Journal of Water Reuse and Desalination*. 2015: jwrd2015061. DOI: 10.2166/wrd.2015.061

[22] Lemarchand K, Lebaron P. Occurrence of Salmonella spp. and Cryptosporidium spp. in a French coastal watershed: relationship with fecal indicators. *FEMS Microbiology Letters*. 2003;**218**: 203–209. DOI: 10.1111/j.1574-6968.2003.tb11519.x

[23] Harakeh S, Yassine H, El-Fadel M. Antimicrobial-resistant patterns of Escherichia coli and Salmonella strains in the aquatic Lebanese environments. *Environmental Pollution*. 2006;**143**: 269–277. DOI: 10.1016/j.envpol.2005.11.027

[24] Amagliani G, Brandi G, Schiavano G. Incidence and role of Salmonella in seafood safety. *Food Research International*. 2012;**45**: 780–788. DOI: 10.1016/j.foodres.2011.06.022

[25] Winfield MD, Groisman EA. Role of nonhost environments in the lifestyles of Salmonella and Escherichia coli. *Applied and Environmental Microbiology*. 2003;**69**: 3687–3694. DOI: 10.1128/AEM.69.7.3687-3694.2003

[26] Johnson JY, Thomas J, Graham T, Townshend I, Byrne J, Selinger L, Gannon VP. Prevalence of Escherichia coli O157: H7 and Salmonella spp. in surface waters of southern Alberta and its relation to manure sources. *Canadian Journal of Microbiology*. 2003;**49**: 326–335. DOI: 10.1139/w03-046

[27] Wattiau P, Boland C, Bertrand S. Methodologies for Salmonella enterica subsp. enterica subtyping: gold standards and alternatives. *Applied and Environmental Microbiology*. 2011;**77**: 7877–7885. DOI: 10.1128/AEM.05527-11

[28] Oubrim N, Ennaji MM, Badri S, Cohen N. Removal of antibiotic-resistant Salmonella in sewage water from wastewater treatment plants in Settat and Soualem, Morocco. *European Journal of Scientific Research*. 2012;**68**: 565–573.

[29] Simental L, Martinez-Urtaza J. Climate patterns governing the presence and permanence of salmonellae in coastal areas of Bahia de Todos Santos, Mexico. *Applied and Environmental Microbiology*. 2008;**74**: 5918–5924. DOI: 10.1128/AEM.01139-08

[30] Grimont P, Weill F. Antigenic Formulas of the Salmonella Serovars, WHO Collaborating. Centre for Reference and Research on Salmonella. 2007. *Forschungsbericht.–9. Ausgabe*. 2009.

[31] Nataro JP, Bopp CA, Fields PI, Kaper JB, Strockbine NA (2011). Escherichia, Shigella, and Salmonella. Manual of Clinical Microbiology, 10th Edition, Washington, DC: American Society of Microbiology: 603–626. Book DOI: 10.1128/9781555816728.ch35

[32] Kuhns M, Zautner AE, Rabsch W, Zimmermann O, Weig M, Bader O, Groß U. Rapid discrimination of Salmonella enterica serovar Typhi from other serovars by MALDI-TOF mass spectrometry. *PLoS One*. 2012;**7**. DOI: 10.1371/journal.pone.0040004

[33] Berge A, Dueger E, Sischo W. Comparison of Salmonella enterica serovar distribution and antibiotic resistance patterns in wastewater at municipal water treatment plants in two California cities. *Journal of Applied Microbiology*. 2006;**101**: 1309–1316. DOI: 10.1111/j.1365-2672.2006.03031.x

[34] Polo F, Figueras M, Inza I, Sala J, Fleisher J, Guarro J. Prevalence of Salmonella serotypes in environmental waters and their relationships with indicator organisms. *Antonie van Leeuwenhoek*. 1999;**75**: 285–292. DOI: 10.1023/A:1001817305779

[35] Bouchrif B, Paglietti B, Murgia M, Piana AF, Cohen N, Ennaji MM, Rubino S, Timinouni M. Prevalence and antibiotic-resistance of Salmonella isolated from food in Morocco. *The Journal of Infection in Developing Countries*. 2009;**3**: 35–40.

[36] Setti I, Rodriguez-Castro A, Pata MP, Cadarso-Suarez C, Yacoubi B, Bensmael L, Moukrim A, Martinez-Urtaza J. Characteristics and dynamics of Salmonella contamination along the coast of Agadir, Morocco. *Applied and Environmental Microbiology*. 2009;**75**: 7700–7709. DOI: 10.1128/AEM.01852-09

[37] Dupray E, Derrien A. Influence of the previous stay of *Escherichia coli* and Salmonella spp. in waste waters on their survival in seawater. *Water Research*. 1995;**4**: 1005–1011.

[38] Mimouni R. Microbiological study of wastewater in Greater Agadir: Purification by infiltration-percolation, impact on the marine environment and reuse in agriculture. Thesis, University of Ibn Zohr, Faculty of Sciences. Agadir Morocco. 2004.

[39] Batt AL, Kim S, Aga DS. Comparison of the occurrence of antibiotics in four full-scale wastewater treatment plants with varying designs and operations. *Chemosphere*. 2007;**68**: 428–435. DOI: 10.1016/j.chemosphere.2007.01.008

[40] Rizzo L, Manaia C, Merlin C, Schwartz T, Dagot C, Ploy M, Michael I, Fatta-Kassinos D. Urban wastewater treatment plants as hotspots for antibiotic resistant bacteria and genes spread into the environment: a review. *Science of the Total Environment*. 2013;**447**: 345–360. DOI: 10.1016/j.scitotenv.2013.01.032

[41] Duong HA, Pham NH, Nguyen HT, Hoang TT, Pham HV, Pham VC, Berg M, Giger W, Alder AC. Occurrence, fate and antibiotic resistance of fluoroquinolone antibacterials in hospital wastewaters in Hanoi, Vietnam. *Chemosphere*. 2008;**72**: 968–973. DOI: 10.1016/j.chemosphere.2008.03.009

[42] Novo A, André S, Viana P, Nunes OC, Manaia CM. Antibiotic resistance, antimicrobial residues and bacterial community composition in urban wastewater. *Water Research*. 2013;**47**: 1875–1887. DOI: 10.1016/j.scitotenv.2013.01.032

[43] Adams C, Wang Y, Loftin K, Meyer M. Removal of antibiotics from surface and distilled water in conventional water treatment processes. *Journal of Environmental Engineering*. 2002;**128**: 253–260. DOI: 10.1061/(ASCE)0733-9372(2002)

[44] Czekalski N, Berthold T, Caucci S, Egli A, Bürgmann H. Increased levels of multiresistant bacteria and resistance genes after wastewater treatment and their dissemination into Lake Geneva, Switzerland. *Role and prevalence of antibiosis and the related resistance genes in the environment*. 2007; **27**: 1–18.

[45] Karthikeyan K, Meyer MT. Occurrence of antibiotics in wastewater treatment facilities in Wisconsin, USA. *Science of the Total Environment*. 2006;**361**: 196–207. DOI: 10.1016/j.scitotenv.2005.06.030

[46] Chen S, Zhao S, White DG, Schroeder CM, Lu R, Yang H, McDermott PF, Ayers S, Meng J. Characterization of multiple-antimicrobial-resistant Salmonella serovars isolated from retail meats. *Applied and Environmental Microbiology*. 2004;**70**: 1–7. DOI: 10.1128/AEM.70.1.1-7.2004

[47] Brands DA, Inman AE, Gerba CP, Maré CJ, Billington SJ, Saif LA, Levine JF, Joens LA. Prevalence of Salmonella spp. in oysters in the United States. *Applied and Environmental Microbiology*. 2005;**71**: 893–897. DOI: 10.1128/AEM.71.2.893-897.2005

Section 3

Salmonellosis in Animals

Chapter 9

Dynamics of *Salmonella* Infection

Fathalla A. Rihan

Additional information is available at the end of the chapter

http://dx.doi.org/10.5772/67284

Abstract

In this chapter, we propose a mathematical epidemic model, with integer and fractional order to describe the dynamics of *Salmonella* infection in animal herds. We investigate the qualitative behaviors of such model and find the conditions that guarantee the asymptotic stability of disease-free and endemic steady states. To assess the severity of the outbreak, as well as the strength of the medical and/or behavioral interventions necessary for control, we estimate basic reproduction number $\mathcal{R}_0$. This threshold parameter specifies the average number of secondary infections caused by one infected individual during his/her entire infectious period at the start of an outbreak. We also provide an unconditionally stable implicit scheme for the fractional-order epidemic model. The theoretical and computational results give insight into the modelers and infectious disease specialists.

Keywords: basic reproduction number, *Salmonella* infection, SIRC epidemic model, stability

1. Introduction

Mathematical epidemic models, for *Salmonella* infections, provide a comprehensive framework for understanding the disease transmission behaviors and for evaluating the effectiveness of different intervention strategies [1, 2]. We recall here that the *Salmonella* infection, a major zoonotic disease, is transmitted between humans and other animals. Reports conducted by the National Center for Emerging and Zoonotic Infectious Diseases (NCEZID) revealed that the number of people infected by *Salmonella*, over the past few years, has remained increasing. The most commonly developed symptoms of *Salmonella* include diarrhea, fever, and abdominal cramps that appear 12–72 hours after infection. The infected people usually recover without medical aid within a period of 4–7 days [3, 4]. However, hospitalization may be needed for some infected people in the case of severe diarrhea. *Salmonella* is found living in the intestinal tracts of not only humans but also other creatures such as birds. The transmission of bacterium to humans occurs through the ingestion of food that has been contaminated with animal feces. These contaminated foods are commonly from an animal source, such as beef, poultry, milk, or eggs [5]. However, vegetables and other foods may also become contaminated. Additionally, foods that have been contaminated are almost impossible to detect while eating, due to their normal taste and smell. Therefore, *Salmonella* is considered as a serious problem for the public health throughout the world. There are no doubts that mathematical modeling of *Salmonella* infection plays an important role in gaining understanding of the transmission of the disease in a specific environment and to predict the behavior of any outbreak. Furthermore, mathematical analysis leads to determining the nature of equilibrium states and to suggest recommended actions to be taken by decision makers to control the spreading of the disease. The objective of this work is to adopt the fractional-order epidemic model to describe the dynamics of *Salmonella* infections in animal herds.

Fractional-order (or free-order) differential models have been successfully applied to system biology, physics, chemistry, and biochemistry, hydrology, medicine, and finance (see, e.g., [6–12] and the references therein). In many cases, they are more contestant with the real phenomena than the integer-order models, because the fractional derivatives and integrals enable the description of the memory and hereditary properties inherent in various materials and processes. Hence, there is a growing need to study and use the fractional-order differential and integral equations in epidemiology and biological systems with memory [13]. However, analytical and closed solutions of these types of fractional equations cannot generally be obtained. As a consequence, approximate and numerical techniques are playing an important role in identifying the solution behavior of such fractional equations and exploring their applications (see, e.g., [14–16] and the references therein).

A large number of work done on modeling biological systems have been restricted to integer-order ordinary (or delay) differential equations (see, e.g., [17–22]). In Ref. [23], the authors proposed the classical *Susceptible-Infected-Recovered* (SIR) model. The authors in Ref. [24] introduced a new compartment into the SIR model, which is called cross-immune compartment to be called SIRC model. The added compartment cross-immune $C(t)$ describes an intermediate state between the fully susceptible $S(t)$ and the fully protected $R(t)$ one. A fractional-order SIRC model of influenza, a disease in human population, was discussed in Ref. [25]. In the present chapter, we consider the fractional-order SIRC model associated with evolution of *Salmonella* infection in animal herds. However, we will take into account the disease-induced mortality rate m in the model. Qualitative behavior of the fractional-order SRIC model is then investigated. Numerical simulations of the fractional-order SRIC model are provided to demonstrate the effectiveness of the proposed method by using implicit Euler's method.

Definitions of fractional-order integration and fractional-order differentiation/integration are given in Appendix.

2. Construction of the model

Assume that the *Salmonella* infection spreads in animal herds which are grouped as four compartments, according to their infection status: $S(t)$ is the proportion of susceptible at time t (individuals that do not have the infection), $I(t)$ is the proportion of infected individuals (that have the infection), $R(t)$ is the proportion of recovered individuals (that recovered from the infection and have temporary immunity), and $C(t)$ is the proportion of cross-immune individuals at time t. The total number of animals in the herd is given by $N = S + I + R + C$. We consider that initially all the animals are susceptible to the infection. Once infected, a susceptible individual leaves the susceptible compartment and enters the infectious compartment where it then becomes infectious. The infected animals pass into the recovered compartment. After recovery from an infection animals, the individuals enter a new class $C(t)$. Therefore, we consider the disease transmission model consists of nonnegative initial conditions together with system of equations.

$$\begin{aligned} \dot{S}(t) &= \mu N + \eta C(t) - (\beta I(t) + \mu)S(t), \\ \dot{I}(t) &= \beta S(t)I(t) + \sigma\beta C(t)I(t) - (\theta + m + \mu)I(t), \\ \dot{R}(t) &= (1-\sigma)\beta C(t)I(t) + \theta I(t) - (\mu + \delta)R(t), \\ \dot{C}(t) &= \delta R(t) - \beta C(t)I(t) - (\eta + \mu)C(t). \end{aligned} \tag{1}$$

Here $'.' = D = \frac{d}{dt}$. The parameter μ denotes the mortality rate in every compartment and is assumed to equal the rate of newborns in the population. β is the contact rate and also called the transmission rate for susceptible to be infected. η^{-1} is the cross-immune period, while θ^{-1} is the infectious period and δ^{-1} is the total immune period. σ represents the fraction of the exposed cross-immune individuals who are recruited in a unit time into the infective subpopulation [24, 26]. The presented model (1) differs from existing model, we assume a disease induced mortality rate m; see the diagram of **Figure 1**.

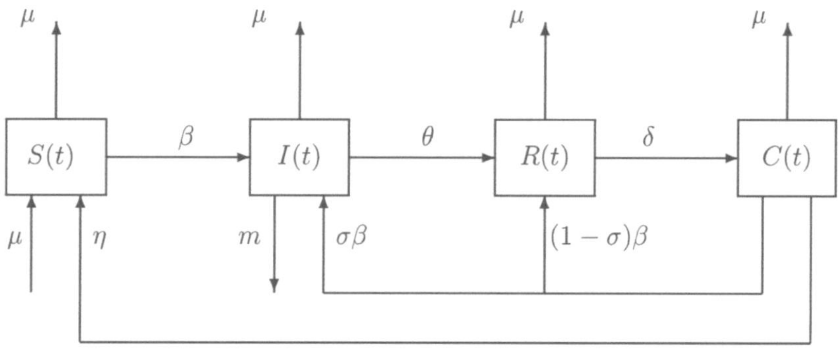

Figure 1. Schematic diagram of SIRC epidemic model for *Salmonella* infection.

2.1. Fractional-order SIRC epidemic model

Most of biological systems have long-range temporal memory. Modeling of such systems by fractional-order (or arbitrary order) models provides the systems with long-time memory and gains them extra degrees of freedom [27]. A large number of mathematical models, based on ordinary and delay differential equations with integer-orders, have been proposed in modeling the dynamics of epidemiological diseases [18, 20, 28, 29]. In recent years, it has turned out that many phenomena in different fields can be described very successfully by models using *fractional-order differential equations* (FODEs) [13, 6, 27]. This is due to the fact that fractional derivatives enable the description of the memory and hereditary properties inherent in various processes. Herein, we replace the integer-order of the model (1) into a fractional-order (or free-order) and assume that $s(t) = S(t)/N$, $i(t) = S(t)/N$, $r(t) = R(t)/N$, $c(t) = C(t)/N$, where N is the total number of population. Then the model with a fractional-order α $(0 < \alpha \leq 1)$ takes the form

$$\begin{aligned} D^\alpha s(t) &= \mu + \eta c(t) - (\beta i(t) + \mu)s(t), \\ D^\alpha i(t) &= \beta s(t)i(t) + \sigma\beta c(t)i(t) - (\theta + m + \mu)i(t), \\ D^\alpha r(t) &= (1-\sigma)\beta c(t)i(t) + \theta i(t) - (\mu + \delta)r(t), \\ D^\alpha c(t) &= \delta r(t) - \beta c(t)i(t) - (\eta + \mu)c(t). \end{aligned} \tag{2}$$

Here,

$$D^\alpha f(t) = \frac{1}{\Gamma(n-\alpha)}\left(\frac{d}{dt}\right)^n \int_0^t (t-s)^{\alpha-n-1} f(s)ds. \tag{3}$$

When $0 < \alpha \leq 1$,

$$D^\alpha f(t) = \frac{1}{\Gamma(1-\alpha)}\int_0^t \frac{f'(s)}{(t-s)^\alpha} ds. \tag{4}$$

(The initial conditions $s(0) = s_0$, $i(0) = i_0$, $r(0) = r_0$ should be given.) We note that the fractional derivatives involve an integration and are nonlocal operators, which can be used for modeling systems with memory; see the Appendix.

2.2. Stability criteria for the epidemic SIRC model (2)

To find the equilibria of the model (2), we put $D^\alpha s(t) = D^\alpha i(t) = D^\alpha r(t) = D^\alpha c(t) = 0$. We have disease-free (infection-free) equilibrium state $\mathcal{E}_0$ and endemic equilibrium state $\mathcal{E}_+$:

$$\mathcal{E}_0 = (1, 0, 0, 0) \text{ and } \mathcal{E}_+ = (s^*, i^*, r^*, c^*), \tag{5}$$

where

$$\begin{aligned} s^* &= \frac{\theta + m + \mu}{\beta} - \sigma\left(\frac{\delta\theta i^*}{(\mu + \delta\sigma)\beta i^* + (\mu + \delta)(\mu + \eta)}\right), \\ r^* &= \frac{\theta i^*(\beta i^* + \eta + \mu)}{(\mu + \delta\sigma)\beta i^* + (\mu + \delta)(\mu + \eta)}, \\ c^* &= \frac{\theta\delta i^*}{(\mu + \delta\sigma)\beta i^* + (\mu + \delta)(\mu + \eta)}. \end{aligned} \tag{6}$$

The positive endemic equilibrium $\mathcal{E}_+ = (s^*, i^*, r^*, c^*)$ satisfies Eq. (2) and i^* is the positive root of $A_1 i^{*2} + A_2 i^* + A_3$, where

$$
\begin{aligned}
A_1 &= -\beta^2[m(\mu+\delta\sigma)+\mu(\theta+\mu+\delta\sigma)],\\
A_2 &= \beta[\beta\mu(\mu+\delta\sigma)+\eta\theta\delta-(\theta+m+\mu)[(\mu+\delta)(\mu+\eta)+(\mu+\delta\sigma)]+\mu\delta\theta],\\
A_3 &= \beta\mu(\mu+\delta)(\mu+\eta)\left[1-\left(\frac{\theta+m+\mu}{\beta}\right)\right].
\end{aligned} \tag{7}
$$

The Jacobian matrix of the model (2) is

$$
J=\begin{pmatrix}
-\beta i(t)-\mu & -\beta s(t) & 0 & \eta\\
\beta i(t) & \beta s(t)+\sigma\beta c(t)-(\theta+m+\mu) & 0 & \sigma\beta i(t)\\
0 & (1-\sigma)\beta c(t)+\theta & -(\mu+\delta) & (1-\sigma)\beta i(t)\\
0 & -\beta c(t) & \delta & -\beta i(t)-(\eta+\mu)
\end{pmatrix}. \tag{8}
$$

2.3. The reproduction number $\mathcal{R}_0$

The basic reproduction number[1] $\mathcal{R}_0$ that includes the indirect transmission may be obtained using next-generation matrix method [30]. The spectral radius of the next generation matrix (FV^{-1}), which is the dominant eigenvalue of the same matrix, gives the value of $\mathcal{R}_0$. Then, the basic reproductive number $\mathcal{R}_0$ is obtained by the form

$$
\mathcal{R}_0=\rho(FV^{-1}), \tag{9}
$$

where the matrices $F=\left[\frac{\partial\mathcal{F}_i(x)}{\partial x_j}\right]_{x=x_0}$ and $V=\left[\frac{\partial\mathcal{V}_i(x)}{\partial x_j}\right]_{x=x_0}$. $\mathcal{F}_i(x)$, where x is the set of all disease-free states in the compartment i, is the rate of appearance of new infections in the compartment i, and $V_i(x)$ is the net transfer rate (other than infections) of the compartment i. The net transfer rate is given by $\mathcal{V}_i=\mathcal{V}_i^{-}-\mathcal{V}_i^{+}$, where $\mathcal{V}_i^{-}$ is the rate of transfer of individuals out of the compartment i and $\mathcal{V}_i^{+}$ is the rate of transfer of individuals into the compartment i by all other means. Therefore, the disease transmission model consists of nonnegative initial conditions, $x_i(0)$, together with the following system of equations:

$$
x'_j=f_j(x)\equiv\mathcal{F}_j(x)-\mathcal{V}_j,\quad j\geq 1. \tag{10}
$$

From the model (2), we have

$$
\begin{aligned}
F&=\begin{pmatrix}\frac{\partial\mathcal{F}_1}{\partial i(t)} & \frac{\partial\mathcal{F}_1}{\partial r(t)}\\ \frac{\partial\mathcal{F}_2}{\partial i(t)} & \frac{\partial\mathcal{F}_2}{\partial r(t)}\end{pmatrix}=\begin{pmatrix}\beta s & 0\\ 0 & 0\end{pmatrix},\\
V&=\begin{pmatrix}\frac{\partial\mathcal{V}_1}{\partial i(t)} & \frac{\partial\mathcal{V}_1}{\partial r(t)}\\ \frac{\partial\mathcal{V}_2}{\partial i(t)} & \frac{\partial\mathcal{V}_2}{\partial r(t)}\end{pmatrix}=\begin{pmatrix}\theta+m+\mu & 0\\ -\theta & \mu+\delta\end{pmatrix}.
\end{aligned} \tag{11}
$$

Since we have only two distinct stages namely $I(t)$ and $R(t)$; it follows that both F and V are 2×2 square matrices. Furthermore, it can be noticed that F is nonnegative and V is nonsingular. The

[1]The number of individuals infected by a single infected individual placed in a totally susceptible population.

basic reproductive number $\mathcal{R}_0$ is the dominant eigenvalue of the matrix FV^{-1}, which is obtained by solving the characteristic equation $(FV^{-1})I - \Lambda I = 0$ where Λ is the eigenvalue and $I(t)$ is the identity matrix. At the disease-free equilibrium, $\mathcal{E}_0 = (1, 0, 0, 0)$, we have

$$\mathcal{R}_0 = \frac{\beta}{\theta + m + \mu}. \tag{12}$$

The following theorem states that $\mathcal{R}_0$ is a threshold parameter for the stability of the model (2).

Theorem 1 *The disease-free equilibrium is locally asymptotically stable and the infection will die out if $\mathcal{R}_0 < 1$ and is unstable if $\mathcal{R}_0 > 1$. Conversely, the endemic equilibrium $\mathcal{E}_+$ is stable when $\mathcal{R}_0 > 1$ and*

$$a_i > 0,\ i = 1, 2, 3, 4,\ \ a_1 a_2 - a_3 > 0 \ \text{ and } \ a_1 a_2 a_3 - a_1^2 a_4 - a_3^2 > 0, \tag{13}$$

where

$$\begin{aligned} a_1 &= (D_1 + D_3 + D_5), \\ a_2 &= (D_1 D_3 - D_4 \delta + D_1 D_5 + D_3 D_5 + \beta^2 i^* s^* + \sigma \beta^2 c^* i^*), \\ a_3 &= (D_1 D_3 D_5 - D_1 D_4 \delta + D_3 \beta^2 i^* s^* + D_5 \beta^2 i^* s^* + \beta^2 c^* \eta i^* - D_2 \sigma \beta \delta i^* + \\ &\qquad \sigma \beta^2 D_1 c^* i^* + \sigma D_3 \beta^2 c^* i^*), \\ a_4 &= D_3 D_5 \beta^2 i^* s^* - D_2 \beta \delta \eta i^* + D_3 \beta^2 c^* \eta i^* - D_4 \beta^2 \delta i^* s^* - \sigma \beta \delta D_1 D_2 i^* + \sigma D_1 D_3 \beta^2 c^* i^*, \end{aligned} \tag{14}$$

and

$$\begin{aligned} D_1 &= \beta i + \mu, \\ D_2 &= (1 - \sigma) \beta c^* + \theta, \\ D_3 &= (\mu + \delta), \\ D_4 &= (1 - \sigma) \beta i^*, \\ D_5 &= \beta i^* + (\eta + \mu), \\ D_5 &= \beta i^* + \mu. \end{aligned} \tag{15}$$

Proof The disease-free equilibrium is locally asymptotically stable if all the eigenvalues, λ_i $i = 1, 2, 3, 4.$ of the Jacobian matrix, $J(\mathcal{E}_0)$ satisfy the following condition

$$|\arg(\lambda_i)| > \frac{\alpha \pi}{2}. \tag{16}$$

where

$$J(\mathcal{E}_0) = \begin{pmatrix} -\mu & -\beta & 0 & \eta \\ 0 & \beta - (\theta + m + \mu) & 0 & 0 \\ 0 & 0 & -(\mu + \delta) & 0 \\ 0 & 0 & \delta & -(\eta + \mu) \end{pmatrix}. \tag{17}$$

The eigenvalues of the Jacobian matrix $J(\mathcal{E}_0)$ are

$$\lambda_1 = -\mu,\ \lambda_2 = \beta - (\theta + m + \mu),\ \lambda_3 = -(\mu + \delta),\ \lambda_4 = -(\eta + \mu). \tag{18}$$

Hence $\mathcal{E}_0$ is locally asymptotically stable if $\mathcal{R}_0 < 1$ and is unstable if $\mathcal{R}_0 > 1$.

Now, we extend the analysis to endemic equilibrium $\mathcal{E}_+$. The Jacobian matrix $J(\mathcal{E}_+)$ evaluated at the endemic equilibrium is

$$J(\mathcal{E}_+) = \begin{pmatrix} -\beta i^* - \mu & -\beta s^* & 0 & \eta \\ \beta i^* & \beta s^* + \sigma\beta c^* - (\theta + m + \mu) & 0 & \sigma\beta i^* \\ 0 & (1-\sigma)\beta c^* + \theta & -(\mu+\delta) & (1-\sigma)\beta i^* \\ 0 & -\beta c^* & \delta & -\beta i^* - (\eta+\mu) \end{pmatrix}, \quad (19)$$

with characteristic equation

$$\lambda^4 + a_1\lambda^3 + a_2\lambda^2 + a_3\lambda + a_4 = 0. \quad (20)$$

Using Routh-Hurwitz stability criteria [31], the endemic equilibrium $\mathcal{E}_+$ is locally asymptotically stable provided that

$$a_i > 0, i = 1,2,3,4, \;\; a_1a_2 - a_3 > 0 \;\text{ and }\; a_1a_2a_3 - a_1^2a_4 - a_3^2 > 0. \quad (21)$$

This completes the proof.

3. Numerical method and simulations

Since most of the FODEs do not have exact analytic solutions, so approximation and numerical techniques must be used. In addition, most of resulting biological systems are stiff,[2] therefore, efficient use of a reliable numerical method for dealing with such problems is necessary. In this section, we provide an implicit scheme to approximate the solutions of the fractional-order epidemic model. We also verify that the approximate solution is stable and convergent.

Consider a biological system, with fractional-order, of the form

$$\begin{array}{lll} D^\alpha y(t) = f(t, y(t)), & t \in [0,T], & \\ y^{(k)}(0) = y^{(k)}(0), & k = 0,1,2,\ldots,m-1. & 0 < \alpha \le 1 \end{array} \quad (22)$$

Here, $y(t) = [y_1(t), y_2(t), \ldots, y_n(t)]^T$ and $f(t, y(t))$ satisfy the Lipschitz condition

$$\|f(t, y(t)) - f(t, x(t))\| \le K\|y(t) - x(t)\|, \quad K > 0, \quad (23)$$

where $x(t)$ is the solution of the perturbed system.

Theorem 2 *The FODE (22) has a unique solution if Lipschitz condition (23) is satisfied and*

[2]One definition of the stiffness is that the global accuracy of the numerical solution is determined by stability rather than local error and implicit methods are more appropriate for it.

$$M = \frac{KT^{\alpha}}{\Gamma(\alpha+1)} < 1. \tag{24}$$

Proof One can apply the fractional integral operator (given in the Appendix) to the differential Eq. (22) and incorporate the initial conditions. Thus, Eq. (22) can be expressed as

$$y(t) = \sum_{k=0}^{m-1} y_0^{(k)} \frac{t^k}{k!} + \frac{1}{\Gamma(\alpha)} \int_0^t (t-s)^{\alpha-1} f(s,y(s))ds. \tag{25}$$

which is a Volterra equation of the second kind. Define the operator $\mathscr{L}$, such that

$$\mathscr{L}y(t) = \sum_{k=0}^{m-1} y_0^{(k)} \frac{t^k}{k!} + \frac{1}{\Gamma(\alpha)} \int_0^t (t-s)^{\alpha-1} f(s,y(s))ds.. \tag{26}$$

Then, we have

$$\begin{aligned} \|\mathscr{L}y(t)-\mathscr{L}x(t)\| &\le \frac{1}{\Gamma(\alpha)} \int_0^t (t-s)^{\alpha-1} \|f(s,y(s))-f(s,x(s))\| ds \\ &\le \frac{K}{\Gamma(\alpha)} \int_0^t (t-s)^{\alpha-1} \sup_{s\in[0,T]} |y(s)-x(s)| ds \\ &\le \frac{K}{\Gamma(\alpha)} \|y-x\| \int_0^t s^{\alpha-1} ds \\ &\le \frac{KT^{\alpha}}{\Gamma(\alpha+1)} \|y-x\| T^{\alpha}. \end{aligned} \tag{27}$$

Then, we have

$$\|\mathscr{L}y(t)-\mathscr{L}x(t)\| \le M\|y-x\|. \tag{28}$$

Using the Banach contraction principle, we can prove that that $\mathscr{L}$ has a unique fixed point which means that the problem has a unique solution. □

Many efficient numerical methods have been proposed to solve the FODEs [14, 32]. Among them, the so-called predictor-corrector algorithm is a powerful technique for solving the FODEs, and considered as a generalization of the Adams-Bashforth-Moulton method. The modification of the Adams-Bashfourth-Moulton algorithm is proposed by Diethelm [14, 33–34] to approximate the fractional-order derivative. However, the converted Volterra integral equation (25) is with a weakly singular kernel, such that regularization is not necessary anymore. In our case, the kernel may not be continuous, and therefore the classical numerical algorithms for the integral part of Eq. (25) are unable to handle the solution of Eq. (22). Therefore, we implement the implicit Euler's scheme to approximate the fractional-order derivative.

Given fractional-order model (Eq. (22)) and mesh points $\mathcal{T} = \{t_0,t_1,\ldots,t_N\}$, such that $t_0 = 0$ and $t_N = T$. Then a discrete approximation to the fractional derivative can be obtained by a simple quadrature formula, using the Caputo fractional derivative (42) of order α, $0 < \alpha \le 1$, and using *implicit* Euler's approximation as follows (see [15]):

$$D_*^\alpha x_i(t_n) = \frac{1}{\Gamma(1-\alpha)} \int_0^t \frac{dx_i(s)}{ds} (t_n-s)^{-\alpha} ds$$

$$\approx \frac{1}{\Gamma(1-\alpha)} \sum_{j=1}^{n} \int_{(j-1)h}^{jh} \left[\frac{x_i^j - x_i^{j-1}}{h} + O(h) \right] (nh-s)^{-\alpha} ds$$

$$= \frac{1}{(1-\alpha)\Gamma(1-\alpha)} \sum_{j=1}^{n} \left[\frac{x_i^j - x_i^{j-1}}{h} + O(h) \right] [(n-j+1)^{1-\alpha} - (n-j)^{1-\alpha}]\} h^{1-\alpha} \quad (29)$$

$$= \frac{1}{(1-\alpha)\Gamma(1-\alpha)} \frac{1}{h^\alpha} \sum_{j=1}^{n} [x_i^j - x_i^{j-1}][(n-j+1)^{1-\alpha} - (n-j)^{1-\alpha}] +$$

$$\frac{1}{(1-\alpha)\Gamma(1-\alpha)} \sum_{j=1}^{n} [x_i^j - x_i^{j-1}][(n-j+1)^{1-\alpha} - (n-j)^{1-\alpha}] O(h^{2-\alpha}).$$

Setting

$$\mathcal{G}(\alpha,h) = \frac{1}{(1-\alpha)\Gamma(1-\alpha)} \frac{1}{h^\alpha}, \text{and } \omega_j^\alpha = j^{1-\alpha} - (j-1)^{1-\alpha}, \quad (\text{where } \omega_1^\alpha = 1), \quad (30)$$

then the first-order approximation method for the computation of Caputo's fractional derivative is then given by the expression

$$D_*^\alpha x_i(t_n) = \mathcal{G}(\alpha,h) \sum_{j=1}^{n} \omega_j^\alpha (x_i^{n-j+1} - x_i^{n-j}) + O(h). \quad (31)$$

From the above analysis and numerical approximation, one arrives at the following Remark.

Remark 1 *The presence of a fractional differential order in a differential equation can lead to a notable increase in the complexity of the observed behavior, and the solution continuously depends on all the previous states.*

3.1. Stability and convergence

Here, we prove that the suggested numerical scheme of implicit difference approximation (Eq. (31)) is unconditionally stable. It follows then that the numerical solution converges to the exact solution as $h \to 0$.

In order to study the stability of the numerical method, let us consider a test problem of linear scaler fractional differential equation

$$D_*^\alpha u(t) = \rho_0 u(t) + \rho_1, \quad u(0) = u_0. \quad (32)$$

such that $0 < \alpha \le 1$, and $\rho_0 < 0$, $\rho_1 > 0$ are constants.

Theorem 3 *The fully implicit numerical approximation (31), to test problem (32) for all $t \geq 0$, is consistent and unconditionally stable.*

Proof We assume that the approximate solution of Eq. (32) is of the form $u(t_n) \approx U^n \equiv \zeta_n$, then Eq. (32) can be reduced to

$$\left(1-\frac{\rho_0}{G_{\alpha,h}}\right)\zeta_n = \zeta_{n-1} + \sum_{j=2}^{n} \omega_j^{(\alpha)} (\zeta_{n-j}-\zeta_{n-j+1}) + \rho_1/G_{\alpha,h}\,, \qquad n \geq 2. \tag{33}$$

Or

$$\zeta_n = \frac{\zeta_{n-1} + \sum_{j=2}^{n} \omega_j^{(\alpha)} (\zeta_{n-j}-\zeta_{n-j+1}) + \rho_1/G_{\alpha,h}}{(1-\frac{\rho_0}{G_{\alpha,h}})}, \qquad n \geq 2. \tag{34}$$

Since $\left(1-\frac{\rho_0}{G_{\alpha,h}}\right) \geq 1$ for all $G_{\alpha,h}$, then

$$\zeta_1 \leq \zeta_0, \tag{35}$$

$$\zeta_n \leq \zeta_{n-1} + \sum_{j=2}^{n} \omega_j^{(\alpha)} (\zeta_{n-j}-\zeta_{n-j+1}), \qquad n \geq 2. \tag{36}$$

Thus, for $n = 2$, the above inequality implies

$$\zeta_2 \leq \zeta_1 + \omega_2^{(\alpha)} (\zeta_0-\zeta_1). \tag{37}$$

Using the inequality (35) and the positivity of the coefficients ω_2, one gets

$$\zeta_2 \leq \zeta_1. \tag{38}$$

Repeating the process, we have from Eq. (36)

$$\zeta_n \leq \zeta_{n-1} + \sum_{j=2}^{n} \omega_j^{(\alpha)} (\zeta_{n-j}-\zeta_{n-j+1}) \leq \zeta_{n-1}. \tag{39}$$

Since each term in the summation is negative. Thus $\zeta_n \leq \zeta_{n-1} \leq \zeta_{n-2} \leq \ldots \leq \zeta_0$. With the assumption that $\zeta_n = |U^n| \leq \zeta_0 = |U^0|$, which entails $\|U^n\| \leq \|U_0\|$ and we have stability.

The above numerical technique can then be used both for both linear and nonlinear problems, and it may be extended to multiterm FODEs.

3.2. Numerical simulations

The approximate solutions of epidemic model (2) are displayed in **Figures 2–4**, and sensitivity of $\mathcal{R}_0$ to transmission coefficients is displayed in **Figure 5**. The numerical simulations are performed by Euler's implicit scheme discussed in Section 3. We choose different fractional-order values ($0.5 < \alpha < 1$), and parameter values given in **Table 1**. The displayed solutions in **Figure 4** confirm that the fractional order of the derivative plays the role of time-delay (or memory) in the system.

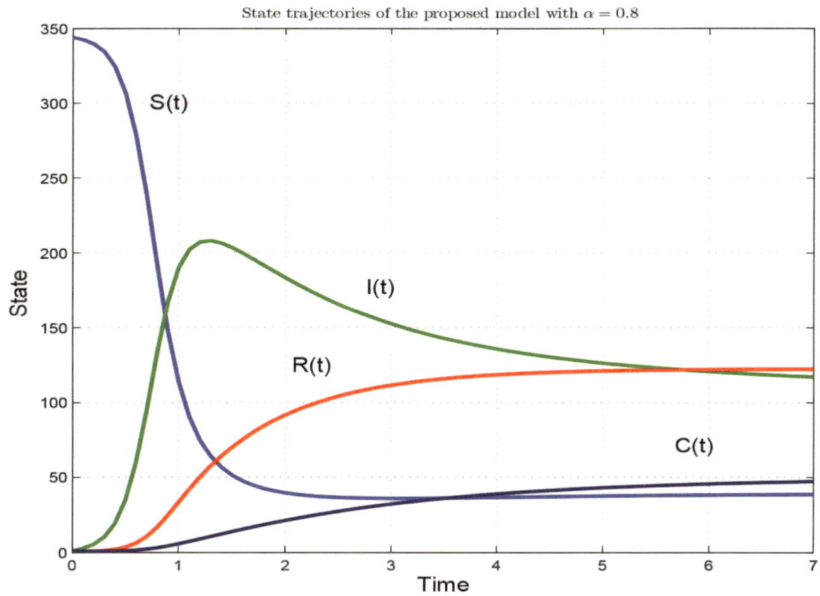

Figure 2. Numerical simulation of the fractional-order epidemic model (2), when $\alpha = 0.8$, and $\mathcal{R}_0 > 1$ (Each infected individual infects more than one other member of the population and a self-sustaining group of infectious individuals will propagate), with parameter values of **Table 1**.

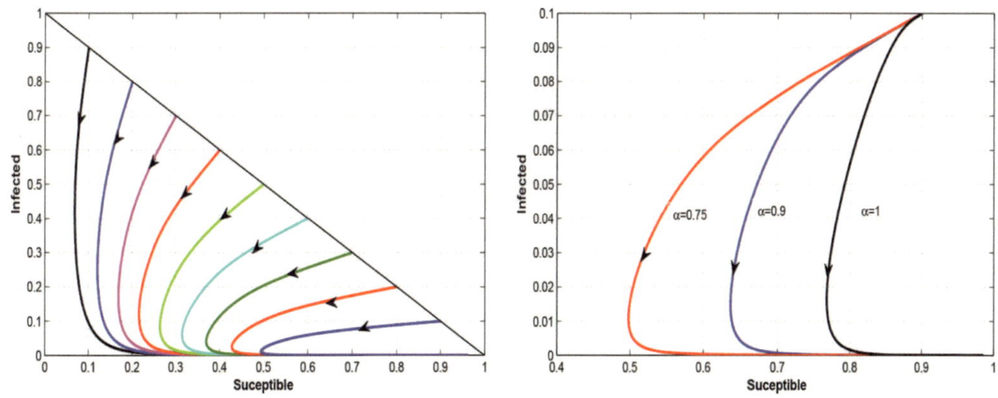

Figure 3. Phase plane portrait for the fractional-order endemic model (2), in absence of $C(t)$ and $R(t)$ components, when $\alpha = 0.7$ (left) and $\alpha = 0.9$ (right) with $\mathcal{R}_0 = 0.5 < 1$. We note that solution paths approach the disease-free equilibrium $\mathcal{E}_0 = (1, 0, 0)$.

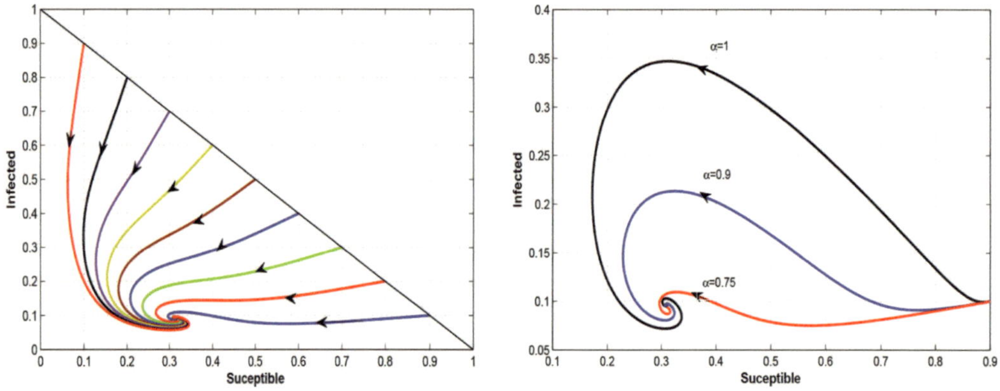

Figure 4. Phase plane portrait for the classic fractional-order endemic model (2) when $\alpha = 1$ (left) and $\alpha = 0.9$ (right) with $\mathcal{R}_0 = 1.2 > 1$. We note that solution paths approach the endemic equilibrium $\mathcal{E}_+$ given by Eq. (5).

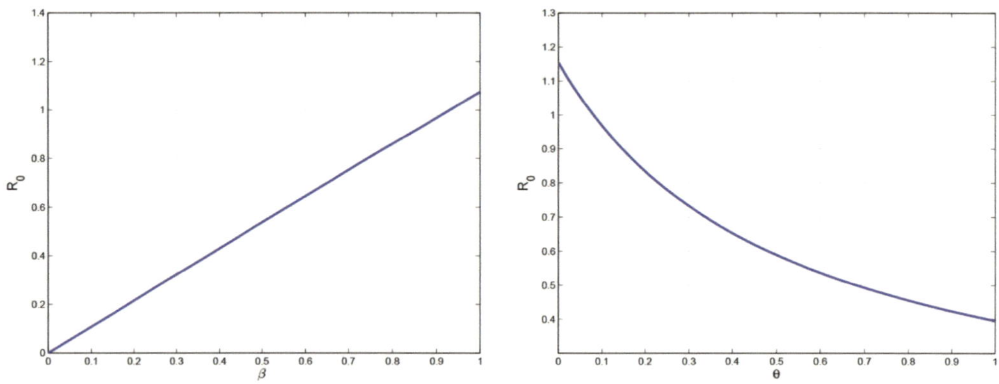

Figure 5. Sensitivity of $\mathcal{R}_0$ with respect to the transmission coefficients β and θ.

Parameter	Description	Value	Reference
μ	Replacement and exit rate (day^{-1})	0.011	[35]
β	Transmission rate of susceptible to be infected (animal^{-1} day^{-1})	0.15	[35]
θ	Recovery rate of infected animals day^{-1}	0.16	Assumed
m	Disease-induced mortality rate (day^{-1})	0.041	Assumed
η	Cross-immune period	0.5	[36]
σ	The average reinfection probability of $C(t)$	0.06	Assumed
δ	The average time of appearance of new dominant clusters	1	Assumed
N	The total number of population	345	Assumed

Table 1. List of parameters.

4. Discussion and conclusion

In this chapter, we provided a fractional-order SIRC epidemic model with *Salmonella* infection. The model provides a comprehensive framework for understanding the disease transmission behaviors, as well as for evaluating the effectiveness of different intervention strategies. We derived the sufficient conditions to preserve the asymptotical stability of disease-free and endemic steady states. The threshold parameter (reproduction number) $\mathcal{R}_0$ has been evaluated in terms of contact rate, recovery rate, and other parameters in the model. The threshold parameter $\mathcal{R}_0$ is very sensitive to transmission coefficients β and θ that reflects that these parameters play an important role to assess the strength of the medical and behavioral interventions necessary for control. We provided an unconditionally stable method, using Euler's implicit method for the fractional-order differential system. The solution of a fractional-order model at any time t^* continuously depends on all the previous states at $t \leq t^*$.

It has been found that fractional-order dynamical models are more suitable to model biological systems with memory than their integer-orders. The presence of a fractional differential order into a corresponding differential equation leads to a notable increase in the complexity of the observed behavior. However, fractional-order differential models are as stable as their integer-order counterpart.

Acknowledgements

This work was supported by UAE University (NRF Project UAEU-NRF-7-20886).

Appendix

Let $L^1 = L^1[a,b]$ be the class of Lebesgue integrable functions on $[a,b]$, $a < b < \infty$.

Definition 1 *The fractional integral of order* $\beta \in \mathbb{R}^+$ *of the function* $f(t)$, $t > 0$ $(f : \mathbb{R}^+ \to \mathbb{R})$ *is defined by*

$$I_a^{\nu} f(t) = \int_a^t \frac{(t-s)^{\nu-1}}{\Gamma(\nu)} f(s) ds, \quad t > 0. \tag{40}$$

The fractional derivative of order $\alpha \in (n-1,n)$ *of* $f(t)$ *is defined by two ways:*

- *Riemann-Liouville fractional derivative: Take fractional integral of order* $(n-\alpha)$ *and then take* n^{th} *derivative,*
- *Caputo fractional derivative: Take* n^{th} *derivative and then take a fractional integral of order* $(n-\alpha)$

$$D_a^{\alpha} f(t) = D_a^n I_a^{n-\alpha} f(t), \quad D_*^n = \frac{d^n}{dt^n}, \quad n = 1, 2, \ldots \tag{41}$$

$$D_a^{\alpha} f(t) = I_a^{n-\alpha} D_a^n f(t), \quad n = 1, 2, \ldots. \tag{42}$$

We notice that the definition of time-fractional derivative of a function $f(t)$ at $t = t_n$ involves an integration and calculating time-fractional derivative that requires all the past history, i.e., all the values of $f(t)$ from $t = 0$ to $t = t_n$. Caputo's definition, which is a modification of the Riemann-Liouville definition, has the advantage of dealing properly with initial value problems. The following Remark addresses some of the main properties of the fractional derivatives and integrals (see [12, 36–39]).

Remark 2 *Let* $v, \gamma \in \mathbb{R}^+$ *and* $\alpha \in (0,1)$. *Then*

i. *If* $I_a^v : L^1 \to L^1$ *and* $f(t) \in L^1$, *then* $I_a^v I_a^\gamma f(t) = I_a^{v+\gamma} f(t)$;

ii. $\lim_{v\to n} I_a^v f(x) = I_a^n f(t)$ *uniformly on* $[a,b]$, $n = 1,2,3,\ldots$, *where* $I_a^1 f(t) = \int_0^t f(s)ds$;

iii. $\lim_{v\to 0} I_a^v f(t) = f(t)$ *weakly;*

iv. *If* $f(t)$ *is absolutely continuous on* $[a,b]$, *then* $\lim_{\alpha\to 1} D_*^\alpha f(t) = \frac{df(t)}{dt}$;

v. *Thus* $D_*^\alpha f(t) = \frac{d}{dt} I_*^{1-\alpha} f(t)$ *(Riemann-Liouville sense) and* $D_*^\alpha f(t) = I_*^{1-\alpha} \frac{d}{dt} f(t)$ *(Caputo sense).*

The generalized mean value theorem and another property are defined in the following Remark [40].

Remark 3

i. *Suppose* $f(t) \in C[a,b]$ *and* $D_*^\alpha f(t) \in C(a,b]$ *for* $0 < \alpha \leq 1$, *then we have*

$$f(t) = f(a) + \frac{1}{\Gamma(\alpha)} D_*^\alpha f(\xi)(t-a)^\alpha, \quad \text{with } a < \xi < t \quad \forall\, t \in (a,b]. \tag{43}$$

ii. *If (i) holds, and* $D_*^\alpha f(t) \geq 0 \ \forall\, t \in [a,b]$, *then* $f(t)$ *is nondecreasing for each* $t \in [a,b]$. *If* $D_*^\alpha f(t) \leq 0$ $\forall\, t \in [a,b]$, *then* $f(t)$ *is nonincreasing for each* $t \in [a,b]$.

Author details

Fathalla A. Rihan

Address all correspondence to: frihan@uaeu.ac.ae

Department of Mathematical Sciences, College of Science, UAE University, Al Ain, United Arab Emirates

References

[1] L. Qin, S. X. Yang, A.-H. Meng, A mathematical model with degree of risk for Salmonella infections, IEEE International Conference on Systems, Man and Cybernetics, Montreal, Que., 2007, pp. 2704–2709.

[2] F. A. Rihan, D. Baleanu, S. Lakshmanan, R. Rakkiyappan, On fractional SIRC model with Salmonella bacterial infection, Abstr. Appl. Anal. 2014 (2014) 1–9.

[3] B. K. Al Ramadi, M. Fernandez-Cabezudo, H. El-Hasasna, S. Al-Salam, G. Bashir, S. Chouaib, Potent anti-tumor activity of systemically-administered IL2-expressing Salmonella correlates with decreased angiogenesis and enhanced tumor apoptosis, Clin. Immunol. 130 (2009) 89–97.

[4] B. K. Al Ramadi, M. Fernandez-Cabezudo, A. Ullah, H. El-Hasasna, R. Flavell, CD154 is essential for protective immunity in experimental Salmonella infection: evidence for a dual role in innate and adaptive immune responses, J. Immunol. 176 (2006) 496–506.

[5] G. Jones, S. Le Hello, N. Jourdan-da Silva, V. Vaillant, H. de Valk, FX Weill, Y. Le Strat. The French human Salmonella surveillance system: evaluation of timeliness of laboratory reporting and factors associated with delays, 2007 to 2011. Euro Surveill. 19(1) 2014, 1–10.

[6] F. A. Rihan, A. Hashish, F. Al-Maskari, M. Sheek-Hussein, E. Ahmed, M. B. Riaza, R. Yafia, Dynamics of tumor-immune system with fractional-order, J. Tumor Res. 2(1) (2016) 109.

[7] F. Mainardi, R. Gorenflo, On mittag-leffler-type functions in fractional evolution processes, J. Comput. Appl. Math. 118 (2000) 283–299.

[8] W.-C. Chen, Nonlinear dynamics and chaos in a fractional-order financial system, Chaos, Solitons Fractals. 36(5) (2008) 1305–1314.

[9] L. Debnath, Recent applications of fractional calculus to science and engineering, Int. J. Math. Math. Sci. 54 (2003) 3413–3442.

[10] A. El-Sayed, Nonlinear functional differential equations of arbitrary orders, Nonlinear Anal. Theo. Methods Appl. 33(2) (1998) 181–186.

[11] A. El-Sayed, A. El-Mesiry, H. El-Saka, On the fractional-order logistic equation, Appl. Math. Lett. 20(7) (2007) 817–823.

[12] E. R. Hilfer, *Applications of Fractional Calculus in Physics*, River Edge, USA: World Scientific, 2000.

[13] F. A. Rihan, Numerical modeling of fractional-order biological systems, Abst. Appl. Anal. 2013 (2013) 11.

[14] K. Diethelm, N. Ford, A. Freed, A predictor-corrector approach for the numerical solution of fractional differential equations, Nonlinear Dynam. 29 (2002) 3–22.

[15] F. A. Rihan, Computational methods for delay parabolic and time fractional partial differential equations, Num. Meth. Partial Diff. Eqns. 26(6) (2010) 1556–1571.

[16] S. Bhalekar, V. Daftardar-Gejji, Synchronization of different fractional order chaotic systems using active control, Commun. Nonlinear Sci. Numer. Simulat. 15 (2010) 3536–3546.

[17] L. Edelstein-Keshet., *Mathematical Models in Biology*, New York: Random House, 1988.

[18] D. S. Jones, M. J. Plank, B. D. Sleeman, Differential Equations and Mathematical Biology, *Mathematical and Computational Biology*, NewYork: Chapman & Hall/CRC, 2008.

[19] D. Kaplan, L. Glass, *Understanding Nonlinear Dynamics*, New York: Springer-Verlag, 1995.

[20] J. Murray, *Mathematical Biology II*, New York: Springer, 2003.

[21] M. Safan, F. A. Rihan, Mathematical analysis of an SIS model with imperfect vaccination and backward bifurcation, Math. Comput. Simul. 96 (2014) 195–206.

[22] F. A. Rihan, *Numerical Treatment of Delay Differential Equations in Bioscience*, PhD. Thesis, University of Manchester (UK), 2000.

[23] W. O. Kermack, A. G. McKendrick, Contributions to the mathematical theory of epidemics, Proc. R. Soc. Lond. 115 (1927) 700–721.

[24] R. Casagrandi, L. Bolzoni, S. A. Levin, V. Andreasen, The SIRC model and influenza A, Math. Biosci. 200 (2006) 152–169.

[25] M. El-Shahed, A. Alsaedi, The fractional SIRC model and influenza A, Math. Probl. Eng. 2011 (2011) 9.

[26] L. Jodar, R. J. Villanueva, A. J. Arenas, G. C. G. alez, Nonstandard finite difference method by nonlocal approximation, Math. Comput. Simul. 79 (2008) 622–633.

[27] F. A. Rihan, S. Lakshmanan, A. Hashish, R. Rakkiyappan, E. Ahmed, Fractional order delayed predator-prey systems with Holling type-II functional response, Nonlinear Dynam. 80 (1) (2015) 777–789.

[28] H. Smith, *An Introduction to Delay Differential Equations with Applications to the Life Sciences*, New York, Dordrecht, Heidelberg, London: Springer, 2011.

[29] G. Marchuk, *Mathematical Modelling of Immune Response in Infectious Diseases*, Dordrecht: Kluwer Academic Publishers, 1997.

[30] O. Diekmann, J. Heesterbeek, J. Metz, On the definition and the computation of the basic reproduction ratio $\mathcal{R}_0$ in models for infectious diseases in heterogeneous populations, J. Math. Biol. 28 (1990) 365.

[31] E. Ahmed, A. El-Sayed, H. A. El-Saka, On some routh–hurwitz conditions for fractional order differential equations and their applications in Lorenz, Rössler, Chua and Chen systems, Phys. Lett. A 356 (2006) 1–4.

[32] R. Anguelov, J. M.-S. Lubuma, Nonstandard finite difference method by nonlocal approximation, Math. Comput. Simul. 61 (2003) 465–475.

[33] K. Diethelm, An algorithm for the numerical solution of differential equations of fractional order, Elec. Trans. Numer. Anal. 5 (1997) 1–6.

[34] K. Diethelm, N. J. Ford, Analysis of fractional differential equations, J. Math. Anal. Appl. 265 (2002) 229–48.

[35] P. Chapagain, J. S. V. Kessel, J. K. Karns, et. al., A mathematical model of the dynamics of salmonella cerro infection in a us dairy herd, Epidemiol. Infect. 136 (2008) 263–272.

[36] I. Podlubny, *Fractional Differential Equations*, New York: Academic Press, 1999.

[37] S. Samko, A. Kilbas, O. Marichev, *Fractional Integrals and Derivatives*, USA: Gordon and Breach Sciences Publishers, 1993.

[38] A. A. Kilbas, H. M. Srivastava, J. J. Trujillo, *Theory and Applications of Fractional Differential Equations, North-HollandMathematical Studies*, Vol. 204, Amsterdam: Elsevier, 2006.

[39] D. Baleanu, K. Diethelm, E. Scalas, J. J. Trujillo, Fractional calculus models and numerical methods, USA: World Scientific, 2012.

[40] Z. Odibat, N. Shawagfeh, Generalized taylor's formula, Appl. Math. Comput. 186 (2007) 286–293.

Section 4

Risk Factors and Control Strategies

Chapter 10

Interaction between *Salmonella* and Plants: Potential Hosts and Vectors for Human Infection

Eva Fornefeld, Jasper Schierstaedt, Sven Jechalke,
Rita Grosch, Kornelia Smalla and Adam Schikora

Additional information is available at the end of the chapter

http://dx.doi.org/10.5772/67061

Abstract

Fruits and vegetables are important for a healthy diet. However, when eaten raw and contaminated with human pathogens (HPs) they may cause a disease outbreak. Contamination with HPs can occur along the entire farm-to-fork production chain and *Salmonella enterica* is one of the most common foodborne pathogens. A range of biotic and abiotic environmental factors can influence the complex interactions between *Salmonella* and plants. Moreover, the outcome of experiments largely depends on the experimental design and parameters or methods employed, and on top, on the accompanying plant microbiome and the genetic equipment of the plant and the *Salmonella* strain. Particularly mobile genetic elements contribute to the diversification and adaptation of *Salmonella* to the plant environment. So far, little is known about the key processes and factors influencing the attachment and potential internalization of *Salmonella* in plants and the plant specific responses. It is therefore important to better understand the ecology of *Salmonella* in the soil and plant environment, in order to propose practicable recommendations for prevention of foodborne diseases. This also requires improved sensitivity and specificity of detection methods. In this chapter, we present the current knowledge, research needs, and methodology regarding the complex interactions between *Salmonella* and plants.

Keywords: *Salmonella enterica*, plant, biofilm, colonization mechanisms, interaction

1. Introduction

The natural microbiome of plants includes a wide diversity of microorganisms and is a key determinant of plant health and productivity, e.g., by supporting the uptake of mineral nutrients in roots or suppressing pathogen growth and inducing the host-immune system [1–3]. Due to its relevance, the plant microbiome (totality of microorganisms associated with the plant) is even called the second plant genome. Because of the tight interplay between plants and their epiphytic and endophytic microorganisms the terms holobiont and meta-organisms are used as well. The plant microbiome is important not only for plant growth and health, but is also positively influencing human health [4]. However, besides positive effects on human health plants can also be carriers of bacterial HPs.

Salmonella is one of the major causal agents of foodborne gastroenteritis and represents a major threat to public health. It is estimated that each year 93.8 million cases of salmonellosis occur globally (86% of which foodborne), with 155,000 deaths [5]. Consumption of raw plants is more and more recognized as a source for HPs and associated with disease outbreaks in several countries. The number of outbreaks linked to fresh produce, spices, and nuts surpassed those linked to foods of animal origin [6]. Sources of HPs in the production chain and factors contributing to the contamination of fruits and vegetables include for example the application of organic fertilizers such as animal manures, contaminated irrigation water, insect and animal vectors but also the use of contaminated seeds [7]. *Enterobacteriaceae* such as *Erwinia, Serratia,* and *Pantoea* belong to bacteria typically associated with the phyllosphere [8–10]. However, it is not completely understood how *Salmonella* persists in the plant environment and which environmental factors trigger its survival. In this chapter, we discuss factors influencing the survival of *Salmonella* in the agricultural environment as well as adaptations that allow successful colonization of plants, such as attachment, biofilm formation, and internalization.

2. Contamination of fresh produce

Besides contaminated animal products, *Salmonella* outbreaks are increasingly associated with fruits and vegetables. Already on the field, plants may be contaminated via soil or irrigation, especially if watered with surface water [11–14]. *Salmonella* has been shown to persist in various ecological niches in soil as well as in irrigation water and fertilizers [15–17]. In this context, the watering system and the agricultural practices seem to play a key role in the prevention of contamination with human pathogens. For instance, lettuce plants were more likely to be contaminated with *Escherichia coli* when watered using overhead sprinklers when compared to subsurface drip or surface furrow irrigation [18]. Besides, even noncontaminated rain-sized water droplets could transfer HPs from contaminated soil or plants to other plants [19].

Organic fertilizers like manure, biogas plant digestates and sewage sludge offer an additional route for contamination of fresh produce. Similarly, animals like birds, game, mice, or insects can contribute to the contamination of fresh produce directly or indirectly via feces or irrigation water [7, 14, 20]. Often underestimated are soil particles, which can be carried by the wind over long distances and contribute to the transient of microbiome between plants [8]. Hence, wind-caused spread of HPs should also be considered. Contaminated plant residues might constitute additional risk if incorporated into soil before the planting of next crop.

The infection of plants is essentially dependent on the ability of HPs to survive and persist in the agricultural environment. *Salmonella*, for example, was shown to survive in soil for more than 200 days if the soil was fertilized [21, 22]. The survival of diverse bacteria newly introduced into soil has been subject of research for many years [23], and the mechanisms that govern this process, compared often to microbial invasion, were described in many studies (recently reviewed by [24]). In order to survive in the soil, HPs need to find an adequate ecological niche in which they can establish. Furthermore, their ability to do so and to survive for extended time increased when the indigenous microbial community was reduced as a result of, for example, sterilization [25]. In addition, the survival of microorganisms that successfully invaded the soil is highly dependent on the environmental heterogeneity [26–28].

Contamination of fresh produce with HPs like *Salmonella,* can occur before the harvest and also along the whole production chain [11, 14]. Since the epidemiological investigations start very often long time after the contamination or the harvest, it is very challenging to assess whether the contamination took place in the field or occurred "post-harvest" during the processing. Consequently in the majority of cases, the information available does not necessarily reveal the real causes of contamination [29].

3. Epidemiology of *Salmonella* in agricultural systems

Fresh produce contaminated with *Salmonella* can easily trigger a salmonellosis outbreak, and despite the difficulties with identification, in the past years fresh produce were repeatedly identified as the outbreak source. Among the outbreaks in the USA, *Salmonella* is the leading cause of the fresh produce-originated foodborne diseases [30]. The available data are depending on the procedures and records in particular countries. At least 12 large, fresh produce-related *Salmonella* outbreaks have been reported since 2010, an overview of international outbreaks with more than 100 associated cases is presented in **Table 1**.

Although fruits and vegetables were identified as source of human pathogens, it is not clear whether the plants were colonized in the field or during processing. *Salmonella* may live epiphytically or be internalized through wounds, the root system, stomata, or hydathodes (see below). Additionally, *Salmonella* can be entrapped in fruits or seeds after contamination of flowers [31, 32]. Moreover, large outbreaks can be destructive to consumer's confidence which results in economic losses [33, 34]. Therefore, the research on the ecology of HPs like *Salmonella* in relation to farming and harvesting practices is very important for human health and also for the economy.

4. Factors influencing the survival of *Salmonella* in soil

Successful establishment of human pathogenic bacteria in soil depends on a variety of biotic and abiotic factors (see **Figure 1** for an overview). Numerous studies, carried out under different conditions, showed that among them are weather or atmospheric conditions like tem-

Salmonella Serovar	Vector	Year	Country	Cases/serovar confirmed	Reference
S. Newport	Tomatoes	2015	USA	115/81	[112]
S. Poona	Cucumbers	2015-16	USA	907/907	[113]
Unknown	Onions, tomatoes	2015	USA	200/0	[114]
S. Enteriditis	Sprouts, beans	2014	USA	115/0	[113]
S. Newport	Cucumbers	2014	USA	275/0	[113]
S. Typhimurium	Cantaloupe	2012	USA	261/261	[115]
S. Braenderup	Mangoes	2012	USA, Canada	127/0	[113]
S. Newport	Mung beans	2011	Germany, The Netherlands	106/32	[116]
Unknown	Produce-based salads, broccoli salad	2011	Japan	1500/0	[117]
S. Agona	Fruit, papaya	2011	USA	106/0	[113]
S. I4,[5],12:i:-	Vegetables, sprouts, alfalfa sprouts	2010	USA	140/0	[118]
S. Hvittingfoss	Vegetables, leafy greens, lettuce, fruit, tomatoes, olives	2010	USA	114/108	[119]

Only large outbreaks with more than 100 associated total or confirmed cases since 2010 are shown.

Table 1. International salmonellosis outbreaks associated with fresh produce.

perature, UV radiation, and moisture content of the soil [7, 35]. In general, temperature has an important effect on growth and decay rates of bacteria. Most studies examined the influence of temperature on survival of enteric bacteria under isothermal conditions, showing a generally reduced survival of *Salmonella* in soil with increasing temperature and, accordingly a better persistence in soil at lower temperatures [36, 37]. Semenov et al. [38] analyzed how temperature fluctuations affect *Salmonella enterica* serovar Typhimurium (*S.* Typhimurium) in cow manure and demonstrated increased decay rates with increasing amplitudes of daily oscillations. Besides temperature, water availability is a key factor for *Salmonella* to survive in the environment. Humidity in soil depends on rainfall and watering as well as on evaporation. Soil moisture also depends on soil properties like clay content or pore size. In general, it seems that survival of *Salmonella* in soil is promoted by high humidity while water shortage has a detrimental influence on persistence, probably due to drought stress [39–41]. The soil type and its physical and chemical characteristics have a strong influence on the fate of bacterial HPs. Those characteristics include texture and particle size distribution, which affect adsorption of *Salmonella* to soil particles. The soil type determines the extent of *Salmonella* leaching, if the bacteria are applied to the soil surface via contaminated slurry or manure as shown by Bech et al. [42]. In this study, percolation of *S.* Typhimurium was more pronounced in loamy

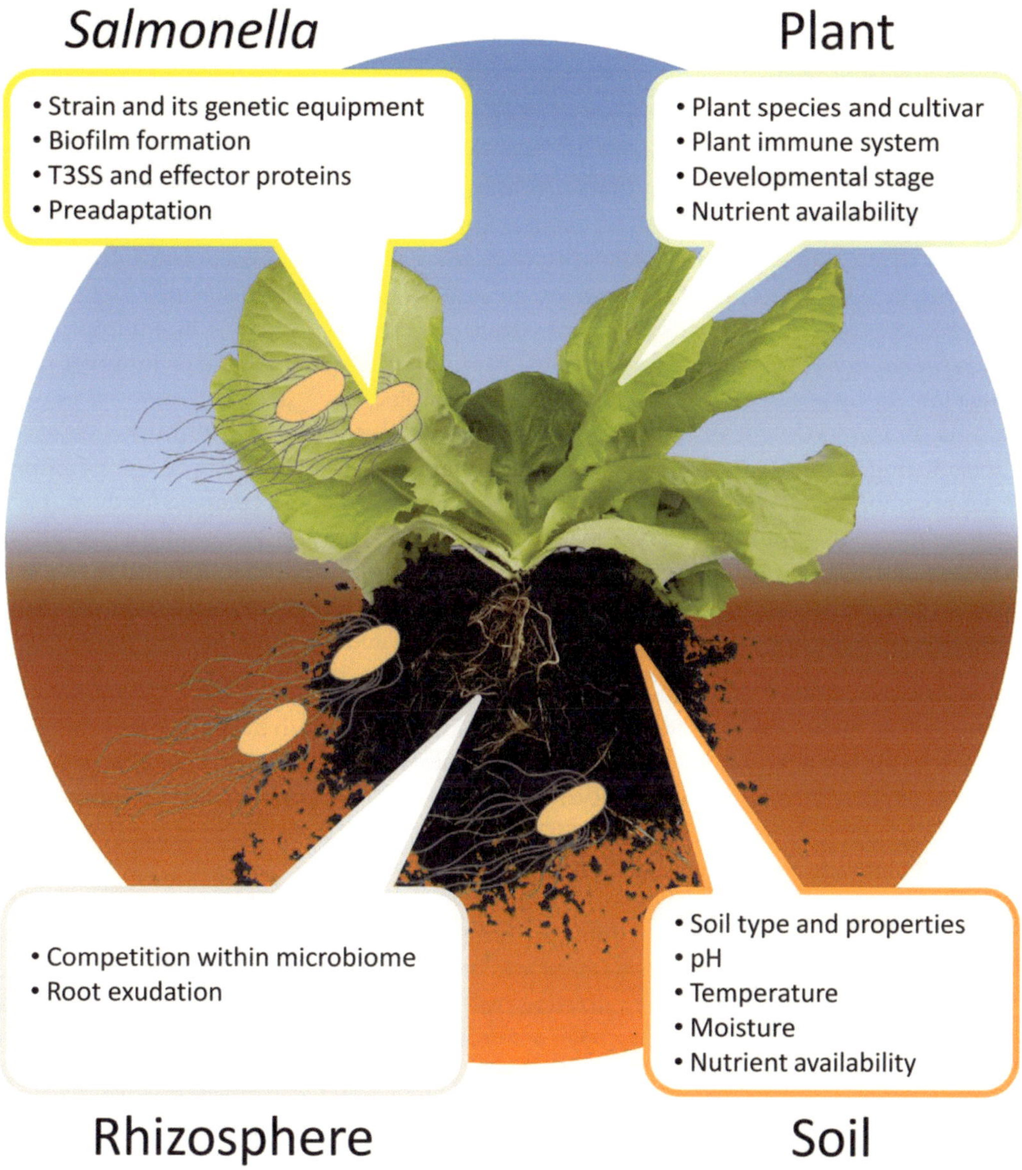

Figure 1. Factors influencing the survival of *Salmonella* in soil and its colonization of plants.

than in sandy soil with leaching bacteria reaching 1 m of depth at 10^5 CFU/ml of leachate. Transport and survival of bacterial pathogens in soil is also influenced by amendment of fertilizers probably because of the presence of organic matter [43]. Leaching of *Salmonella* through soil was observed to reach greater depths after application of slurry than of manure [44]. In the same line, the application method of fertilizers can also have an effect on *Salmonella* survival in soil since an injection of manure or slurry or clumping of the applied fertilizer aboveground protect bacteria in the soil from desiccation, UV, and high temperatures [43, 45, 46]. Agricultural practices like tillage that have an effect on the porosity of soil determine the extent of leaching [47] and the availability of oxygen. While a detrimental influence of aeration on survival of *E. coli* O157:H7 has been demonstrated, the oxygen availability does not influence the survival of *Salmonella* [48]. Soil pH is also an important factor for *Salmonella* survival and *Salmonella* can survive in the environment with neutral to acidic pH while alkaline pH has a detrimental effect on its persistence [49]. Another important determinant of *Salmonella* survival in soil is the availability of nutrients. In this environment, nutrients can only partly be used by bacterial HPs and are generally rather scarce. *Salmonella* is chemoheterotrophic and therefore depends on carbohydrates, lipids, and protein in its environment as sources for energy, nitrogen, and amino acids. Addition of organic fertilizers improves nutrient availability by addition of readily available carbon and nitrogen sources as well as other nutrients. But amendment of fertilizers also changes the microbiological properties of soil by introducing microorganisms to the soil microbial community. Moreover, the additional nutrients stimulate growth of copiotrophic soil bacteria which might compete for the nutrient resources [50]. So far, no clear correlations between the type of fertilizer and survival in soil have been identified [51]. But when survival in manure was compared to survival in manure-amended soil, *Salmonella* usually survived better in soil [22]. This could be due to competition by the microbial flora of manure, which is more concentrated than in soil.

The soil microbial community and its composition have a great influence on the survival of *Salmonella* [52]. In the soil ecosystem, *Salmonella* has to compete with the indigenous microbial community for space and nutrients [24]. For example, it was shown that *Salmonella enterica* serovar Newport (*S.* Newport) survived about 10 weeks longer in sterilized soil compared to nonsterilized manure-amended soil [22]. Similarly, a better survival was found in γ-irradiated than in untreated soil [53]. These results indicate suppression by the native microbial community. Overall, results demonstrate the importance of the microbial community affecting the fate of *Salmonella* in soil. Plant pathogens, fungi, viruses, and animal pests present in the environment can degrade the plant material and increase the content of available nutrients or provide entry sites facilitating internalization into plants [7, 14, 54]. They may also serve as vectors [7, 55]. Effects of protists have been analyzed using protozoa showing that their presence can foster or reduce survival of different species. For example, *Salmonella enterica* serovar Thompson was accumulated in vesicles of *Tetrahymena* [56], while growth of protozoa can also decimate *S.* Typhimurium populations [37].

In addition to the environment in which *Salmonella* is introduced, the bacterial characteristics are crucial for persistence. Firstly, the genetic disposition of the strain, for example, the presence of type III secretion system (T3SS), the ability to form biofilms, chemotaxis, or motility are important. Studies using strains with mutations influencing these characteristics usually resulted in reduced survival [57–59]. *Salmonella* can also produce an *O*-antigen capsule, which improves survival under desiccation stress [60]. Furthermore, the ability to form biofilms enhances environmental persistence of some *Salmonella* serovars [61]. Similarly, a biofilm-producing *Salmonella* strain survived chlorination significantly better than the biofilm-deficient mutant [62]. The conditions under which *Salmonella* are grown before their inoculation in the environment are also important since preadaptation influences the persistence [20]. Finally,

http://dx.doi.org/10.5772/67061

many studies on the survival of HPs in soil employed a relatively high inoculum, which under natural conditions occurs only locally, e.g., by fecal point contaminations. Inoculation resulted in a fast initial decline of inoculated bacterial populations with usually low numbers of *Salmonella* that survive for a long time after the inoculation.

In conclusion, studies analyzing the survival of *Salmonella* demonstrated complex interactions with the environment and a network of factors, which might play an important role in the persistence of *Salmonella*. Therefore, the very often contradictory results reflect the variability of strains, their survival strategies in a complex environment as well as differences in experimental setups used.

5. Attachment to plant surfaces and biofilm formation

Attachment and adhesion of *Salmonella* to plant surfaces are essential steps of plant colonization. Several bacterial elements such as fimbrial structures, nonfimbrial adhesins, flagella, cellulose, and lipopolysaccharides (LPS) are important bacterial factors for colonization [63, 64]. Although previous studies demonstrated that the attachment depends on plant and bacterial factors, no single factor was found to be essential, suggesting that bacteria use several parallel mechanisms to ensure attachment to different plants or to different plant cells under a wide variety of conditions [65]. Furthermore, the attachment of *S. enterica* to plant surfaces appears to be serovar-dependent [66]. For example, the strength of the attachment to basil, lettuce, or spinach leaves differed between *S. enterica* serovars. While *S.* Typhimurium, *Salmonella enterica* serovar Enteritidis, and *Salmonella enterica* serovar Senftenberg were efficient, other serovars including *Salmonella enterica* serovar Agona, *Salmonella enterica* serovar Heidelberg or *Salmonella enterica* serovar *Arizonae* showed less attachment [67]. Clear differences in attachment were also observed in leaves of different age, for example, *S.* Typhimurium showed a better attachment to older compared to younger lettuce leaves [68]. Additionally, *S. enterica* serovars were reported to actively move toward plant roots, attracted by root exudates [69]. There, they are able to efficiently attach and to form biofilms at natural openings or wounds [70, 71].

Several other studies provided evidence for biofilm formation by *Salmonella* on plant surfaces [72]. Within biofilms, bacteria are generally well-protected against environmental stresses, antibiotics, and disinfectants. The importance of biofilms for the attachment of *Salmonella* to plants and their role in the persistence in plants was recently described by Yaron and Romling [65]. Biofilm formation of *Salmonella* is influenced by environmental conditions and is reported to be maximal under reduced nutrient availability, aerobic conditions, low osmolarity, and mid temperatures [73], which are characteristic for the plant surface. In contrast, it was shown *in vitro* that *S.* Typhimurium cells grown at 37°C, the temperature in the animal host, do not produce cellulose and fimbriae [64]. Furthermore, the *red dry and rough* (*rdar*) and the *smooth and white* (*saw*) morphotypes, regulated by the *agfD* promoter and defined by a combination of traits such as the presence of thin aggregative fimbriae (tafi), cellulose, and *O*-antigen capsule, might affect the dispersal of *Salmonella* in an agricultural environment [74]. In contrast to the *saw* morphotype, the *rdar* morphotype, isolated from tomato, showed better attachment to plant surfaces [74, 75]. Biofilm-producing *Salmonella* on parsley showed a higher resistance against disinfectants than the biofilm-deficient mutant. Furthermore, after a storage period of the plant, the cells that were able to produce the biofilm matrix were significantly more resistant to the disinfection treatment [62]. A screening of 6000 transposon mutants of *S.* Newport resulted in the identification of 20 mutants selected for reduced adherence to alfalfa sprouts [70]. Interestingly, these mutants contained insertions associated with genes, for example, for the surface-exposed aggregative fimbriae nucleator (*agfB*) and the general transcriptional regulator *rpoS*. The respective proteins have been reported to regulate the production of curly, cellulose, and other adhesins such as pili. Two other genes (STM0278 and STM0650) were identified as important factors for the colonization of alfalfa seedlings. Both play an important role in the formation of biofilms [76]. Furthermore, bacterial cellulose and curly were involved in the colonization of parsley with *S.* Typhimurium from irrigation water [77].

Although many factors influencing the colonization of plants were identified by *in vitro* experiments, a more detailed investigation of genes of *Salmonella* that are expressed during the colonization of plants is needed. New techniques for the isolation of mRNA from samples containing both plant and bacterial materials as well as for the quantitative PCR allow the analysis of the transcriptome and the identification of genes with related functions [78].

6. Internalization of *Salmonella* into plant tissues

An increasing number of salmonellosis outbreaks associated with plants shows that human pathogenic bacteria use plants as a niche for replication or as hosts and vectors for animal and human infection (**Table 1**). For a long time it was assumed that *Salmonella* rather survives on plant surfaces than colonizes the plant interior. This view has been challenged by recent reports. Today we know that *Salmonella* can actively enter and spread within the plant. Plants offer multiple entry possibilities for HPs; stomata, for example, were identified already a few years ago. Stomata are used for gas exchange between the surroundings and cells of the inner mesophyll layers, this is necessary for proper photosynthetic efficacy. They can close if a pathogen is recognized. Some pathogens, however, produce toxins (coronatine), which reopen stomata and therefore allow their use as gates for colonization of underlying tissues. *Salmonella* was shown to gather around the open stomata and enter the mesophyll tissue of lettuce leaves [58]. Similar to lettuce, a high incidence of internalization was observed in arugula leaves, while romaine and red-lettuce, as well as basil showed significantly lower internalization rates [79]. Interestingly, in this study parsley and tomato leaves showed only marginal internalization [79]. In addition to stomata, also hydratodes and trichomes allow an internalization of *Salmonella* into leaves [31, 80, 81]. Not only *Salmonella* or phytopathogenic bacteria use stomata as entry points, also other *Enterobacteriaceae,* for example *E. coli,* use similar strategies to access the plant's interior [82, 83]. Importantly to note is the fact that the preference to gather around open stomata manifests only in photosynthetically active leaves, and an artificial opening of the stomata at night has no effect on the bacterial behavior [58]. This observation is in line with the proposed hypothesis that those bacteria are in a direct competition for C- and N-sources with the native leaf microbiome [69, 71], and suggests a chemotaxis toward the newly synthesized products of the photosynthesis.

From the consumers' point of view, not only the internalization into leaves but also the translocation within the plant, e.g., toward fruits is important. In some crop plants, e.g., tomato, such translocation was detected [81]. The authors showed internalization into the tomato fruits when the entire plant was systemically colonized. Still, the colonization rates seemed rather low [81]. Nonetheless, in light of the persistent pathogenicity in animals after the passage through a plant host [84], the internalization mechanisms are of high interest. Some detailed mechanisms were already suggested. Erlacher and coworkers proposed one of those possible mechanisms: colonization of the niche below the cuticle layer of the epidermis [9]. Obviously such a behavior protects bacteria from the harsh conditions on the leaf surface (UV light, drought, and quick changes in temperature) but also from surface sterilization agents. Another strategy would be an intracellular lifestyle, which would resemble the strategy in the animal infection model. Until now, this possibility remains unverified, two reports postulated internalization into plant cells using *Arabidopsis* and tobacco systems [84, 85]. Yet, another helpful strategy is the efficient formation of biofilms, this strategy was discussed above and was reviewed by Yaron and Romling [65]. Only recently, it was discovered that particular *Salmonella* strains may avoid the recognition by the plant immune system [86], which would make them very well adapted colonizers (see below).

Many row eaten crop plants plants associated with salmonellosis outbreaks or food poisoning are usually grown in soil (lettuce, basil, parsley, etc.). In such cases the translocation from the potentially contaminated soil (through manure or irrigation water) via roots into the harvested and consumed plant parts is of enormous importance. Several reports assessed already this possibility and pointed at a very diverse picture with regard to pathogenic *E. coli* or *Salmonella*. Here the high heterogeneity with regard to colonization in the plant population is very remarkable [69, 87], usually about 20% of the plant population is colonized, however, this range may vary from 0 to 100% and strongly depends on plant species and bacterial strain [51, 69, 77, 88–90].

7. The function of T3SS and the role of plant immune system during the interactions between plant and *Salmonella*

Bacterial pathogens use T3SS and T4SS to inject so-called effector proteins directly into the cytoplasm of host cells. Those effectors are able to manipulate the host immune system and suppress the otherwise negative effects of defense responses. *Salmonella* uses two T3SS and more than 40 effectors in order to manipulate the immune system (perception mechanisms and signaling cascades) as well as the cytoskeleton of animal cells at different stages of the infection process [91]. Recent discoveries from others and our group imply that the mechanisms used in animal and plant hosts may resemble each other [59, 85, 86, 92–95]. The inoculation with the wild-type *Salmonella* strains and mutants in one or both of the T3SSs showed that functional secretion systems are required for efficient plant colonization [59, 85, 93]. Two observations allow such a conclusion: (1) The mutants had lower proliferation rates when compared to the respective wild type, which suggests that a functional T3SS helps with the colonization of plants; and (2) T3SS mutants induced stronger immune response of the host plant. Similar to animals or humans, plants respond to colonization of pathogenic bacteria inducing numerous immune responses, among others are oxidative burst and enhanced expression of *Pathogenesis Related* (*PR*) genes. Both were observed after inoculation with *Salmonella* and both were stronger if the inoculation was performed using mutants in T3SS [59, 85, 86]. Those results suggest that the wild-type strain is able to suppress the immune response. It is very plausible to think that this suppression is due to functional T3SS-dependent effector proteins. We know only little about their function in plant cells, since only two effectors (SseF and SpvC) were evaluated in this respect. SseF together with SseG are translocated into animal cells and are responsible for the establishment of the reproduction niche [96]. In plants, SseF induces the hypersensitive response (HR) [94]. Important is the fact that silencing of the suppressor of SGT1 eliminates the response to SseF, suggesting that this effector is recognized in R protein-dependent manner, which is the usual recognition method of pathogen effectors during the effector-triggered immunity (ETI). SpvC is a phosphothreonin lyase which dephosphorylates activated MAP kinases. Those kinases build a core compound in the signaling cascade leading from the perception of the pathogen on the cell surface to the transcriptional response at the chromatin level. Especially the trio MPK3, MPK4, and MPK6 plays an important role in plants [97], and is activated (phosphorylated) during the response to *Salmonella* [84]. SpvC interacts actively with the MPK6 and dephosphorylates this kinase, consequently abolishing the signal transduction [95]. A comprehensive overview of the reports regarding the plant immune responses to HPs was published only recently and is an excellent compendium of the current knowledge [98].

8. *Salmonella* changes its physiology in contact with plant host

During the interaction between *Salmonella* and crop plants, not only the plant reacts to the presence of the bacteria, also *Salmonella* adapts to the conditions represented by a plant organism. Recent results show that bacteria modify their physiology and motility in order to adjust to the physiological conditions occurring in plants. Several authors evaluated the transcriptional changes of bacteria when in contact with plants or plant-originated products [99, 100]. Interestingly, the analysis of the transcriptome, revealed a partial overlap between bacteria from macerated lettuce or cilantro leaves and bacteria from intestine, suggesting that those bacteria might be better adapted to the exploitation of plant material than estimated [100]. Similar results were observed for the pathogenic *E. coli* O157:H7, which seem to change its enzymatic and metabolomic equipment in order to utilize plant compounds [101, 102]. In addition, the bacteria upregulate a plethora of genes related to attachment, antimicrobial resistance and response to oxidative stress [101]. Very striking was the fact that although plant filtrates or root exudates contain numerous amino acids, which are available to the bacteria as C and N sources, *E. coli* induced many amino acid synthesis pathways probably to supplement the missing compounds [102].

9. Detection, characterization and quantification of *Salmonella* in environmental samples

Salmonella is rarely detected in crop plants. For example, in a previous study *Salmonella* could not be detected in more than 170 plants but in their environment [103]. This suggests that environmental factors are affecting the prevalence of *Salmonella* in the field, or that the sensitivity of the currently used detection system is not sufficient.

Traditional methods for the detection and identification of HPs often rely on cultivation-dependent techniques followed by biochemical and serological identification, which is typically time-consuming and laborious [104]. Furthermore, in response to environmental stresses *Salmonella* can enter a physiological state where the cells remain viable, but are no longer culturable on typically used growth media. *Salmonella* in this VBNC state are often only detectable by methods depending on nucleic acids. This highlights the importance of the complementary use of cultivation-dependent and -independent detection methods for the diagnosis and prevention of food contamination and foodborne diseases. In the recent decades, there have been increasing efforts to develop and improve molecular methods for the rapid detection and characterization of pathogens in animals and animal products [105–108]. These methods, which include immunological as well as biosensor- and nucleic acid-based assays (e.g., ELISA, PCR, microarrays, next generation sequencing) have an improved sensitivity and specificity but are also time-, cost-, and labor-demanding. Typically, to further increase the sensitivity of these methods nonselective or selective enrichment steps are employed. One of the most challenging problems is the sample preparation, which is strongly depending on the sample matrix, associated inhibitory compounds, and the bacterial load.

So far, knowledge is scarce regarding the specific and reliable detection of *Salmonella* in complex and often heterogenous plant- and environmental-matrices (e.g., vegetables, spices, soil samples, manure, biogas digestates) as well as the appropriate extraction and purification techniques. For iceberg lettuce, carrot- and cucumber-peelings, qPCR detection limits of 10^3 bacterial cells per gram were reported [109]. Since the infectious dose of *Salmonella* was reported to be less than 10^3 cells [110], small numbers have to be detected reliably. Besides direct extraction of total DNA from the sample material, a preceding enrichment step in the respective culture media can be performed. This enrichment has the advantage to increase the sensitivity of detection and additionally to reactivate cells in the dormant VBNC state. After extraction of DNA from the respective samples, *Salmonella* can be detected by qPCR or PCR-Southern blot hybridization, e.g., by detection of the *invA* gene [104, 111]. Alternatively or additionally to DNA-based methods, RNA-based methods can be used. Apart from a more laborious sample preparation, RNA-based methods have the advantage that in contrast to DNA-based methods only living and active *Salmonella* are detected, i.e., *Salmonella* relevant for a potential infection of humans. Especially the detection of mRNA of pathogenicity determinants could be appropriate to prove the viability and potential virulence of HPs.

Microarrays and next-generation sequencing technologies offer intriguing possibilities regarding the rapid and accurate detection as well as genetic characterization of *Salmonella* in environmental matrices. However, the costs and technical requirements for the analysis of large data sets still limit their practicability in the day-to-day qualitative and quantitative detection. The further development of rapid, reliable, and cost-effective high-throughput detection methods will very likely contribute to the understanding of the ecology of *Salmonella* in the plant environment and consequently help to reduce or prevent infections mediated by plant-associated HPs.

10. Conclusions

Today the notion that human pathogenic bacteria such as *Salmonella* might persist on or within plants in low numbers is widely accepted. The research on the interactions between crop or model plants and *Salmonella* is obviously driven by its medical aspects and the need for better prevention methods. We already know various features of the interactions but many are still not fully understood. New techniques that use high-throughput analyses and unbiased approaches are useful. Numerous national survey agencies started to use next-generation sequencing for the epidemiological analysis of salmonellosis outbreaks and have therefore direct access to the genome sequences of particular serovars. They are also able to monitor the genomic changes, for example, reception of new plasmids or pathogenicity islands, which are important prerequisites in virulence of the bacterial strain. Similarly, the full range of "omic" approaches is being used in model systems providing very detailed data on both partners in the *Salmonella*-plant interaction at biochemical, physiological, and transcriptional levels. The study of those interactions harbors even more potential, it permits the characterization of the different infection mechanisms and the different strategies available for *Salmonella* in contact with diverse hosts. New and more efficient prevention strategies greatly depend on our understanding of these mechanisms. Therefore, the new findings might significantly improve our possibilities to diminish the number of future outbreaks.

Acknowledgements

The authors would like to apologize to all colleagues whose work was not cited due to space limitation. This work was supported by the German Federal Environment Agency (Umweltbundesamt; 371271209), the JKI, and the Federal Office for Agriculture and Food (Bundesanstalt für Landwirtschaft und Ernährung, BLE), Grants 13HS026 and 13HS029.

http://dx.doi.org/10.5772/67061

Author details

Eva Fornefeld[1], Jasper Schierstaedt[2], Sven Jechalke[3], Rita Grosch[2], Kornelia Smalla[1] and Adam Schikora[1*]

*Address all correspondence to: adam.schikora@julius-kuehn.de

1 Julius Kühn-Institut, Federal Research Centre for Cultivated Plants (JKI), Institute for Epidemiology and Pathogen Diagnostics, Braunschweig, Germany

2 IGZ, Leibniz Institute of Vegetable and Ornamental Crops, Großbeeren, Germany

3 Institute of Phytopathology, JLU Gießen, Gießen, Germany

References

[1] Berendsen RL, Pieterse CM & Bakker PA. The rhizosphere microbiome and plant health. *Trends Plant Sci* 2012;**17**:478–486.

[2] Buee M, De Boer W, Martin F et al. The rhizosphere zoo: An overview of plant-associated communities of microorganisms, including phages, bacteria, archaea, and fungi, and of some of their structuring factors. *Plant Soil* 2009;**321**:189–212.

[3] Turner TR, James EK & Poole PS. The plant microbiome. *Genome Biol* 2013;**14**:10.

[4] Berg G, Grube M, Schloter M et al. The plant microbiome and its importance for plant and human health. *Front Microbiol* 2014;**5:491**.

[5] Majowicz SE, Musto J, Scallan E et al. The global burden of nontyphoidal *Salmonella* gastroenteritis. *Clin Infect Dis* 2010;**50**:882–889.

[6] Brandl MT, Cox CE & Teplitski M. Salmonella interactions with plants and their associated microbiota. *Phytopathology* 2013;**103**:316–325.

[7] Brandl MT. Fitness of human enteric pathogens on plants and implications for food safety. *Annu Rev Phytopathol* 2006;**44**:367–392.

[8] Rastogi G, Sbodio A, Tech JJ et al. Leaf microbiota in an agroecosystem: spatiotemporal variation in bacterial community composition on field-grown lettuce. *Isme Journal* 2012;**6**:1812–1822.

[9] Erlacher A, Cardinale M, Grube M et al. Biotic stress shifted structure and abundance of *Enterobacteriaceae* in the lettuce microbiome. *PLoS ONE* 2015;**10**:e0118068.

[10] van Overbeek LS, van Doorn J, Wichers JH et al. The arable ecosystem as battleground for emergence of new human pathogens. *Front Microbiol* 2014;**5**:17.

[11] Olaimat AN & Holley RA. Factors influencing the microbial safety of fresh produce: A review. *Food Microbiol* 2012;**32**:1–19.

[12] Allende A & Monaghan J. Irrigation water quality for leafy crops: A perspective of risks and potential solutions. *Int J Environ Res Public Health* 2015;**12**:7457–7477.

[13] Li B, Jackson SA, Gangiredla J et al. Genomic evidence reveals numerous Salmonella enterica serovar Newport reintroduction events in suwannee watershed irrigation ponds. *Appl Environ Microbiol* 2015;**81**:8243–8253.

[14] Jacobsen CS & Bech TB. Soil survival of *Salmonella* and transfer to freshwater and fresh produce. *Food Res Int* 2012;**45**:557–566.

[15] Barak JD & Liang AS. Role of soil, crop debris, and a plant pathogen in Salmonella enterica contamination of tomato plants. *PLoS One* 2008;**3**:e1657.

[16] Duffy EA, Lucia LM, Kells JM et al. Concentrations of *Escherichia coli* and genetic diversity and antibiotic resistance profiling of salmonella isolated from irrigation water, packing shed equipment, and fresh produce in texas. *J Food Protect* 2005;**1**:70–79.

[17] Miles JM, Sumner SS, Boyer RR et al. Internalization of *Salmonella enterica* serovar montevideo into greenhouse tomato plants through contaminated irrigation water or seed stock. *J Food Protect* 2009;**4**:696–914.

[18] Fonseca JM, Fallon SD, Sanchez CA et al. *Escherichia coli* survival in lettuce fields following its introduction through different irrigation systems. *J Appl Microbiol* 2011;**110**:893–902.

[19] Monaghan JM & Hutchison ML. Distribution and decline of human pathogenic bacteria in soil after application in irrigation water and the potential for soil-splash-mediated dispersal onto fresh produce. *J Appl Microbiol* 2012;**112**:1007–1019.

[20] Semenov AM, Kuprianov AA & van Bruggen AH. Transfer of enteric pathogens to successive habitats as part of microbial cycles. *Microb Ecol* 2010;**60**:239–249.

[21] Islam M, Morgan J, Doyle MP et al. Persistence of salmonella enterica serovar Typhimurium on lettuce and parsley and in soils on which they were grown in fields treated with contaminated manure composts or irrigation water. *Foodborne Pathog Dis* 2004;**1**:27–35.

[22] You Y, Rankin SC, Aceto HW et al. Survival of *Salmonella enterica* serovar Newport in manure and manure-amended soils. *Appl Environ Microbiol* 2006;**72**:5777–5783.

[23] Acea MJ, Moore CR & Alexander M. Survival and growth of bacteria introduced into soil. *Soil Biol Biochem* 1988;**20**:509–515.

[24] Mallon CA, Elsas JD & Salles JF. Microbial invasions: the process, patterns, and mechanisms. *Trends Microbiol* 2015;**23**:719–729.

[25] Mallon CA, Poly F, Le Roux X et al. Resource pulses can alleviate the biodiversity–invasion relationship in soil microbial communities. *Ecol Soc Am* 2015;**96**:915–926.

[26] Fierer N & Jackson RB. The diversity and biogeography of soil bacterial communities. *Proc Natl Acad Sci USA* 2006;**103**:626–631.

[27] Martiny JB, Bohannan BJM, Brown JH et al. Microbial biogeography: Putting microorganisms on the map. *Nat Rev Microbiol* 2006;**4**:102–112.

[28] Horner-Devine MC, Lage M, Hughes JB et al. A taxa–area relationship for bacteria. *Nature* 2004;**432**:750–753.

[29] Suslow TV, Oria MP, Beuchat LR et al. Production practices as risk factors in microbial food safety of fresh and fresh-cut produce. *Compr Rev Food Sci Food Saf* 2003;**2**:38–77.

[30] Hanning IB, Nutt JD & Ricke SC. Salmonellosis outbreaks in the united states due to fresh produce: Sources and potential intervention measures. *Foodborne Pathog Dis* 2009;**6**:635–648.

[31] Gu G, Cevallos-Cevallos JM & van Bruggen AH. Ingress of *Salmonella enterica* Typhimurium into tomato leaves through hydathodes. *PLoS One* 2013;**8**:e53470.

[32] Guo X, Chen J, Brackett RE et al. Survival of salmonellae on and in tomato plants from the time of inoculation at flowering and early stages of fruit development through fruit ripening. *Appl Environ Microbiol* 2001;**67**:4760–4764.

[33] WBG. The economic impact of ebola on sub-Saharan Africa: Updated estimates for 2015. 2015;1–17.

[34] Butler D. The next time the world is ill-prepared for the next epidemic or pandemic. But the horror of the ebola outbreak in West Africa may drive change. *Nature* 2015;**524**:22–25.

[35] Santamaría J & Toranzos GA. Enteric pathogens and soil: a short review. *Int Microbiol* 2003;**6**:5–9.

[36] Arrus KM, Holley RA, Ominski KH et al. Influence of temperature on *Salmonella* survival in hog manure slurry and seasonal temperature profiles in farm manure storage reservoirs. *Livest Sci* 2006;**102**:226–236.

[37] García R, Baelum J, Fredslund L et al. Influence of temperature and predation on survival of *Salmonella enterica* serovar Typhimurium and expression of *invA* in soil and manure-amended soil. *Appl Environ Microbiol* 2010;**76**:5025–5031.

[38] Semenov AV, van Bruggen AH, van Overbeek L et al. Influence of temperature fluctuations on *Escherichia coli* O157:H7 and *Salmonella enterica* serovar Typhimurium in cow manure. *FEMS Microbiol Ecol* 2007;**60**:419–428.

[39] Bernstein N, Sela S & Neder-Lavon S. Effect of irrigation regimes on persistence of *Salmonella enterica* serovar Newport in small experimental pots designed for plant cultivation. *Irrigation Sci* 2007;**26**:1–8.

[40] Or D, Smets BF, Wraith JM et al. Physical constraints affecting bacterial habitats and activity in unsaturated porous media—a review. *Adv Water Resour* 2007;**30**:1505–1527.

[41] Holley RA, Arrus KM, Ominski KH et al. *Salmonella* survival in manure-treated soils during simulated seasonal temperature exposure. *J Environ Qual* 2006;**35**:1170–1180.

[42] Bech TB, Johnsen K, Dalsgaard A et al. Transport and distribution of *Salmonella enterica* serovar Typhimurium in loamy and sandy soil monoliths with applied liquid manure. *Appl Environ Microbiol* 2010;**76**:710–714.

[43] Horswell J, Hewitt J, Prosser J et al. Mobility and survival of *Salmonella Typhimurium* and human adenovirus from spiked sewage sludge applied to soil columns. *J Appl Microbiol* 2010;**108**:104–114.

[44] Semenov AV, van Overbeek L & van Bruggen AH. Percolation and survival of *Escherichia coli* O157:H7 and *Salmonella enterica* serovar Typhimurium in soil amended with contaminated dairy manure or slurry. *Appl Environ Microbiol* 2009;**75**:3206–3215.

[45] Hutchison ML, Walters LD, Moore T et al. Fate of pathogens present in livestock wastes spread onto fescue plots. *Appl Environ Microbiol* 2005;**71**:691–696.

[46] Nicholson FA, Groves SJ & Chambers BJ. Pathogen survival during livestock manure storage and following land application. *Bioresour Technol* 2005;**96**:135–143.

[47] Hruby CE, Soupir ML, Moorman TB et al. Effects of tillage and poultry manure application rates on *Salmonella* and fecal indicator bacteria concentrations in tiles draining Des Moines Lobe soils. *J Environ Manage* 2016;**171**:60–69.

[48] Semenov AV, van Overbeek L, Termorshuizen AJ et al. Influence of aerobic and anaerobic conditions on survival of *Escherichia coli* O157:H7 and *Salmonella enterica* serovar Typhimurium in Luria-Bertani broth, farm-yard manure and slurry. *J Environ Manage* 2011;**92**:780–787.

[49] Bennett DD, Higgins SE, Moore RW et al. Effects of lime on *Salmonella enteritidis* survival in vitro. *J Appl Poult Res* 2003;**12**:65–68.

[50] Ding GC, Radl V, Schloter-Hai B et al. Dynamics of soil bacterial communities in response to repeated application of manure containing sulfadiazine. *Plos One* 2014;**9(3)**:e92958.

[51] Franz E, van Diepeningen AD, de Vos OJ et al. Effects of cattle feeding regimen and soil management type on the fate of *Escherichia coli* O157:H7 and *Salmonella enterica* serovar Typhimurium in manure, manure-amended soil, and lettuce. *Appl Environ Microbiol* 2005;**71**:6165–6174.

[52] Moynihan EL, Richards KG, Brennan FP et al. Enteropathogen survival in soil from different land-uses is predominantly regulated by microbial community composition. *Appl Soil Ecol* 2015;**89**:76–84.

[53] Goberna M, Podmirseg SM, Waldhuber S et al. Pathogenic bacteria and mineral N in soils following the land spreading of biogas digestates and fresh manure. *Appl Soil Ecol* 2011;**49**:18–25.

[54] Ge C, Lee C, Nangle E et al. Impact o f phytopathogen infection and extreme weather stress on internalization of *Salmonella* Typhimurium in lettuce. *Int J Food Microbiol* 2014;**168–169**:24–31.

[55] Caldwell KN, Anderson GL, Williams PL et al. Attraction of a free-living nematode, *Caenorhabditis elegans*, to foodborne pathogenic bacteria and its potential as a vector of *Salmonella* Poona for preharvest contamination of cantaloupe. *J Food Protect* 2003;**66**:1964–1971.

[56] Brandl MT, Rosenthal BM, Haxo AF et al. Enhanced survival of *Salmonella enterica* in vesicles released by a soilborne *Tetrahymena* species. *Appl Environ Microbiol* 2005;**71**:1562–1569.

[57] Cooley MB, Miller WG & Mandrell RE. Colonization of *Arabidopsis thaliana* with *Salmonella enterica* and enterohemorrhagic *Escherichia coli* O157:H7 and competition by *Enterobacter asburiae*. *Appl Environ Microbiol* 2003;**69**:4915–4926.

[58] Kroupitski Y, Golberg D, Belausov E et al. Internalization of *Salmonella enterica* in leaves is induced by light and involves chemotaxis and penetration through open stomata. *Appl Environ Microbiol* 2009;**75**:6076–6086.

[59] Schikora M, Neupane B, Madhogaria S et al. An image classification approach to analyze the suppression of plant immunity by the human pathogen *Salmonella Typhimurium*. *BMC Bioinformatics* 2012;**13**.

[60] Gibson DL, White AP, Snyder SD et al. *Salmonella* produces an O-antigen capsule regulated by AgfD and important for environmental persistence. *J Bacteriol* 2006;**188**:7722–7730.

[61] Vestby LK, Moretro T, Langsrud S et al. Biofilm forming abilities of *Salmonella* are correlated with persistence in fish meal and feed factories. *BMC Vet Res* 2009;**5**.

[62] Lapidot A, Romling U & Yaron S. Biofilm formation and the survival of *Salmonella* Typhimurium on parsley. *Int J Food Microbiol* 2006;**109**:229–233.

[63] Wiedemann A, Virlogeux-Payant I, Chausse AM et al. Interactions of *Salmonella* with animals and plants. *Front Microbiol* 2014;**5**:791.

[64] Tan MSF, White AP, Rahman S et al. Role of fimbriae, flagella and cellulose on the attachment of *Salmonella Typhimurium* ATCC 14028 to plant cell wall models. *PLos One* 2016;**11**:13.

[65] Yaron S & Romling U. Biofilm formation by enteric pathogens and its role in plant colonization and persistence. *Microb Biotechnol* 2014;**7**:496–516.

[66] Ongeng D, Geeraerd AH, Springael D et al. Fate of *Escherichia coli* O157:H7 and *Salmonella enterica* in the manure-amended soil-plant ecosystem of fresh vegetable crops: a review. *Crit Rev Microbiol* 2015;**41**:273–294.

[67] Berger CN, Shaw RK, Brown DJ et al. Interaction of *Salmonella enterica* with basil and other salad leaves. *ISME J* 2009;**3**:261–265.

[68] Kroupitski Y, Pinto R, Belausov E et al. Distribution of *Salmonella* Typhimurium in romaine lettuce leaves. *Food Microbiol* 2011;**28**:990–997.

[69] Klerks MM, Franz E, van Gent-Pelzer M et al. Differential interaction of *Salmonella enterica* serovars with lettuce cultivars and plant-microbe factors influencing the colonization efficiency. *ISME J* 2007;**1**:620–631.

[70] Barak JD, Gorski L, Naraghi-Arani P et al. *Salmonella enterica* virulence genes are required for bacterial attachment to plant tissue. *Appl Environ Microbiol* 2005;**71**:5685–5691.

[71] Klerks MM, van Gent-Pelzer M, Franz E et al. Physiological and molecular responses of *Lactuca sativa* to colonization by *Salmonella enterica* serovar Dublin. *Appl Environ Microbiol* 2007;**73**:4905–4914.

[72] Steenackers H, Hermans K, Vanderleyden J et al. *Salmonella* biofilms: An overview on occurrence, structure, regulation and eradication. *Food Res Int* 2012;**45**:502–531.

[73] Gerstel U & Romling U. The *csgD* promoter, a control unit for biofilm formation in *Salmonella* Typhimurium. *Res Microbiol* 2003;**154**:659–667.

[74] Cevallos-Cevallos JM, Gu G, Danyluk MD et al. Adhesion and splash dispersal of *Salmonella enterica* Typhimurium on tomato leaflets: effects of rdar morphotype and trichome density. *Int J Food Microbiol* 2012;**160**:58–64.

[75] Cevallos-Cevallos JM, Gu G, Danyluk MD et al. *Salmonella* can reach tomato fruits on plants exposed to aerosols formed by rain. *Int J Food Microbiol* 2012;**158**:140–146.

[76] Barak JD, Gorski L, Liang AS et al. Previously uncharacterized *Salmonella enterica* genes required for swarming play a role in seedling colonization. *Microbiology* 2009;**155**:3701–3709.

[77] Lapidot A & Yaron S. Transfer of *Salmonella enterica* serovar Typhimurium from contaminated irrigation water to parsley is dependent on curli and cellulose, the biofilm matrix components. *J Food Prot* 2009;**72**:618–623.

[78] Holmes A, Birse L, Jackson RW et al. An optimized method for the extraction of bacterial mRNA from plant roots infected with *Escherichia coli* O157:H7. *Front Microbiol* 2014;**5**:286.

[79] Golberg D, Kroupitski Y, Belausov E et al. *Salmonella Typhimurium* internalization is variable in leafy vegetables and fresh herbs. *Int J Food Microbiol* 2011;**145**:250–257.

[80] Barak JD, Kramer LC & Hao LY. Colonization of tomato plants by *Salmonella enterica* is cultivar dependent, and type 1 trichomes are preferred colonization sites. *Appl Environ Microbiol* 2011;**77**:498–504.

[81] Gu G, Hu J, Cevallos-Cevallos JM et al. Internal colonization of *Salmonella enterica* serovar Typhimurium in tomato plants. *PLoS One* 2011;**6**:e27340.

[82] Berg G, Erlacher A, Smalla K et al. Vegetable microbiomes: Is there a connection among opportunistic infections, human health and our 'gut feeling'? *Microb Biotechnol* 2014;**7**:487–495.

[83] Erlacher A, Cardinale M, Grosch R et al. The impact of the pathogen *Rhizoctonia solani* and its beneficial counterpart *Bacillus amyloliquefaciens* on the indigenous lettuce microbiome. *Front Microbiol* 2014;**5**:175.

[84] Schikora A, Carreri A, Charpentier E et al. The dark side of the salad: *Salmonella Typhimurium* overcomes the innate immune response of Arabidopsis thaliana and shows an endopathogenic lifestyle. *PLoS One* 2008;**3**:e2279.

[85] Shirron N & Yaron S. Active suppression of early immune response in tobacco by the human pathogen *Salmonella Typhimurium*. *PLoS One* 2011;**6**:e18855.

[86] Garcia AV, Charrier A, Schikora A et al. *Salmonella enterica* flagellin is recognized via FLS2 and activates PAMP-triggered immunity in *Arabidopsis thaliana*. *Molecular Plant* 2014;**7**:657–674.

[87] Gorbatsevich E, Sela Saldinger S, Pinto R et al. Root internalization, transport and in-planta survival of *Salmonella enterica* serovar Newport in sweet basil. *Environ Microbiol Rep* 2013;**5**:151–159.

[88] Erickson MC, Webb CC, Diaz-Perez JC et al. Infrequent internalization of *Escherichia coli* O157:H7 into field-grown leafy greens. *J Food Prot* 2010;**73**:500–506.

[89] Bernstein N, Sela S & Neder-Lavon S. Assessment of contamination potential of lettuce by *Salmonella enterica* serovar Newport added to the plant growing medium. *J Food Prot* 2007;**70**:1717–1722.

[90] Franz E, Visser AA, Van Diepeningen AD et al. Quantification of contamination of lettuce by GFP-expressing *Escherichia coli* O157:H7 and *Salmonella enterica* serovar Typhimurium. *Food Microbiol* 2007;**24**:106–112.

[91] Niemann GS, Brown RN, Gustin JK et al. Discovery of novel secreted virulence factors from *Salmonella enterica* serovar Typhimurium by proteomic analysis of culture supernatants. *Infect Immun* 2011;**79**:33–43.

[92] Hernandez-Reyes C & Schikora A. *Salmonella*, a cross-kingdom pathogen infecting humans and plants. *FEMS Microbiol Lett* 2013; 343(1):1–7.

[93] Schikora A, Virlogeux-Payant I, Bueso E et al. Conservation of *Salmonella* infection mechanisms in plants and animals. *PLoS One* 2011;**6**:e24112.

[94] Ustun S, Muller P, Palmisano R et al. SseF, a type III effector protein from the mammalian pathogen *Salmonella enterica*, requires resistance-gene-mediated signalling to activate cell death in the model plant *Nicotiana benthamiana*. *New Phytol* 2012;**194**:1046–1060.

[95] Neumann C, Fraiture M, Hernandez-Reyes C et al. The *Salmonella* effector protein SpvC, a phosphothreonine lyase is functional in plant cells. *Front Microbiol* 2014;**5**:548.

[96] Deiwick J, Salcedo SP, Boucrot E et al. The translocated Salmonella effector proteins SseF and SseG interact and are required to establish an intracellular replication niche. *Infect Immun* 2006;**74**:6965–6972.

[97] Pitzschke A, Schikora A & Hirt H. MAPK cascade signalling networks in plant defence. *Curr Opin Plant Biol* 2009;**12**:421–426.

[98] Melotto M, Panchal S & Roy D. Plant innate immunity against human bacterial pathogens. *Front Microbiol* 2014;**5**:411.

[99] Deng X, Li Z & Zhang W. Transcriptome sequencing of *Salmonella enterica* serovar Enteritidis under desiccation and starvation stress in peanut oil. *Food Microbiol* 2012;**30**:311–315.

[100] Goudeau DM, Parker CT, Zhou Y et al. The *Salmonella* transcriptome in lettuce and cilantro soft rot reveals a niche overlap with the animal host intestine. *Appl Environ Microbiol* 2013;**79**:250–262.

[101] Kyle JL, Parker CT, Goudeau D et al. Transcriptome analysis of *Escherichia coli* O157:H7 exposed to lysates of lettuce leaves. *Appl Environ Microbiol* 2010;**76**:1375–1387.

[102] Crozier L, Hedley PE, Morris J et al. Whole-transcriptome analysis of verocytotoxigenic *Escherichia coli* O157:H7 (Sakai) suggests plant-species-specific metabolic responses on exposure to spinach and lettuce extracts. *Front Microbiol* 2016;**7**:1088.

[103] Micallef SA, Rosenberg Goldstein RE, George A et al. Occurrence and antibiotic resistance of multiple Salmonella serotypes recovered from water, sediment and soil on mid-Atlantic tomato farms. *Environ Res* 2012;**114**:31–39.

[104] Hein I, Flekna G, Krassnig M et al. Real-time PCR for the detection of *Salmonella* spp. in food: An alternative approach to a conventional PCR system suggested by the FOOD-PCR project. *J Microbiol Methods* 2006;**66**:538–547.

[105] Park SH, Aydin M, Khatiwara A et al. Current and emerging technologies for rapid detection and characterization of *Salmonella* in poultry and poultry products. *Food Microbiol* 2014;**38**:250–262.

[106] Mandal PK, Biswas AK, Choi K et al. Methods for rapid detection of foodborne pathogens: an overview. *Am J Food Technol* 2011;**6**:87–102.

[107] Law JWF, Ab Mutalib NS, Chan KG et al. Rapid methods for the detection of foodborne bacterial pathogens: principles, applications, advantages and limitations. *Front Microbiol* 2015;**5**:19.

[108] Zhao X, Lin CW, Wang J et al. Advances in rapid detection methods for foodborne pathogens. *J Microbiol Biotechnol* 2014;**24**:297–312.

[109] Vojkovska H, Kubikova I & Kralik P. Evaluation of DNA extraction methods for PCR-based detection of *Listeria monocytogenes* from vegetables. *Lett Appl Microbiol* 2015;**60**:265–272.

[110] Blaser MJ & Newman LS. A review of human salmonellosis: I. Infective dose. *Rev Infect Dis* 1982;**4**:1096–1106.

[111] Nastasi A, Mammina C & Mioni R. Detection of *Salmonella* spp. in food by a rapid PCR-hybridization procedure. *Microbiologica* 1999;**22**:195–202.

[112] MDH. Update: Tomatoes identified as source of Salmonella outbreak in restaurant chain. 2015.

[113] CDC. *Salmonella* outbreaks. Available at http://www.cdc.gov/Salmonella/outbreaks.html. Accessed July 2016:177–188.

[114] CDHD. Health department investigating recent salmonella cases. 2015.

[115] ISDH. Chamberlain farm produce, inc. 2012.

[116] RKI. Salmonella Newport-Ausbruch in Deutschland und den Niederlanden, 2011. *Epidemiologisches Bulletin* 2012;**20**:177–188.

[117] TJP. Available at http://www.japantimes.co.jp/news/2011/02/24/news/salads-caused-hokkaido-food-scare. Accessed July 2016. 2011.

[118] FDH. Fei number 1000515256. 2011.

[119] IDPH. Summary of *S.* ser. Hvittingfoss outbreak April-June 2010. 2010.

Chapter 11

Preharvest *Salmonella* Risk Contamination and the Control Strategies

Rebeca Zamora-Sanabria and
Andrea Molina Alvarado

Additional information is available at the end of the chapter

http://dx.doi.org/10.5772/67399

Abstract

Salmonella is present in most food production environments and can enter the food supply at any stage of food production from farm to fork. Control strategies for *Salmonella* include preharvest and postharvest aspects. Preharvest approach is very important because as a result of large-scale production, many animals could be infected with *Salmonella* serotypes during the primary production, causing human salmonellosis by consuming meat, milk, and eggs or foods containing ingredients of animal origin. The first step for prevention approaches is to determinate the source of infection; *Salmonella* serovars should be founded, and control strategies must be executed. Infection sources include vertical transmission, feed, pest (rodents and insects), wild birds, water, humans, manure, transportation coops, tractors or vehicles, and farm environment. Preventive and control strategies involve many factors, including hygiene, biosecurity procedures, animal feed surveillance, litter, manure and carcasses disposed, cleaning and disinfection programs, food interventions, diagnostic, and vaccination.

Keywords: *Salmonella*, preharvest, farm to fork approach, surveillance, sources of infection, biosecurity, feedstuffs, cleaning and disinfection, pest control, water safety, vaccination, litter and carcasses disposal

1. Introduction

Salmonellosis is one of the most common food-borne bacterial diseases in the world. In most food animal species, *Salmonella* can establish a clinically unapparent infection of variable duration, which is significant as a potential zoonosis.

Human food-borne salmonellosis has increased in association with the development of food industry. Food industry is based on large-scale animal production. Food processing plants have grown larger, and when there is a salmonellosis outbreak, it will infect many more people than in the past. In addition, there has been a change in dining habits of consumers, and a high proportion of meals are eaten at institutions, restaurants, and fast food places. These establishments are often a significant link and amplifier of *Salmonella* infections.

Salmonella is present in most food production environments and can enter the food supply at any stage of food production from *farm to fork*. Control strategies for *Salmonella* include preharvest and postharvest aspects. Most control strategies for *Salmonella* are focused on specific aspects of food production or processing and are generally assessed on their ability to reduce levels of *Salmonella* spp. at the processing stage.

Nevertheless, preharvest approach is very important because as a result of large-scale production, many animals are placed in small area producing a lot of feces. Several *Salmonella* serovars that are not host specific may colonize the digestive tract of animals, provoking human salmonellosis by consuming meat, milk, and egg or food containing ingredients of animal origin.

Animal feed (and ingredients therein) has been described as a source of *Salmonella* infection for animals and humans, through the contamination of food products of animal origin. This threat is aggravated due to the bacteria capability to persist for long periods in a wide variety of feedstuffs. Therefore, animal feed may serve as vehicle to introduce *Salmonella* serovars into the food chain and could contribute to the circulation and spreading of antimicrobial-resistant bacteria or antimicrobial-resistant genes.

At the farm, level food safety programs involve many factors such as hygiene, biosecurity procedures, animal feed surveillance, litter and carcasses disposal, depopulation, cleaning, disinfection programs, food interventions, diagnostic, and vaccination. The source of infection should be determined. At the end of the production, animals should be sent to slaughter with special precaution, and they should be healthy to prevent contamination during the processing.

Other strategies should be taken during the transport and time of slaughter to decrease *Salmonella* contamination. A good food safety program should include the entire food chain of production; however, the aim of this chapter is to describe preharvest *Salmonella* risk contamination factors including *Salmonella* prevalence in animal feedstuffs and the control strategies and interventions.

1.1. Farm-to-fork concept

"Farm to fork" is a strategy to prevent food-borne hazards. This approach is based in many measures to trace the different stages of the food chain. "Farm-to-fork" system examines the practices and procedures that ensure food safety.

The procedures to prevent *Salmonella* contamination in the food chain comprise many events, from the primary production to the final consumer. *Salmonella* contamination events can occur during different parts of the food chain which included primary production, processing, distribution, preparation, and dining habits of consumers.

http://dx.doi.org/10.5772/67399

In 2003, Food and Agriculture Organization (FAO) of the United Nations [1] showed the importance about a new approach in food-borne hazards which it had called "food chain approach." Its objective is to ensure that the food is free from borne hazards: pesticides, chemicals, bacteria, and others contaminants. Every food chain step has to be analyzed: growing, raising, production, collecting, processing, packing, commercialization, and consumption.

The FAO and World Health Organization (WHO) [2] have produced guidance documents for use by governmental authorities on food-borne outbreak investigation [3]. They suggest that good control measurements at the farm level are likely to correspond with lower prevalence of *Salmonella* infection and, subsequently, a reduction of cross contamination of carcasses processed at the slaughterhouse and a reduction in human salmonellosis.

1.2. One health

Also, Codex Alimentarius (CA) standards and risk analysis methodologies are recognized in the area for food safety. The CA and the World Organization for Animal Health (OIE) are working together to develop their respective standards for food-borne zoonosis so that they are non-duplicative, cohesive, and will cover the whole food chain [3].

Primary production is focused in animal health, livestock, housing management, animal food quality, animal welfare, and transportation regarding for food processing.

Farming practices or primary production vary widely according to soil and climatic conditions, social conditions, cost of the feedstuffs, potential marketability of specific farm products, and the economic objectives of the farmer. However, there are general control strategies to prevent the entrance of *Salmonella* in primary production.

In spite of those production measurements, bacteria can enter anywhere in the food chain, causing animal disease and food contamination. One of the major sources of *Salmonella* in the food chain has been animal feed, especially swine and poultry. It is a major cause of economic loss in swine production [4] and has a great economic significance to the poultry industry around the world.

Salmonella could be a risk to public health through consumption of contaminated eggs and meat. These bacteria causes diarrheal diseases in humans [5] and high mortality in animals, like chickens. Other farm animals as cattle and sheep suffer disease, could become *Salmonella* reservoirs, and contribute as vector in the transmission.

2. Sources of infection

Salmonella genus is a group of microorganisms that are successfully adapted to live in very different environmental conditions [6]. For this reason, it is easy to find many potential sources of contamination, and control could be complicated. These sources include vertical transmission, feed, pest (rodents and insects), wild birds, water, humans, manure, transportation coops, tractors or vehicles, and farm environment. There are also some variables that contribute *Salmonella* contamination, such as age of the animal, survival of the bacteria through the gastric barrier, competing bacteria in the intestinal tract, availability of a hospitable colonization site, the diet, physiological status, health, disease, and medications [7].

Identifying animal sources of infection, target interventions, and control measurements is the correct approach for preventing *Salmonella*; every source should be considered. Risk assessment studies have recommended an intervention for a productive overall approach.

2.1. Transmission

Salmonella is extremely widespread and very persistent in the environment. It is recovered from many vertebrates which included many farm animal species. Serovars of *Salmonella enterica* have varied hosts and reservoirs, cause disease in animals and humans, and can move between host species [5] because most of them are nonhost specific (**Table 1**).

Farm animal	*S. enterica* subsp. *enterica* serovar	Clinical signs	Authors
Sheep	Brandenburg Abortusovis Dublin Arizonae Typhimurium	Adults: abortion, gastroenteritis, pneumonia Lams: gastroenteritis, pneumonia, polyarthritis	[59]
Cattle	Dublin Typhimurium Montevideo Brandenburg Enteritidis Panamá Heidelberg Kentucky	Frequently is a subclinical disease Adults: diarrhea, enteritis abortion, depressed milk yield Calves: enteritis, arthritis, meningoencephalitis, respiratory signs	[59] [60] [61]
Poultry	Enteritidis, Typhimurium Paratyphi B Heidelberg Kentucky Infantis Gallinarum, pullorum	Frequently is a subclinical disease Gallinarum and pullorum (nonmotile): septicemia Others strains: asymptomatic	[62] [63]
Pig	Typhimurium Choleraesuis Derby Enteritidis Istanbul Mbandaka Agona Heidelberg	Septicemia and enterocolitis, pigs 6–8 weeks	[10] [26] [59] [64]
Horse	Typhimurium Newport Enteritidis St Paul Agona Anatum Heidelberg	Abortion, diarrhea, typhlitis, colitis, arthritis, nosocomial infections	[19] [64]

Table 1. *Salmonella enterica* subsp. *enterica* common serovars in farm animals.

In farm animals *Salmonella* cause clinical disease, and there are also asymptomatic animals called carriers, e.g., *Salmonella* subclinical infections persist in hens more than 22 weeks [8]. Carrier pigs are important as the initial source of contamination of the environment, other animals, and carcasses in the harvest [9]. Monitoring programs in the USA suggest that 20% of broiler chickens are contaminated with harmful *Salmonella* strains [6] and 27% incidence was found in feces in organic pig farms [10]. They are very important in the transmission because they can shed *Salmonella* in feces continuously and intermittently in the absence of clinical signs. Pets such as dogs and cats [11] show asymptomatic infections and could shed *Salmonella* and contaminated food-producing animals.

There is a different *Salmonella* susceptibility in farm animals. Stressors can aggravate *Salmonella* shedding, including mixing, climate, transportation, and food deprivation. Some results suggest that the duration of *Salmonella* shedding might depend on serotypes, strain, animal age, farm, or others risk factors [10].

Horizontal transmission also occurs by fecal-oral route or by aerogenous transmission. In pigs oropharyngeal secretions can contaminate and spread the disease via nose to nose [12]. *Salmonella* can be introduced in a herd through new purchased and infected pigs. There is evidence of bacterial spread by feed, drinking water, fomites, asymptomatic carriers, and dry feces from infected animals with clinical disease.

Vertical transmission is crucial in poultry related infected with *S. enterica* subspecies *enterica* serovars Enteritidis, Typhimurium, Gallinarum, Heidelberg, and Infantis [13]. *Salmonella* produces persistent infection in birds, located in the ovary [13]. Transmission to progeny occurs by transovarian infection, when the ovary and the developing eggs became infected in the oviduct. Bacteria migrate inside the yolk before shell deposition. *Salmonella* enteritidis can also get access to eggs by migrating from the cloaca to the reproductive organs. *S. enterica* subsp. *enterica* serovar Heidelberg was the most common serovar founded in ovaries in layers in Canada [8]; there is evidence supporting vertical transmission of *Salmonella* in dairy cattle [14]. *Salmonella* might be transmitted vertically from the dam to her fetus in utero. Calves might be infected with *Salmonella* at birth or post birth.

If progeny persists infected, there is no chance of eradication, and the control becomes complicated. From a public health point of view, the number of eggs and animals affected by *Salmonella* is a risk for a human disease or infection.

2.2. Feed

Animal feed is a recognized source of *Salmonella* for farm livestock. Bacteria can be introduced into the feed by contaminated feedstuffs, processing, transport, storage, distribution, and administration due to dirty feeders.

Salmonella can be isolated frequently from animal-feed ingredients, such as meat bone meals and fish meals. Few quantities of *Salmonella* cause infection, less than one *Salmonella* per gram of feed has been shown to establish colonization in 1- to 7-day-old chicks [15].

Salmonella could be isolated from feedstuff in 17.6% of pig herds among five EU countries and from 6.9% of all feed samples [16], and also it can survive at least 26 months in artificially contaminated poultry food [17].

2.3. Farm environment

Farm *Salmonella* eradication is a complicated strategy, and its control could be difficult because there are numerous potential source environment. It is able to grow between 7 and 45°C, is destroyed at 65°C during 10–15 minutes, and resists every acid pH and salt added in food up to 20% [6].

Animals are the major reservoir of *Salmonella*; dissemination into environment has resulted from the human practices and animal behavior. *Salmonella* may be present in any waste from human or animal activities; it survives in frozen food and remains viable during years in the environment. In broiler houses, microorganisms could persist for at least 1 year [18]. *Salmonella* is shed efficiently in feces, persists within the environment, and is spread readily between food-producing animals in the farm environment. *Salmonella* can survive desiccation and persist for many months in association with dust particles on fans, floors, and feed deposits.

This microorganism can survive and replicate for long periods in different environments, although the original fecal source may be remote in time. For instance, *S. enterica* subsp. *enterica* serovar Choleraesuis persists in dry feces 13 months post shedding and after disinfection process and survives in soil between 25 and 200 days [5].

Bailey et al. [7] found that the environment was the primary source of contaminating *Salmonella* in chicken houses not treated with competitive exclusion microflora. They recovered high rates of *Salmonella* from feces, litter, and near the entrance doors to the poultry houses. Hatchery transport paper pads were the most frequently observed *Salmonella* positive in this research. Salmonellosis is also commonly observed in contaminated facilities in veterinary hospitals [19]. Barns, pens, dust, egg belts, feeders, fans, feed bins, vehicles, and equipment can be contaminated.

Survival capacity, environment persistence, and infection may be influenced by different genetic, productive, and environmental factors such as intensification of handling practices, reduction in genetic diversity of breeding stock, and increasing standardization of food types [5].There is a differential distribution of specific serovars and genotypes between animals and environments. Certain serovars have a greater ability to establish infection, shedding patterns, and concentration. In pigs, *S. enterica* subsp. *enterica* serovar Typhimurium was more frequently isolated from the manure compared to other bacteria [20].

2.4. Water

Contaminated water supplies have been implicated in the introduction and persistence of *Salmonella*. Contaminated waters might contribute through direct ingestion of the water or via indirect contamination of the surfaces. In a review [21], they found *Salmonella* in different countries and in very diverse water sources. *Salmonella* contamination occurred in surface water used for recreational purposes, as source of drinking water and for irrigation. They detected a mixed of human and animal origin of *Salmonella* serovars in drinking water sources.

In artificial freshwater systems, *Salmonella* and *Escherichia coli* survived for at least 56 days [5]. Factor contributes to *Salmonella* resistance, and persistence in water is its capacity to attach to different types of plastic, glass, cement, rubber, and stainless steel or biotic surfaces (plant surfaces, epithelial cells, and gallstones) [6]. *Salmonella* forms a complex called biofilm inside drinkers and pipes. This biofilm is a bacteria surface-associated formation that allows bacteria to resist against different stress factors such as desiccation, disinfectants, and antibiotics [22].

2.5. Pest

2.5.1. Rodents

Mice and rats are involved in the transmission and the perpetuation of the infection in the farm buildings and facilities. Rodents can be long-term sources of *Salmonella* infection. Their droppings can be contaminated for up to 3 months for infection. A study found that 3 weeks old chicks became infected via mice artificially contaminated with *S. enterica subsp. enterica* serovar Enteritidis 5 months before [23].

Mice travel from one farm to another; they leave empty farms or facilities and return after cleaning and disinfection activities. They have also good reproductive capacity and can spread *Salmonella* for one flock to other flocks or herds. They contribute to perpetuate infections. Rodents are important vectors and amplifiers of *Salmonella* infection in farm animals, e.g., mouse fecal pellets have been shown to contain up to 10^4 CFU of *Salmonella* [23, 24]. One single mouse can shed 100 fecal pellets per day [24]. Fecal pellets are seed shaped; pigs and chicken eat these pellets and become infected. On a clean pig farm, 5–10% rodents can be found infected with *Salmonella* [25, 26]. Isolates from contaminated mice contained three times more *Salmonella* than isolates from environment of contaminated house samples [24]. The presence of a mouse-infected population is an important risk for animal and product contamination. Layer farms with high rodent densities showed more *S. enterica* subsp. *enterica* serovar Enteritidis and serovar Infantis isolations and hens infected than farms with low rodent densities [27].

Rats, mice, and cats are associated with contamination of water, food, and grains stored. They carry bacteria in their intestinal tracts without clinical symptoms and disease and cause transmission of pathogens to farm animal feed and environment. Rodents acquire the infection from feces of sick animals, wild animals, and members of their family [23]; they also get infected from outdoor paddocks and inaccessible feces-contaminated parts of the livestock houses.

The environment conditions around facilities attract rodent, e.g., waste, spilled food and feedstuffs, sources of water, and abilities to build dens. Dead mice also can be a contamination source if they remain in the barns of houses after cleaning and disinfection procedures.

2.5.2. *Darkling beetles, flies, mites, ticks, and cockroaches*

Salmonella is widely distributed in flies and less in beetle and mites of affected livestock units. Farms offer great and suitable niches as manure, dust, spilled food, and long production periods of time without cleaning.

Flies act as mechanical vector; the *Musca domestica* is most prevalent in farms and associates with zoonosis. They perform diurnal excursions around animal houses and can fly many miles from the farms contributing with *Salmonella* dissemination. Heavy fly populations have been identified as a risk factor for *Salmonella* in poultry, dairy cattle, swine, and feedlot cattle [28]. Authors report that flies carry *S. enterica* subsp. *enterica* serovar Typhimurium for up to 10 days [26]. Flies become contaminated from environment, and animals ingesting contaminated flies get infected. There is not enough evidence of flies as biological vector (*Salmonella* multiplication inside the flies).

Darkling beetle *Alphitobius diaperinus* is a very common pest in poultry houses. They carry and shed by defecation variety of microorganisms which included *Salmonella*. Beetles survive cleaning and disinfection because they hide in inaccessible poultry house structures and outside of the poultry buildings. They drill wall cavities complicating insecticides access. Chickens can ingest contaminated beetle larvae and adults and become infected. *Salmonella* isolates from beetles are usually lower than isolates from flies [29].

Mites can acquire and transmit *Salmonella*. The most frequently mites founded in poultry are *Dermanyssus gallinae* (red mite), *Ornithonyssus sylviarum*, and *Ornithonyssus bursa.* They are usually present in manure, litter, and feed. Adults and nymphs of ticks visit poultry houses only to feed; adults can survive for months or years at swine or poultry facilities. A *Salmonella* vector role for ticks remains speculative.

Cockroaches will opportunistically colonize animal facilities and carry bacteria. They have been reported to carry *Salmonella* [30] and can transmit these bacteria to other cockroaches and to eggshells.

2.6. Wild animals

Wild bird and little mammals are regarded as the main reservoir for *Salmonella* in the environment. Wildlife vectors may be responsible for the introduction of some Salmonellae to farms.

Birds as pigeons, sparrows [5], foxes [31], shrews, reptiles, and other wild animals have a potential role in the *Salmonella* dissemination [29]. The spread or recycling of *Salmonella* infection among livestock may occur through the contamination of water or feed or the direct contamination of the environment. Building, houses, and barns should be constructed to block wild animal access. Birds cannot nest and reproduce in the houses to prevent bacterial contamination.

2.7. Humans

Human traffic on the farm increases the risk of infection in pigs, chickens, and hens. The entrance of visitors was associated with higher *Salmonella* prevalence [32].

People transport pathogens from their nose, hair, throat, pharynx, clothes, and shoes. They also could have *Salmonella* in their intestine; therefore, having access to toilets and washing facilities have a protective effect against *Salmonella* [9].

3. Surveillance and prevalence of *Salmonella* in animal feedstuffs

Animal feedstuff could serve as vehicle for *Salmonella* serovars into the farm environment and cause animal infection that could reach the human consumer through animal food products. As we already mentioned above, *Salmonella* has the capability to survive in a vast variety of commodities and to resist desiccation among other adverse conditions. During our work and research in *Salmonella* surveillance in animal feed, we have seen that *Salmonella* has the ability to remain in different animal feedstuffs for long time periods; this has been also confirmed by other research groups [33, 34].

Animal feedstuffs have been found to be a cause of *Salmonella* infection in animals and humans [17, 35, 36]. In spite of this, there is controversy in the roll or relevance of animal feed in food-borne infections since the serovars frequently isolated from animal feed do not correlate with the serovars frequently associated with human infections. Through animal feed new *Salmonella* serovars and resistance bacteria could enter and spread into the food chain [37, 38]. The surveillance and control of *Salmonella* in animal feed and feed ingredients should be an important part of animals and food safety programs aimed to counteract *Salmonella* food-borne infections.

In many countries around the world, *Salmonella* surveillance feedstuff programs are being executed; each program has its own specific objectives and specifications. For example, in Costa Rica all finished feed and feed ingredients must be registered and inspected by the Ministry of Agriculture and Livestock. These feedstuffs are also analyzed for *Salmonella*, and this must be absent regardless the serovar. In contrast with the FDA guidance for control of *Salmonella* in food for animals, the FDA recommended regulatory actions depending on the serovar found and the animal species that would receive the feed [39]. The serovars that have been reported to cause disease in the animal species for which the feed is for should be absent, for example [39]:

Poultry feed: *S. enterica* subsp. *enterica* serovar Gallinarum and Enteritidis

Swine feed: *S. enterica* subsp. *enterica* serovar Choleraesuis

Sheep feed: *S. enterica* subsp. *enterica* serovar Abortusovis

Horse feed: *S. enterica* subsp. *enterica* serovar Abortusequi

Dairy and beef feed: *S. enterica* subsp. *enterica* serovar Newport or Dublin

These differences between the *Salmonella* control programs could hamper international trade. Furthermore, in a previous research [40] in which we analyzed 1725 samples of feed and feed ingredient between the years 2009 and 2014, we found *Salmonella* serovars which do not frequently cause disease in animals but have been involved in food-borne outbreaks.

In our study, the overall *Salmonella* prevalence in animal feedstuff was 6.4%. Finished feeds such as: poultry, pet, and swine and feed ingredients such as: meat and bone meal (MBM), fish meal and poultry meal were tested.

Meat and bone meal and poultry feed presented the higher *Salmonella* relative prevalence 26,7 and 5,4%, respectively [40]. **Figure 1** shows the most frequently found serovars in MBM and poultry feed in this study [40, 41]: in MBM: *S. enterica* subsp. *enterica* serovar Give (13.8%) and serovar Rissen (4.6%) and in poultry feed: *S. enterica* subsp. *enterica* serovar Havana (10.8%), serovar Rissen, serovar Soerenga, and serovar Schwarzengrund (6.2%). These serovars have been associated with animal and human infections and outbreaks [42–44].

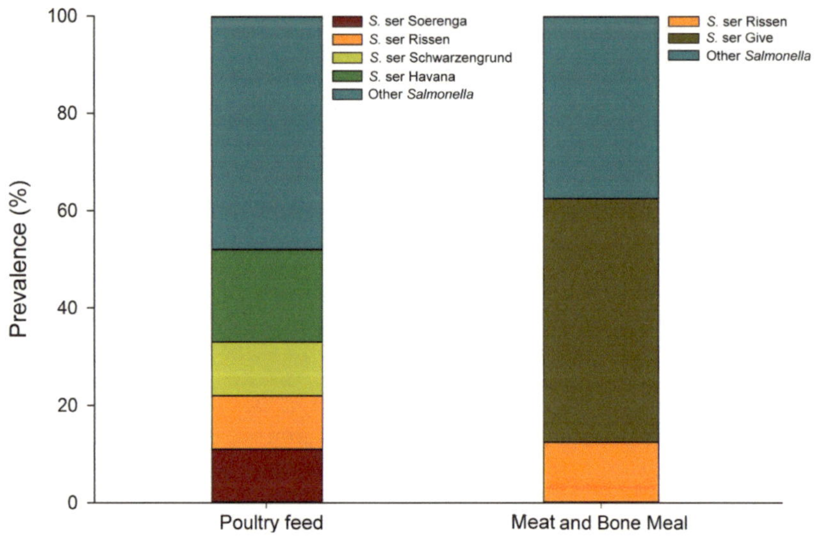

Figure 1. Distribution of *Salmonella enterica* serovars among the isolates found in feed and feed ingredients in Costa Rica [41].

The high *Salmonella* prevalence found in MBM in our previous study [40] is worrying given that MBM is used in some countries as a relative cheap protein source to feed pets and monogastric animals [38, 45].

In the EU, there is also no common sampling plan for *Salmonella* surveillance in animal feed; in the EFSA report for 2014, the overall level of *Salmonella* contamination in feedstuff was 3.8% [46] similar to our previously reported prevalence for Costa Rica [40].

4. Detection and surveillance of *Salmonella* in food production systems

Owing to the fact that *Salmonella* is ubiquitous and has the capability to survive in a great variety of commodities, it is important to control it in each step of the food chain in order to minimize the risk of human infections and food-borne outbreaks and achieve safer food to consumers. It is crucial to maintain a *Salmonella* surveillance program in food-producing animals

http://dx.doi.org/10.5772/67399

in order to reduce food-borne Salmonellosis and infections in animals causing economic loss to the livestock sector. The fact that *Salmonella* in animals causes frequently subclinical infections that could go unnoticed favors the *Salmonella* spread in a herd or flock [47].

Table 2 shows the *Salmonella* prevalence in farm animals, and the serovars most commonly found in animals and in their meat according to the last EFSA and ECDC [46] report. In this report, the authors demonstrated that the most prevalent serovars were shared between food producing animals and the meat for consumption. In contrast, other researchers (including ourselves) found no relation among the strains encountered in feed, live animals and processed meat [40].

Farm animal	Overall EU prevalence of *Salmonella* (2014)	Most commonly serovars in flock	Most commonly serovars in meat
Breeding and fattening turkey flocks	3.3%	*S. enterica* subsp. *enterica* ser. Infantis (22.2% of isolates)	*S. enterica* subsp. *enterica* ser. Stanley, *S. enterica* subsp. *enterica* ser. Infantis, and *S. enterica* subsp. *enterica* ser. Typhimurium
Breeding and fattening pigs	7.9%	*S. enterica* subsp. *enterica* ser. Typhimurium (54.7%) and *S. enterica* subsp. *enterica* ser. Derby (17.5%) (of 2037 isolates)	*S. enterica* subsp. *enterica* ser. Typhimurium (27.8%), *S. enterica* subsp. *enterica* ser. Derby (24.4%), and monophasic strains of *S. enterica* subsp. *enterica* ser. Typhimurium (18%)
Cattle (breeding animals, dairy cows or calves, or were unspecified)	3.9%	*S. enterica* subsp. *enterica* ser. Typhimurium (46.8%), *S. enterica* subsp. *enterica* ser. Dublin (31.3%), and *S. enterica* subsp. *enterica* ser. Enteritidis (4.6%) (of 3243 reported isolates)	*S. enterica* subsp. *enterica* ser. Derby (24.7%), *S. enterica* subsp. *enterica* ser. Typhimurium (20.6%) and *S. enterica* subsp. *enterica* ser. Enteritidis (17.8%)

Table 2. *Salmonella* prevalence in farm animals and their meat in the Europe Union [46].

5. Control measures for *Salmonella* in food production

The objective of preharvest approach is to minimize opportunities for the introduction, persistence, and transmission of *Salmonella* infections and other animal pathogens. Strategies should be directed against all *Salmonella* serovars, but sometimes more specific strategies against particular *Salmonella* serovars are required when one of them has high public health impact or economic significance.

Most of the time, general strategies are sufficient to control all *Salmonella* serovars; nevertheless, sometimes it is necessary to apply specific tools, e.g., vaccination against specific serovars. Prevention programs or strategies included risk reduction, risk management, and verification by implementation of biosecurity programs.

Biosecurity is known as a group of procedures or prevention measurements to protect farm animals against biological agents, such as bacteria, viruses, fungi, parasites, protozoa, and any other agents able to induce infectious diseases into a farm. Biosecurity programs identify risk, origin, reservoirs, vector, and carriers, preventing the access to the farm. It includes strategies as control of wild birds and flies, obligatory disinfection of boots, clothes, and equipment for farm workers and visitors. Cleaning and disinfection of houses, litter, and dead animal's management and vaccination are also important in a prevention program.

5.1. Cleaning and disinfection

High level of *Salmonella* persisting for months in surfaces and contaminated facilities demonstrates the importance of cleaning organic matter and dust from the environment and animal houses. Empty houses should be cleaned and disinfected between flocks and herds.

Cleaning has to be detailed, using water and appropriate detergents. In poultry houses, cleaning should be focused in difficult access places as ceilings, cages, egg-conveyor belts, egg-grading equipment, manure belts, feed troughs, hoppers, feed bins, louvers, curtains, brush blades, air inlets, fans, and other ventilation equipment. Feather removal is an important measure in poultry facilities. Also, frequently visited rooms should be cleaned; anterooms, egg-packing rooms, and egg-storage rooms, offices, storage rooms, and restrooms can be contaminated.

After washing and cleaning, administration of disinfectants by high-pressure spray, foam, and fumigation reduce environmental contamination. Disinfectant dilutions and application directions should be strictly followed. A suitable disinfectant against *Salmonella* should have residual properties and activity in the presence of organic matter. Drying of houses immediately after application of disinfectants is highly advisable to reduce water activity, which allows *Salmonella* multiplication.

Disinfectants as sodium hypochlorite or quaternary ammonium compounds are able to eliminate *Salmonella* bacteria. Other studies showed that the use of glutaraldehyde, formaldehyde, and peroxygen at a concentration of 1% in field conditions was inadequate for the elimination of *Salmonella* in the farm [48]. Higher doses should be used. Povidone-iodine, potassium permanganate, ethanol, chlorhexidine digluconate, and hydrogen peroxide exhibited high efficacy in other studies [49, 50].

Recontamination after cleaning and disinfecting may occur. Houses recently cleaned should be closed before animals arrive to prevent organic matter and dust contamination. Equipment should be washed and disinfected before entering a house to prevent recontamination.

5.2. Vaccination

Vaccination is a specific control tool against *Salmonella*. Vaccines are used to increase the infection resistance. It can enhance the short-term responsiveness of control programs but does not completely eliminate problems. A combination of biosecurity procedures, *Salmonella*-free replacement of flocks and herds, and vaccination should be a suitable control approach. Farm management programs need integrated interventions to be satisfactory.

Immunization has been shown to significantly reduce the number of hens infected by *S. enterica* subsp. *enterica* serovar Enteritidis and the rate of egg transmission [51]. Live-attenuated vaccines and nonliving vaccines (bacterins) of *S. enterica* subsp. *enterica* serovar Enteritidis vaccines are used to immunize chickens. Live vaccines are used against *S. enterica* subsp. *enterica* serovar Gallinarum and Typhimurium.

Live vaccines reduce intestinal and internal organ (spleen, liver, ovary, and oviducts) infection and stimulate mucosal immunity in the digestive tract [52]. Bacterins (killed vaccines) induce high levels of circulation antibodies and reduce colonization of internal organs and the number of bacteria in egg content [53]. However, they have a limited effect in feces shedding; for this reason, they may not contribute to prevent environment contamination. Therefore, a combination of both lives and bacterins are commonly used in layers and showed to be effective in *Salmonella* control in poultry [51].

Vaccination of sows and piglets can be helpful. Both vaccines are used, live and bacterins. Live vaccines are considered to provide good protection in pigs. However, some live vaccines in pigs show risks as reversion to virulence and excretion to the environment. And also, there is no differentiation between naturally infected and vaccinated animals [12]. Inactivated vaccines in sows could reduce transmission to the progeny and enhance maternal immunity. An effective, safe, and efficient vaccine program should prevent clinical symptoms, colonization, and development of carriers and reduce shedding.

5.3. Pest control

5.3.1. Rodents

Reduction or elimination of these vectors is an important part of the prevention strategies or control. An effective control program should be keep rodents number to the lowest level possible.

Chemicals and baits are the most common methods of rodent control. Farmers use frequently traps and cats. The use of cats as exterminator is not recommended. A study in a pig farm founded 12% of farm cat *Salmonella* [20] and *Toxoplasma gondii* positive [25].

A rodent control should have an integral approach, and it should include:

- Monitoring of rodent populations by visualization, traps, and creation of an index.
- Removal of old stored material and waste.
- Repairing facility structure.
- Do not allow rodents to enter the houses (repair holes, door seals, etc.).
- Removal of habitat elements and shelters for rodents near animal buildings, barns, and stables.
- Limiting access to water and feed.
- Limit the development of high rodent densities.

- Cleaning of outdoor paddocks.
- Removal of vegetation around the houses.
- The use of effective rodenticides.
- Secure disposal of died animals, litter, and waste.
- Do not maintain spilled feed.
- Follow strict biosecurity procedures.

It has been demonstrated that rodent integral control programs that follow these guidelines, has effectively decreased *Salmonella* in livestock animal houses.

Sometimes when high rodent densities are found, a program such as the mentioned is required.

5.3.2. Insects

For a successful insect control is required to keep litter dry and well ventilated, preventing wet areas and leaks is a must. Frequent removal of litter and replacement of fresh shavings in poultry houses can help to reduce beetle populations [54].

The use of insecticides such as :pyrethrins, carbamates and phosphates is a common practice. Sometimes, mite control could be complicated, because of the resistance from the insects to the acaricide; and also technical limitations like the usage in the lay period in hens. Rotation of insecticides reduces development of resistance.

Biological control methods should be used especially in animal production periods. Fly parasites, depredators, and insect growth regulators could be good options. Wettable powders are used with chemical insecticides in the beetle control.

5.4. Water safety

Water sanitation at the farm is essential in a biosecurity program. Drinking water sanitation can prevent initial contamination and recontamination of animals with *Salmonella.* Water filtration is a critical component of a water sanitation program. Dirty water cannot be effectively sanitized. Frequent washed and cleaned tanks are also required.

Chlorine is the most common disinfectant used in drinking water. It is a strong oxidizing agent and used to sanitize drinking water in farms. It is effective against Gram-positive and Gram-negative bacteria, viruses, fungal, and protozoa. When added to the water, a chemical reaction occurs, formation of Hypochlorous acid (HOCL) (weak acid) and Hypochlorite ion (OCL^-). Both are referred as free chlorine or available free chlorine. HOCL is more efficient as sanitizer. HOCL is necessary to keep low water pH, under 6.5 [55]. Chlorine is available in liquid form as sodium hypochlorite and in solid form as calcium hypochlorite. Sodium hypochlorite is usually available at a concentration of 10–12%.

http://dx.doi.org/10.5772/67399

Other halogens as iodine and bromine are used. Hydrogen peroxide, peracetic acid, ozone, and ultraviolet light showed to be successful to sanitize drinking water. Addition of organic acids to the drinking water showed variable results [56]. The antibacterial effects of acids depend on the type of organic acid, the bacterial species, the concentration used, and the physical form in which it is administered to the animals.

Strategies to reduce drinkers and pipe biofilm should be implemented. Biofilm causes resistance to free chlorine residuals, which can lead to persistence of bacteria in chlorine-treated water. Surfactin, glucose, halogenated furanones, 4(5)-aryl 2-aminoimidazoles, furocoumarins, and salicylates are used as biofilm inhibitors and disinfectant combinations of triclosan and quaternary ammonium salts or halogenated furanones and treatment antibiotics/disinfectants and microemulsions such as soybean oil in water [6]. It is essential that the effectiveness of sanitization program can be monitored.

5.5. Litter and carcasses disposed

Manure is one of the most important sources of *Salmonella* contamination. Pig slurry and poultry litter should not be spread, sprayed, or reused before a disinfection treatment. Land spreading of manure can lead to contamination of soil and water, which can potentially lead to bacteria transmission to animals and humans.

Transportation and disposal of slurry and manure from pig and poultry houses and barns, the transportation of slaughter offal to rendering plants, the cross contamination of rendered meat meal, and other poultry and animal byproducts contribute to spreading *Salmonella* in the environment [5].

If *Salmonella* is present in the litter and manure, the birds and pigs could be exposed at a time when they are highly susceptible and get sick. Well-designed facilities should avoid contact between animals and their feces. There are many manure treatments or disinfection procedures. Manure methods can be physical, chemical, biological, or a combination of all three and include technologies such as anaerobic digestion, composting, and separation. It has been shown that stored separate pig manure fractions under controlled conditions (10.5°C for 84–112 days) reduced *Salmonella* [57].

Salmonella may also be introduced into soil and the adjacent environment by decomposition of infected carcasses [5]. Dead animals should be disposed into a secured container, which is regularly washed and disinfected. Burying, composting, incineration, and dropping off at designated sites are the most commonly recommended and utilized methods for carcass disposed [58].

5.6. Transportation

Pigs and chickens and other animals increased shedding of *Salmonella* during transport from the farm to the slaughterhouse. Long transportation duration, high stock density, weather conditions, and long feed withdrawal are causes of bacteria increase shedding.

Feed tracks can also act as mechanical vectors and can transfer bacteria from one farm to another. Pig and poultry vehicles and drivers represent a considerable risk; therefore, they should not be allowed into the clean areas of the farm. Transport vehicles, feed trucks, and chicken coops should to be cleaned and appropriately disinfected to prevent *Salmonella* contamination in harvest. In layers decontaminated and sanitized coops or cages and vehicles should be used to transport pullets from grow-out houses to the layer farm.

5.7. Feed additives and heat treatment

Organic acids and their salts, essential oils, formaldehyde, bacteriophages, probiotics, prebiotics, and symbiotics can be used to modify the gut environment to prevent *Salmonella* colonization, invasion, multiplication, and shedding. Probiotics consist of single or multiple beneficial bacteria strains that colonize intestinal tract; they compete with pathological bacteria as *Salmonella* for attachment sites, nutrients in the luminal surface of enterocytes. Probiotics also produce antibacterial compounds as bacteriocins and volatile fatty acids. Prebiotics are food ingredients as oligosaccharides that stimulate intestinal bacteria and probiotic growth. Symbiotics are products that contain both prebiotics and probiotics. Bacteriophages are viruses that infect and replicate in bacteria and have an effect against *Salmonella*.

Organic acids reduce *Salmonella* in contaminated feed. Formic and propionic acids and their salts are commonly included in feed, but the effect varies by the inclusion rate, food level contamination, feed´s moisture and the type of acid. Formaldehyde is permitted in some countries; therefore, it is corrosive and potentially harmful for humans and animals.

Appropriate pelleting process can eliminate *Salmonella* by heat treatment; it is performed at 93°C for 90 s [17]. Combinations of several of these treatments have been shown effective in recontaminated feed. Measures to prevent recontamination of finished feed should to be taken.

Author details

Rebeca Zamora-Sanabria and Andrea Molina Alvarado*

*Address all correspondence to: andrea.molina@ucr.ac.cr

Center for Research in Animal Nutrition (CINA), University of Costa Rica, Ciudad Universitaria Rodrigo Facio, San José, Costa Rica

References

[1] FAO. www.fao.org [Internet]. 2003. Available from: www.fao.org/english/newsroom/news/2003/15903-en.html

[2] FFAO/WHO Food and Agriculture Organization of the United Nations/World Health Organization. *Salmonella* and *Campylobacter* in chicken meat: Meeting report. Microbiological Risk Assessment Series. 2009. No.19. Rome, 56 pp.

[3] Slorach S. Coordinating surveillance policies in animal health and food safety "from farm to fork". Scientific and Technical Review OIE. 2013;32(2):313-317.

[4] Griffith R.W., Schwartz K.J., Meyerholz D.K. Diseases of Swine. 9th ed. Oxford, United Kingdom: Blackwell Publishing; 2006.

[5] Barrow P.A., Methner U., *Salmonella* in Domestic Animals. 2nd ed., edited by Paul A. Barrow and U. Methner. Oxfordshire, Wallingsford, CABI, United Kingdom; 2013. 547 pp.

[6] Terzolo H. Bacteriological study of avian salmonellosis (*S. pullorum, S. gallinarum, S. enteritidis* and *S. typhimurium*) in Latin America. In: Alberto R., editor. International Seminar on Avian Salmonellosis; 28–30 June 2011; Rio Jainerio. Brazil: Latin America Poultry Association; 2011.

[7] Bailey J.S., Stern, N.J., Fedorka-Cray P., Craven S.E., Cox N.A., Cosby D.E., Ladely S., Musgrove T.M. Sources and movement of *Salmonella* through integrated poultry operations: A multistate epidemiological investigation. Journal of Food Protection. 2001;64(11):1690-1697.

[8] Poppe C., Johnson R., Forsberg C., Irwin R. *Salmonella* enteritidis and other *Salmonella* in laying hens and eggs from flocks with *Salmonella* in their environment. Canadian Journal of Veterinary Research. 1992;56:226-232.

[9] Andres V., Davies R. Biosecurity measures to control *Salmonella* and other infections agents in pig farms: A review. Comprehensive reviews. In Food Science and Food Safety. 2015;4:317-335.

[10] Pires A.F.A., Funk J.A., Bolin C.Risk factors associated with persistence of *Salmonella* shedding in finishing pigs. Preventive Veterinary Medicine. 2014;116:120-128.

[11] Gow A.G., Gow D.J., Hall E.J., Langton D., Clarke C., Papasouliotis K. Prevalence of potentially pathogenic enteric organisms in clinically healthy Kittens in the UK. Journal of Feline Medicine and Surgery. 2009;11:655-622.

[12] De Busser E., De Zutter L., Dewulf J., Houf K., Maes, D. *Salmonella* control in live pigs and at slaughter. The Veterinary Journal. 2013;196:20-27.

[13] Berchieri A., Murphy C.K., Marston K., Barrow P.A. Observations on the persistence and vertical transmission of *Salmonella enterica* serovars Pullorum and Gallinarum in chickens: Effect of bacterial and host genetic background. Avian Pathology. 2001;30:221-231.

[14] Hanson D.L., Loneragan G.H., Brown R.T., Nisber D.J., Hume M.E., Edrington T.S. Evidence supporting vertical transmission of *Salmonella* in dairy cattle. Epidemiology and Infection. 2016;144:962-967.

[15] Schleifer J.J., Juven B.J., Beard C.W., Cox N.A. The susceptibility of chicks to *Salmonella* Montevideo in artificially contaminated poultry feed. Avian Disease. 1984;28:497-503.

[16] Lo Fo Wong D.M.A., Hald T., Van der Wolf P.J., Swanenburg M. Epidemiology and control measures for *Salmonella* in pigs and pork. Livestock Production Science. 2002;76:215-222.

[17] Jones F.T. A review of practical *Salmonella* control measures in animal feed. Journal of Applied Poultry Research. 2011;20:102-113.

[18] Aphis. www.aphis.usda.gov [Internet]. 25 March 2005. Available from: www.aphis.usda.gov/vs/ceah/ncahs/nahms/poultry/Layers99/lay99se.pdf

[19] Ekiri A.B., Morton A.J., Long M.T., MacKay R.J., Hernandez J.A. Review of the epidemiology and infection control aspects of nosocomial *Salmonella* infections in hospitalized horses. Equine Veterinary Education. 2010;22:631-641.

[20] Barber D.A., Bahnson P.B., Jones C.J., Weigel R.M. Distribution of *Salmonella* in swine production ecosystems. Journal of Food Protection. 2002;65(12):1861-1868.

[21] Levantesi C., Bonadonna L., Briancesco R., Grohmann E., Toze S., Tandoi V. *Salmonella* in surface and drinking water: Occurrence and water-mediated transmission. Food Research International. 2012;45:587-602.

[22] Jacques M., Aragon V., Tremblay Y.D. Biofilm formation in bacterial pathogens of veterinary importance. Animal Health Research Review. 2010;11(2):97-121.

[23] Davies R.H., Wray C. Mice and carriers of *Salmonella* enteritidis on persistently infected poultry units. Veterinary Record. 1995;137(14):337-341.

[24] Henzler D.J., Opitz H.M. The role of mice in the epizootiology of *Salmonella* enteritidis infection on chicken layer farms. Avian Diseases. 1992;336:625-631.

[25] Meeburg, B.G., Van Riel J.W., Cornelissen J.B., Kijlstra A., Mul M.F.. Cats and goat whey associated with *Toxoplasma gondii* infection in pigs. Vector Borne Zoonot. 2006;6:266-274.

[26] Wales A.D., Carrique-Mas J.J., Ranquin M., Bell B., Thind B.B., Davies R.H. Review of the carriage of zoonotic bacteria by Arthropods, with special reference to *Salmonella* in mites, flies and litter beetles. Zoonosis and Public Health. 2010;57:299-314.

[27] Lapuz R.R.S., Umali D., Suzuki T., Shirota K., Katoh H. Comparison of prevalence of *Salmonella* infection in layer hens from commercial layer farms with high and low rodent densities. Avian Diseases. 2012;56:29-34.

[28] Vanselow B.A., Hornitzky M.A., Walker K.H., Eamens G.J., Bailey G.D., Gill P.A., Coates K., Corney B., Cronin J.P., Renilson S. *Salmonella* on-farm risk factors in healthy slaughterage cattle and sheep in eastern Australia. Australian Veterinary Journal. 2007;85:498-502.

[29] Tessier C., Parama A.L., Lagadec E., Le Minter G., Denis M., Cardinale E. Wild fauna as a carrier of Salmonella in Reunion Island: Impact on pig farms. Acta Tropica. 2016;158: 6-12. doi:10.1016/j.actatropica.2016.01.027

[30] Fathpour H., Emtiazi G., Ghasemi E.. Cockroaches as reservoirs and vectors of drug resistant *Salmonella* spp. Fresenius Environmental Bulletin. 2003;12:724-727.

[31] Handeland K., Nesse L.L., Lillehaugh A., Vokore T., Djonne B., Bergsjo B. Natural and experimental *Salmonella* Typhimurium infections in foxes. Veterinary Microbiology. 2008;132:129-134.

[32] Kich J.D., Mores N., Piffer I.A., Coldebella A., Amaral A., Ramminger L.,Cardoso M. Factor associated with seroprevalence of *Salmonella* in commercial pig herds. Ciencia Rural. 2005;35:398-405.

[33] Andino A., Pendleton S., Zhang N., Chen W., Critzer F., Hanning I.. Survival of *Salmonella enterica* in poultry feed is strain depended. Poultry Science. 2014;93:441-447.

[34] Chen W., Golden A.D., Critzer F.J.. *Salmonella* survival and differential expression of fatty acid biosynthesis-associated genes in a low-water-activity food. Letters in Applied Microbiology. 2014;59:133-138.

[35] EFSA. European Commission on Microbiological Risk Assessment in feedingstuffs for food-producing animals. EFSA Journal. 2009;720:1-84.

[36] Hald, T., Wingstrand, A., Pires, S. M., Vieira, A., Coutinho Calado Domingues, A. R., Lundsby, K. L.,Thrane,C. Assessment of the human-health impact of *Salmonella* in animal feed. Copenhagen: Technical University of Denmark (DTU); 2012. 73 p.

[37] Silbergeld E.K., Graham J., Price L.B.. Industrial food animal production, antimicrobial resistance, and human health. Annual Review of Public Health. 2009;29:151-169.

[38] Granados-Chinchilla F., Alfaro M., Chavarría G., Rodríguez C.. Unravelling a vicious circle: Animal feed marketed in Costa Rica contains irregular concentrations of tetracyclines and abundant oxytetracycline-resistant Gram-positive bacteria. Food Additives & Contaminants. Part A, Chemistry, Analysis, Control, Exposure & Risk Assessment. 2014;31:1017-1025.

[39] Food and Drug administration. Compliance Policy Guide 690.800 *Salmonella* in Food for Animals. FDA. 2013.

[40] Molina A., Granados-Chinchilla F., Jiménez M., Acuña-Calvo M.T., Alfaro M., Chavarría G. Vigilance for *Salmonella* in feedstuffs available in Costa Rica: Prevalence, serotyping and tetracycline resistance of isolates obtained from 2009 to 2014. Foodborne Pathogens and Disease. 2016; 13(3):119-127. doi:10.1089/fpd.2015.2050

[41] Molina-Alvarado A., Granados-Chinchilla F. Microbiological safety of animal feed in Costa Rica. Revista Nutrición Animal Tropical. 2015; 9(3):13-31.

[42] Center for Disease Control (CDC). Multiple-serotype *Salmonella* gastroenteritis outbreak after a reception – Connecticut, 2009. Morbidity and Mortality Weekly Report (MMWR). 2010;59(34):1093-1097.

[43] Rebolledo J., Garvey P., Ryan A., O'Donnell J., Cormican M., Jackson S., et al. International outbreak investigation of *Salmonella* Heidelberg associated with in-flight catering. Epidemiology and Infection. 2014;142(4):833-842. doi: 10.1017/S0950268813001714

[44] Almeida I.A., Peresi J.T., Alves E., Marques D.F., Teixeira I.S., Silva S.I. *Salmonella* Alachua: Causative agent of a foodborne disease outbreak. Brazilian Journal of Infectious Diseases. 2015;19:233-238.

[45] Adedokun S.A., Adeola O. Metabolizable energy value of meat and bone meal for pigs. Journal of Animal Science. 2005;83:2519-2526.

[46] EFSA (European Food Safety Authority) and ECDC (European Centre for Disease Prevention and Control). The European Union Summary Report on Antimicrobial Resistance in Zoonotic and Indicator Bacteria from Humans, Animals and Food in 2014. EFSA Journal. 2016;14(2):4380,207p. doi:10.2903/j.efsa.2016.4380

[47] Hugas M., Beloeil P.A. Controlling *Salmonella* along the food chain in the European Union – progress over the last ten years. Eurosurveillance. 2014;19(19):20804. Doi: 10.2807/1560-7917.ES2014.19.19.20804

[48] Marin C., Hernandez A., Lainez M. Biofilm development capacity of *Salmonella* Stains isolated in poultry risk factors and their resistance against disinfectants. Poultry Science. 2009; 88:424-431.

[49] Martínez-Martínez S.,Yubero-Delgado S., Rodríguez-Ferri E.F., Frandoloso R., Alvarez-Estrada A., Gutiérrez-Martín C.B. In vitro efficacy of several disinfectants against *Salmonella enterica* serovar Enteritidis and *Escherichia coli* strains from poultry. Ciencia Rural, Santa María. 2016;45:1438-1442.

[50] Soliman E. Taha E.G., Sobiehand M.A.A., Reddy P.G. Efficacy of some commercial chemical disinfectants on *Salmonella enterica* serovar Typhimurium. American Journal of Animal and Veterinary Sciences. 2009;4:58-64.

[51] Dorea F., Cole D.J., Hofacre C., Zamperini K., Mathis D., Doyle M.P., Lee M., Maurer J.J. Effect of *Salmonella* vaccination of breeder chickens on contamination of broiler chicken carcasses in integrated poultry operations. Applied and Environmental Microbiology. 2010;76:7820-7825.

[52] Horacio T.. Model of *Salmonella* live vaccine safety management program. In: Alberto R., editor. International Seminar on Avian Salmonellosis; 28-30 June 2011; Rio Janeiro. Brazil: Latin America Poultry Association; 2011.

[53] Villareal Laura. Model of *Salmonella* Killed vaccine (bacterins) safety management programme. In: Alberto R., editor. International Seminar on Avian Salmonellosis; 28-30 June 2016; Rio Janeiro. Brazil: Latin America Poultry Association; 2011.

[54] Dunford J., Kaufman P. University of Florida. Lesser Mealworm, Litter Beetle, *Alphitobius diaperinus* [Internet]. March 2006. Available from: http://edis.ifas.ufl.edu [Accessed: August 2016]

[55] Tahseen A. Chlorinating drinking water on poultry farms. World Poultry. 2005;21(5):24-25.

[56] De Ridder L., Maes D., Dewulf J., Pasmans F., Boyen F., Méroc E., Butaye P., Van der Stede Y. Transmission study of *Salmonella* in pigs with 3 intervention strategies. Proceedings of the 9th International Conference on the Epidemiology and Control of Biological, Chemical and Physical Hazards in Pigs and Pork. 2011. Iowa State University, June 19–22, Maastricht, Netherlands; 30-33. Available from: www.lib.dr.iastate.edu/safepork/

[57] Mccarthy G., Lawflor P., Gutiérrez M., OSulivan L., Muphy A., Zhan X., Gardiner G. An assessment of *Salmonella* survival in pig manure and its separated solid and liquid fractions during storage. Journal of Enviromental Science and Health. Part B. 2015;50:1532-4109.

[58] Tobin M., Goldhear J.L., Price L.B., Graham J.P., Leibler J.H. A framework to reduce infectious disease risk from urban poultry in the United States. Public Health Reports. 2015; 130 (4): 380-391.

[59] Sternberg S., Skog L., Frossling J., Wahlstrom H. Geographical distribution of *Salmonella* infected pig, cattle and sheep herds in Sweden 1993–2010. Acta Veterinaria Scandinavica. 2011;53:51.

[60] Harhay D., Bono J., Smith T., Fields P., Dinsmore B., Santovenia M. Complete closed genome sequences of *Salmonella enterica* subsp. *enterica* serotypes Anatum, Montevideo, Typhimurium and Newport, isolated from beef, cattle and humans. Genome Announcemements. 2016;4(1):1-2.

[61] Fegan N., Vanderline P., Higgs G., Desmarchelier P., Quantification and prevalence of *Salmonella* in beef cattle presenting at slaughter. Journal of Applied Microbiology. 2004;97:892-898.

[62] Rivera W., Barquero E., Zamora R.. *Salmonella* contamination risk points in broiler carcasses during slaughter line processing. Journal of food protection. 2014;77:2031-2034.

[63] Barbour E., Ayyash D., Alyahiby A., Yaghmoor S., Yaghmoor S., Lyer A., Yousef J., Kumosani T., Harakeh S. Impact of sporadic reporting of poultry *Salmonella* serovars from selected developing countries. Journal of Infection in Developing Countries. 2015;9(1):001-007.

[64] Branka V., Savic S., Prica N., Suvajdzic L. Epizootiology and control measures for *Salmonella* in pigs. Procesdia Food Science. 2015;5:312-315.

Chapter 12

Prevalence, Risks and Antibiotic Resistance of Salmonella in Poultry Production Chain

Niki Mouttotou, Shakeel Ahmad, Zahid Kamran and Konstantinos C. Koutoulis

Additional information is available at the end of the chapter

http://dx.doi.org/10.5772/67438

Abstract

Salmonella spp. are bacteria that cause salmonellosis, a common form of foodborne illness with major impact on human health and huge financial losses in poultry industry. The incidence of notified cases of salmonellosis has declined from a peak of 24 per 100,000 in 2009 to 20.4 reported cases per 100,000 population in 2013, with *S. enteritidis* and *S. typhimurium* being the most commonly reported serovar in EU. *Salmonella* spp. has been detected in a range of foods, and outbreaks have predominantly been associated with animal products such as eggs, poultry and dairy products, but also with plant origin food such as salad dressing, fruit juice and sesame. At the time of slaughter, *Salmonella*-infected poultry may have high numbers of organisms in their intestines as well as on the outside of the bird and are therefore an important source of contamination. Nowadays, food safety has become an important concern for the European society and governments; therefore, more strict and harmonized regulations are being implemented throughout the poultry production chain with the aim to guarantee and increase the consumer confidence in foodstuffs of animal origin. Furthermore, increasing antimicrobial resistance in non-typhoid *Salmonella* species has been a serious problem for public health worldwide.

Keywords: salmonellosis, foodborne, prevalence, poultry, antibiotic resistance

1. Introduction

Salmonella has been declared by the World Health Organization (WHO) and the Food Agriculture Organization (FAO) as the most common and important zoonosis since 1950.

This has led to its inclusion in the terrestrial animal health code of the World Animal Health Organization In humans, typhoid disease manifests one to 2 weeks following bacterial inoculation with generalized fever and malaise, abdominal pain with or without other symptoms including headache, myalgias, nausea, anorexia and constipation [1]. An estimation of the annual non-typhoid *Salmonella* gastroenteritis suggests that there are around 94 million cases, resulting in 155,000 deaths, and that the majority of the disease burden, according to this study, is in the South-East Asian Region and the Western Pacific Region [2]. Most human salmonellosis cases are foodborne, but each year, infections are also acquired through direct or indirect animal contact in homes, veterinary clinics, zoos, farm environments or other public, professional or private settings. It has been estimated that approximately 80.3 million of 93.8 million human *Salmonella*-related gastroenteritis cases—that are diagnosed globally each year—are foodborne, thus representing approximately 86% of human salmonellosis cases [2]. Another study estimated that approximately 55% of human *Salmonella* cases were foodborne, 14% were travel-related, 13% are acquired through environmental sources, 9% occurred due to direct human-to-human transmission and 9% were attributable to direct animal contact [3, 4].

2. *Salmonella* species classification

The bacteria of the genus *Salmonella* are responsible for illnesses in human beings and animals. The genus is divided into two species: *Salmonella enterica* and *Salmonella bongori* [5]. *S. enterica* is divided into six subspecies (*enterica, salamae, arizonae, diarizonae, houtenae* and *indica*) and each one of them has several serovars or serotypes. Nowadays, more than 2500 serotypes are known and almost 1500 of them belong to the subspecies enterica [6]. Most pathogenic isolates from humans and other mammals belong to *S. enterica* subspecies enterica. Other *S. enterica* subspecies and *S. bongori* are more common in cold-blooded animals and the environment, with lower pathogenicity to humans and livestock [7, 8].

A few serotypes are host specific; i.e. *S. typhi* is implicated in typhoid fever in human beings, while *Salmonella pullorum* and *gallinarum* are responsible for bacillary white diarrhoea and fowl typhoid in poultry, respectively [9]. *Salmonella choleraesuis* is host restricted to pigs, *Salmonella* ser. *abortusovis* is involved in sheep abortions and *Salmonella dublin* infects bovines [10]. There are a number of non-host-specific serotypes that may infect several animal species, including humans, and these are generally responsible for foodborne diseases with foods of animal origin being the main source. From the early years, the most common agent of human foodborne disease was *Salmonella typhimurium*, but in the last few decades the frequency of *Salmonella enteritidis* has dramatically increased [11]. Almost 80 out of 2500 serovars are thought to be frequently involved in animal and human salmonellosis. *S. typhimurium* and *S. enteritidis* are the most common agents of disease in human beings and animals, but lately, there is also increasing concern about *S. typhimurium monophasic, S. derby, infantis, agona, hadar, heidelberg* and *virchow* serotypes.

3. Transmission routes, public health and economic cost associated with *Salmonella* infection

The gastrointestinal tracts of humans and animals are the primary sources of *Salmonella*. The bacteria are carried asymptomatically in the intestines or gall bladder of many animals and are continuously or intermittently shed in the faeces. Also, these can be carried latently in the mesenteric lymph nodes or tonsils [12], which are not then shed, but can become reactivated after stress or immunosuppression [13]. Although most infections cause mild to moderate self-limiting disease, serious infections leading to deaths do occur [14]. Its widespread presence in the environment is considered to be due to the direct or indirect faecal contamination [15]. The transmission to humans usually occurs through the consumption of food or water contaminated with animal faeces, but it can also happen through direct contact with infected animals or their environment and directly between humans. In the same way, animals can become infected from contaminated feed (including pastures), drinking water or close contact with an infected animal (including humans).

Transovarian (vertical transmission) or trans-shell (horizontal transmission) occurs in poultry. In the first case, a contamination of the vitelline membrane, albumen and possibly the yolk of eggs occurs. Following this route, *Salmonellae* are introduced from infected reproductive tissues to eggs prior to shell formation. *Salmonella* serotypes with high importance to public health, associated with poultry reproductive tissues, include *S. enteritidis, S. typhimurium* and *Salmonella heidelberg*. Among all the different serotypes, *S. enteritidis* may be more invasive and, consequently, may be found more frequently in reproductive tissues. Faecal contamination of egg shell is the primary cause of horizontal transmission [16]. This can also include contamination through environmental vectors, such as farmers, pets and rodents, feed, water, fluff, dust, shavings and straw, insects, equipment, and thus, many different serotypes of the genus *Salmonella* can be involved [17, 18]. Bacteria can contaminate egg contents by migration through the egg shell and membranes. Such a route is facilitated by factors such as moist egg shells, storage at ambient temperature and shell damage. Faecal shedding of *S. enteritidis* was detected for up to 8-week post-inoculation by hens housed in enriched colony cages and 10 weeks by hens housed in conventional cages, which were experimentally infected with *S. enteritidis* [19]. Studies on the survival of *S. enteritidis* in poultry units and food were carried out over a 2-year period and showed that the organism persisted for at least 1 year in an empty trial house at the laboratory in which naturally infected broiler breeder birds had previously been housed [20]. In the same study, a similar survival period was found in a building which had housed an infected layer breeder flock, although infection was not detected in a subsequent pullet flock. *Salmonella* contamination appeared to persist preferentially in association with dust particles swept from the floor and in food troughs, and *S. enteritidis* survived at least 26 months in artificially contaminated poultry food [20].

Salmonella spp. can also be transmitted *in utero* in other mammals. Wild birds, rodents, fomites and mechanical vectors (insects) can spread *Salmonella* to livestock. In general, *Salmonella* serotypes have a broad host range and clinical manifestations that result from the combination between serotype and host species involved [21] are prevalent in a whole range of warm-blooded animal population [22] but also in snakes [23], and free-living terrestrial and aquatic turtles [24].

Salmonella spp. can survive for long periods in the environment, particularly, where it is wet and warm. They can be isolated from many sources including farm effluents, human sewage and water. Persistence of *Salmonella* in acid soils is facilitated by their ability to adapt to low-pH environments [25]. There is also some evidence that *Salmonella* may survive in soils in a viable but non-culturable state [26], although significance of this state is not yet understood. *S. choleraesuis* has been isolated for up to 450 days from pig meat and for several months from faeces or faecal slurries [27]. *Salmonella typhimurium* and *Salmonella dublin* have been found for over a year in the environment.

Plant origin material can be contaminated through direct deposition of *Salmonella*-containing animal faeces or through deposition of soil or dust previously contaminated with animal faecal material. In some circumstances, there has been an increasing evidence that *Salmonella* may be internalized in plant tissues [28]. This, however, was quite uncertain whether it was relevant to crops commonly used as components of animal feed.

Person-to-person transmission of *Salmonella* is well-recognized, and secondary transmission of *Salmonella* in outbreaks has been demonstrated [29]. Carriage in faeces in convalescent cases can be quite substantial with numbers approximating 10^6 to 10^7 Salmonella/g persisting up to 10 days after initial diagnosis according to the authors. Reduction in numbers with time seems to be variable; most people will have count of less than 100 Salmonella/g after 35–40 days, but a count of 6×10^3/g has been recorded in one patient 48 days post-illness [30]. Asymptomatic carriage may also occur, as it was mentioned for a British outbreak of hospital-acquired infection [31] and another case where asymptomatic food handlers have been responsible for an outbreak in a catering establishment in Jerusalem [32].

Non-typhoidal *Salmonella* are a leading cause of bacterial diarrhoea worldwide; they are estimated to cause 94 million cases of gastroenteritis and 115,000 deaths globally each year [2]. Of these, 80.3 million cases were estimated as foodborne origin. In one analysis [33] using data from the Foodborne Diseases Active Surveillance Network (FoodNet), the risk of *Salmonella* infection among travellers returning to the USA varied by region of the world visited. Travellers with salmonellosis were most likely to report visiting the following countries: Mexico (38% of travel-associated salmonellosis), India (9%), Jamaica (7%), the Dominican Republic (4%), China (3%) and the Bahamas (2%). Travel-associated infections were related to *Salmonella* in 36.7% of the cases reported, of which non-typhoidal *Salmonella* accounted for 88.3%, typhoidal *Salmonella* 7.7%, and paratyphoidal *Salmonella* 3.9%.

In the latest EFSA's report, a total of 82,694 confirmed salmonellosis cases were reported by 27 European Union (EU) member states in 2013, resulting in an EU notification rate of 20.4 cases per 100,000 population [11].

A decrease of 7.9% in the EU notification rate compared with 2012 was shown in the above report, which supports the declining trend of salmonellosis in the EU/European Economic

Area (EEA) in the 5-year period of 2009–2013 (**Figure 1**). However, the above was not statistically significant when analysed by month. Nine out of 14 EU member states reported a total of 59 fatal cases, which gave an EU case-fatality rate of 0.14% among the 40,976 confirmed cases. Some researchers claim that human salmonellosis represents a considerable economic impact and the estimated costing can be as €3 billion/year [34]. As in previous years, *S. enteritidis* and *S. typhimurium* represented 39.5 and 20.2%, respectively, in confirmed human cases, and they were the two most commonly reported *Salmonella* serovars in 2013 [11]. An interesting finding in the same report was that in the 2-year period from 2011 to 2013, cases of *S. typhimurium*, including the variant monophasic *S. typhimurium* 1,4,[5],12:i:-, decreased by 11.1%, while cases of *S. infantis* (which was the fourth most common serovar observed), increased by 26.5%. The fifth most common serovar observed in 2013, was *S. derby*, and this could partly be explained by a local outbreak in Berlin, Germany and surrounding areas in December 2013/January 2014. The outbreak occurred in hospitals and nursing homes with 145 elderly patients affected and one fatal case. The suspected vehicle of infection was rawfermented pork spread ('teewurst') [11].

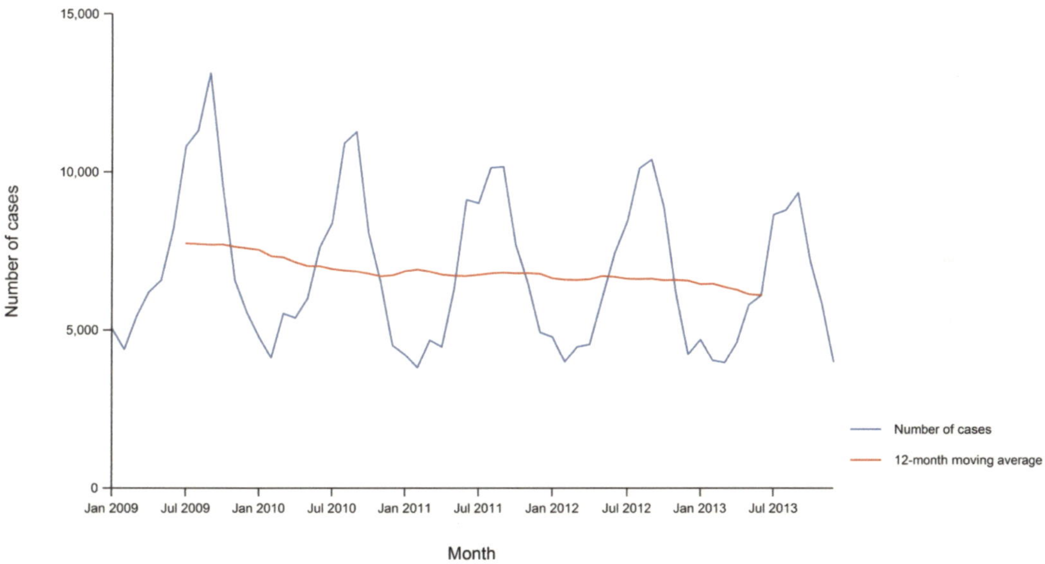

Figure 1. Trend in reported confirmed cases of human non-typhoidal salmonellosis in the EU/EEA, 2009–2013. Source: Austria, Belgium, Cyprus, Czech Republic, Denmark, Estonia, Finland, France, Germany, Greece, Hungary, Iceland, Ireland, Lithuania, Luxembourg, Malta, Netherlands, Norway, Portugal, Romania, Slovakia, Slovenia, Spain, Sweden and United Kingdom. Bulgaria, Croatia, Italy, Latvia, Poland and Romania did not report data over the whole period in the level of detail needed for the analysis.

In a recent report published by USDA in 2015 [35], a comparison of the economic burden showed that *Salmonella* ranks first among the 15 pathogens included in the study and sixth on a per-case basis. It imposes an estimated $3.7 billion in economic burden in a typical year. Almost 90% of this burden, thus $3.3 billion, is due to deaths; 8%, $294 million, is due to hospitalization and the remaining 2% is due to non-hospitalized cases (hospitalization rate of 27.2% and a death rate of 0.5%).

According to Decision No. 2119/98/EC and 2000/96/EC, surveillance of foodborne salmonellosis in humans is mandatory in the EU member states as well as setting up a network for the epidemiological surveillance and control of communicable diseases in the Community [36, 37]. Data on humans, animals and food are compiled and analysed jointly by the European Food Safety Agency (EFSA) and the European Centre for Disease Prevention and Control (ECDC) and presented annually in the EU Summary Report on trends and sources of zoonoses, zoonotic agents and foodborne outbreaks [37].

4. *Salmonella* spp. in poultry and poultry products

Salmonella species that colonize the intestinal tract of poultry can persist throughout the bird's lifespan in a poultry-producing environment and are shed with faeces [9, 16]. Faecal shedding allows *Salmonella* to be transmitted among birds in a flock. *Salmonella* spp. is widespread in poultry production in Europe. Prevalence varies considerably depending on country and type of production as well as the detection methods applied. Results showed that prevalence is at the lowest level at the top of the production pyramid, i.e. the breeding stock. As mentioned above poultry meat and eggs represent an important source of human infection with *Salmonella* spp. *with S. enteritidis* and *S. typhimurium* been the most commonly reported serovars involved.

In the primary production, there are numerous activities that influence the introduction, growth or elimination of *Salmonella* species for poultry and poultry products, and therefore, many opportunities are given to *Salmonella* to enter the food chain, even though other steps will prevent growth or inactivate the pathogen. Several studies have studied the risk factors [38–40] associated with *Salmonella* contamination in broiler chickens. The most important risk factors included contaminated chicks, size of the farm (>3 poultry sheds—presumably related to increased human traffic among multiple sheds) and contaminated feed (the risk of Salmonella contamination of the flock was increased when feed trucks were parked near the entrance of the workers' change room and when feed meal, instead of small pellets). A systematic review of the risk factors associated with *Salmonella* in laying hens [41] concluded that the presence of previous *Salmonella* infection, absence of larger flock size (>30,000 hens), multi-age management, cage housing systems, rearing pullets on the floor, induced molting and in-line egg processing were factors associated with Salmonella infection. Also, cleaning and disinfection, presence of rodents, pests with access to feed prior to movement to the feed trough, visitors allowed in the layer houses and trucks near farms and air inlets were risks identified to be associated with *Salmonella* contamination of laying hen premises. However, high level of manure contamination, middle and late phase of production, high degree of egg-handling equipment contamination, flock size of >30,000, and egg production rate of >96% were identified as the risk factors associated with *Salmonella* contamination of shell eggs.

These were risks which showed strong to moderate evidence of association with *Salmonella* contamination of laying hens and shell eggs. In the same study, eggshells testing positive for *Salmonella* were 59 times higher when faecal samples were positive and nine times higher when floor dust samples were positive. Furthermore, the presence of *Salmonella enteriditis* infection in laying hens was associated with risk factors such as flock size, housing system and farms with hens of different ages.

The Panel on Biological Hazards [42] recommended that the application of hazard analysis critical control point (HACCP) principles, including good manufacturing practices and general hygiene procedures are recognized as important measures for *Salmonella* control in feed production. However, prevalence data for Salmonella in feed ingredients or compounded feed are usually very difficult to compare between different studies due to differences in sampling and analytical methods applied. The existing community legislation on food hygiene and control of zoonosis [43] constitutes a number of provisions that aim to control and prevent the *Salmonella* contamination of foodstuffs. Targets for *Salmonella* spp. were set progressively in different animal populations: breeding flocks of Gallus gallus, laying hens, broilers and turkeys. As an obligation, member states have developed and submitted national control programs to the commission which include recommendation on establishing strict biosecurity measures at farm level (including *Salmonella*-free poultry feed and water), vaccination programs in the parent flocks [44] as well as testing and removal of positive flocks from production. Except of encouraging immunity or resistance to *Salmonella* infection in birds through the use of antibodies, other strategies to prevent infection include the use of feed additives or acidified food. It is expected that acid treatments have a residual protective effect on feed, which reduces both the recontamination of feed as well as the contamination of milling and feeding equipment and the general environment [45]. However, the efficacy of organic acids against *Salmonella* depends on the level of bacterial contamination [46]. The same author recommends that, except feed treatment, water acidification can help prevent *Salmonella*, as the supplementation of acids in drinking water reduces the pH level and bacterial counts.

Nowadays, the trend seems to be towards production becoming more integrated, and many small farms will be replaced in the future by fewer, bigger farms, which will allow a greater integration and consequently to a better control of *Salmonella*. Furthermore, comparisons of *Salmonella* species contamination of free range or organic production systems with 'conventional' systems have produced varied results and more statistically valid surveys are required to ascertain if differences do occur [47]. In addition, the transportation of poultry between farms and from the farm to the processing plant offers an environment where *Salmonella* species might be spread between birds [48–50]. Shedding of large numbers of pathogens in faecal material during transport is believed to be related to increased stress in birds [48, 49].

Sewage and farm effluents, which can contaminate pasture, soil and water with *Salmonella*, tend to be handled more consciously lately, due to the pressure of environmental law requirements. However, the breeding stocks used all over the world are produced by a small number of companies, meaning that these sell to purchasers worldwide and this can lead to the wide-scale spread of *Salmonella*, if the breeding stocks are infected. One should also take into consideration that where the aim is to control specific serotypes, a zero-tolerance policy with respect to these organisms may give a false sense of security, because the predominant serotypes in poultry flocks are likely to change over time.

5. Primary and secondary poultry processing and retail

The most important control measure at primary production, apart from those focusing in the elimination of *Salmonella* in grandparent and parent flocks by vaccination and an all-in-all-out production at the broiler farm, is to avoid any carry over during processing which is achieved by a logistic slaughter planning scheduled to avoid pathogens being transferred from contaminated processing equipment to another flock, and finally the satisfactory cleaning of transport crates. The operations that are thought to increase the contamination while in the processing line are scalding, plucking and evisceration. The most important critical control point in the process in relation to contamination is the feather plucker. Also, evisceration can be considered as an important risk due to a consequence of gut rupture. The evisceration machinery may play a role in damaging poultry carcasses while these are not entirely uniform in size. Most studies so far have shown that the prevalence of *Salmonella* species is usually higher on poultry carcasses at the end of primary processing than at the start [51, 52], although the concentrations of organisms on carcasses tend to decrease [17].

To reduce carcass contamination, decontamination measures can be applied. Many countries after the adoption of the 'Code of hygienic practice recommended for poultry processing' by the Codex Alimentarius in 1994, adopted their own code of practices for poultry processing. The requirements for cleaning of de-feathering equipment and recommended list of used disinfectants and practices of physical separation of de-feathering from later primary processing steps, requirements for processors to define acceptable levels of visible faecal contamination following evisceration and monitoring requirements for faecal contamination and practices of spaying or rinsing/dipping are included in this code. As far as these decontamination measures is concerned, one should take into consideration that, there are some regional differences, since chemical treatment is not accepted in the EU at the moment, but is widely used in other parts of the world, e.g. in the USA and New Zealand.

Poultry secondary processing includes portioning and processing of carcasses or portions into value-added products. During secondary processing, *Salmonella* prevalence may increase due to cross-contamination, while concentrations of *Salmonella* may increase if temperature control is not properly maintained [53]. Both poultry muscle and skin are excellent substrates for a wide variety of microorganisms [54], but the potential shelf life of raw poultry is quite short (e.g. chicken samples had spoiled after 4 days at 9°C) [55]. Unless frozen, raw poultry has a rapid turnover at retail, often 24–48 hours with a best before date of 3–4 days [56].

Salmonella species can survive well at refrigeration temperatures and will grow on fresh poultry under warmer, more favourable, temperatures (e.g. during transportation from a retail outlet to a consumer's home). *Salmonella* numbers are reduced under frozen storage conditions but salmonellosis outbreaks from 1998 to 2008 due to consumption of frozen products showed that bacteria can survive freezing and *Salmonella* may pose an infection risk if the product is improperly cooked [57]. Thus, freezing cannot be considered as an adequate control step.

In a New Zealand consumer survey, the times and temperatures of purchased poultry products during transportation by consumers were examined [58]. It showed that thawing poultry at room temperature for up to 12 hours was a common practice and that any *Salmonella* present on the surface of the poultry could be able to grow once the surface reached room temperature [59]. Other studies have shown that the time required for frozen poultry (–18°C) to reach minimum growth temperature (7°C) would be in the range 3–16 hours, depending on the freezer temperature and ambient (air) temperatures [60]. As growth is greatly reduced up to 15°C (requiring another 3 hours thawing), and not optimal until 35–37°C, normal thawing periods before cooking are unlikely to permit much growth, although situations involving warm freezer temperatures (–7°C) and high ambient temperatures may increase the amount of growth that occurs.

The detection of *Salmonella* in poultry products leads to rejection of large consignments of raw poultry meat, thus affecting poultry trade with huge economic impacts as a consequence. Of course, on top of that, the impact on human health and the associated costs, the trade disruptions and the cost of implementing effective control measures explains why the Codex Alimentarius Commission (CAC) in 2010 [61] agreed that the development of guidelines for the control of *Salmonella* in poultry was a priority. Even though information on the prevalence of *Salmonella* on poultry meat at the end of processing or at retail were available, very few surveys have been undertaken where the number of organisms has been quantified [62] because enumeration of *Salmonella* proved to be very laborious.

Furthermore, interventions at the processing stages are assessed using growth models. These take into consideration several factors such as the levels of contamination when carcasses leave the processing plant, storage time in retail stores, transport time, storage times in homes and the temperatures carcasses were exposed to during each of these periods. It should be mentioned that the presence and level of *Salmonella* in this step is very much country specific, since the level of infection when leaving the processing step varies between the countries in relation to the methods which are used at the processing plant. In any case, national data must be used when estimating levels of contamination therefore [16].

6. Food of animal and plant origin as a source of *Salmonella* serovars for humans

Both plant and animal product-based animal feed ingredients may be contaminated with *Salmonella*. Red and white meat, meat products, milk, cheese and eggs are considered the major food sources of human salmonellosis, although a wide variety of other foods have been associated with outbreaks [8]. Other researchers reported that lamb's liver was responsible for an outbreak of *S. typhimurium* phage-type 197 in Australia [63]. In Germany, from 2001 to 2005, microbiological testing, trace-back investigations and epidemiological studies showed that pork and pork products were involved in human salmonellosis outbreaks [64]. In Italy, an outbreak of *S. typhimurium* phage-type DT 104A involving 63 cases suggested that the consumption of pork salami was associated with this outbreak, underlining the importance of good manufacturing practices for ready-to-eat foods [65]. Many other reports involving human salmonellosis outbreaks associated with consumption of red meat have been recorded in the literature [66, 67], and in most of cases, the disease was associated with the consumption of contaminated meat or was a result of incorrect or inadequate cooking.

In the European Union (EU), contaminated foodstuffs serving as a source of *Salmonella* infection for humans include table eggs closely followed by pig meat, whereas the risks associated with broiler and turkey meat are similar and approximately two-fold lower [68]. As far as the distribution of serovars is concerned, in the EU, *S. enteritidis* and *S. typhimurium* are the serovars most commonly associated with human illness. Human cases of *S. enteritidis* are most frequently associated with the consumption of contaminated eggs and poultry meat, while *S. typhimurium* cases are associated with the consumption of contaminated pig meat or bovine meat [69]. It is estimated that around 10.6, 17, 56.8 and 2.6% of the human salmonellosis cases in the EU are attributable to broilers, laying hens (eggs), pigs and turkeys, respectively [70]. Of the broiler-associated human salmonellosis cases, around 82 and 6.5% are estimated to be due to the serovars *S. enteritidis* and *S. infantis*, respectively [71]. In the EU, approximately 9% of turkey carcasses are *Salmonella*-positive and the top six serovars that contribute to human cases are *S. enteritidis, S. kentucky, S. typhimurium, S. newport, S. virchow* and *S. saintpaul* [70]. While there are few data on the prevalence of pathogens on trimmings and meat cuts used for minced meat products, in [71] *Salmonella* spp. was detected on up to 5.3% of beef trimmings. The highest levels of non-compliance with *Salmonella* criteria generally occurred in foods of meat origin that are intended to be cooked before consumption in 2014, as in the last years [11]. Minced meat and meat preparations from poultry intended to be eaten cooked showed the highest level of non-compliance (category 1.5; 8.7% of single samples and 5.7% of batches). One should consider that growth of *Salmonella* should be absent or very slow in correctly chilled meat intended for preparation of mince since the organism show a reported minimum growth temperature of 5°C and an optimum temperature of 35–43°C [72], a pH growth range of 4.5–9.0.

A long list of foods that have been contaminated by *Salmonella* includes: seafood (shellfish, salmon), cereal and cereal products (barley, cereal powder), oilseeds and oilseed products (cottonseed, soybean sauce, sesame seeds), nuts and nut products (desiccated coconut, peanut butter), spices (white and black pepper, paprika), vegetables (watercress, tomatoes, lettuce, potato and other salads and bean sprouts), fruit and fruit products (watermelon, melon and cider) and other miscellaneous products (chocolate, cocoa powder, dried yeast and candy). *Salmonella* contaminated tahini (a product made from crushed sesame seeds) has caused a number of outbreaks worldwide, including New Zealand and Australia [73]. In 2002, an outbreak of *S. montevideo* occurred in New South Wales, Australia showing that imported 'tahini' was rapidly identified as the source of infection.

In foods from vegetable origin, detection of *Salmonella* serovars is a matter of increasing concern. Recent literature highlights the importance of foods of vegetable origin as potential vehicles of gastrointestinal infection nowadays. *Salmonella* serovars may contaminate vegetables during production, storage or even in retail outlets. Furthermore, fruits and juices, as they are usually consumed raw, may also be implicated in human salmonellosis.

In 2002, tomatoes, grown and packed in Virginia state (USA), contaminated with *S. newport*, caused illness in 510 patients in 26 other states [74]. Later, in July–November 2005, the same strain (confirmed by PFGE) caused illness in at least 72 patients in 16 states of the USA. *S. newport* strain was responsible for the outbreak which was isolated from pond water used to irrigate tomato fields, suggesting persistent contamination of the fields [75]. Also, during 2005–2006, in the USA and Canada three more outbreaks of *Salmonella* infections associated with eating tomatoes were detected. These outbreaks resulted in 387 culture-confirmed cases of salmonellosis, with isolation of *S. newport*, *S. braenderup* and *S. typhimurium* [76].

Unpasteurized orange juice was responsible for foodborne salmonellosis in 152 people in six states in the USA between May and July 2005 [77]. From 1995 to 2005, some researchers reviewed fruit juice-associated outbreaks of illness reported to Centres for Disease Control and Prevention (CDC), in Atlanta, USA [78]. Twenty-one juice-associated outbreaks were reported to CDC; 10 implicated apple juice or cider, eight were linked to orange juice and three implicated other types of fruit juice. These outbreaks caused 1366 illnesses, with an average of 21 cases per outbreak (range, 2–398 cases). Five out of 13 outbreaks of known aetiology, were caused by *Salmonella* serovars.

Human salmonellosis due to *S. thompson* infection were reported in Norway as a result of the consumption of rucola lettuce and mixed salad [79]. Prepared salads were also responsible for infectious intestinal disease outbreaks in England and Wales from 1992 to 2006 [80] as a result of international trade. Cross-contamination, infected food handler or inappropriate storage were the most common factors associated with this vegetable contamination.

7. Antibiotic resistance in *Salmonella* serovars: a serious problem in public health

Since 2003, according to the U.S. Food and Drug Administration, antimicrobial resistance in *Salmonella* spp., as well as in other bacterial species, has been recognized as a global threat and an increasing public health matter. Salmonellae have evolved not only virulence mechanisms to interact with host defence mechanisms at various tissues in different stages of infection resulting in significant host immunopathology, morbidity and mortality [1] but have evolved resistance mechanisms against antimicrobial agents, thus triggering host responses.

Individual organisms may transfer mutations that render antibiotics ineffective, passing on a survival advantage to the mutated strain, resulting in a normal genetic variation in bacterial populations. Advantageous mutations can also be conveyed via plasmid exchange within the bacterial colony, in the presence of antibiotics, resulting in proliferation of the resistance trait in the bacterial populations. Natural selection leads to an inherent consequence of exposure to antibiotic compounds and then antibiotic resistance arises.

On the other hand, the spread of particularly resistant clones and the occurrence of resistance genes within these clones can be exacerbated by the use of antimicrobials in human and animal populations and its selective pressure [81]. Many factors may also influence the spread of resistant clones, such as foreign travel by humans, international food trade, animal movements, farming systems, animal husbandry and the pyramidal structure of some types of animal primary production. During the late 1990s and early 2000s, several clones of multi-drug-resistant (MDR) *Salmonella* emerged, and since then, they have expanded worldwide. Multi-drug-resistant *S. enterica* serotype *typhimurium* has been associated with a higher risk of invasive infection, higher frequency and duration of hospitalization, longer illness and increased risk of death as compared to infections caused by susceptible strains [82]. The spread of this resistance in other serotypes is of great concern as well. A very characteristic example is the behaviour of *S. typhimurium*, the genomic element that carries resistance to five antimicrobials (ampicillin, chloramphenicol, streptomycin, sulphonamides and tetracycline), which can be spread horizontally among other serotypes and acquire additional resistance determinants. Genes conferring antimicrobial resistance in *Salmonella* are often carried on integrons and plasmids and could be transmitted through conjugation. These are mobile DNA elements and play an important role in transmission and dissemination of antimicrobial resistance determinants among *Salmonella* strains [83].

2013/652/EU Commission Decision sets an enhanced monitoring of antibiotic resistance (AMR) in bacteria from food and food-producing animals, which has been successfully implemented in all reporting and non-reporting member states. In accordance with the above legislation, the AMR monitoring started in 2014 and collected data referred on food and food-producing animals specifically targeted in different poultry populations and meat derived thereof. Two agents are responsible in performing the analyses of the data: EFSA and ECDC. The results are published in the first EU Summary Report on AMR [81] derived from 28 member states which reported data on AMR in zoonotic bacteria to the EFSA and 21 member states which submitted data to the ECDC. In the above report, the results showed that high proportions of human *Salmonella* isolates were resistant to tetracyclines (30.3%), sulphonamides (28.6%) and ampicillin (28.2%) and more than half (54.8%) of all isolates from humans were susceptible to the complete range of antimicrobial classes tested. A total of 8.8 and 1.1% of *Salmonella* isolates were resistant to ciprofloxacin to cefotaxime, respectively, which is thought to be an overall relatively low proportion of resistance to these clinically important antimicrobials. In the same report, resistance to third-generation cephalosporins was more common in *S. infantis* and *S. kentucky* with particularly high levels observed in Italy, most likely due to the circulation of a multiresistant and ESBL-producing (cefotaximase (CTX-M) type) clone of S. infantis. Also, an extremely high proportion (84.0%) of *S. kentucky* which showed high resistance to ciprofloxacin was mentioned. This is consistent with the dissemination of the ciprofloxacin-resistant *S. kentucky* ST198 strain in Europe and elsewhere since 2010 [84]. Overall, MDR in the EU was high (26.0%), with very high prevalence in some countries. It must be mentioned that some serovars exhibited very high to extremely high MDR. These were *S. kentucky* (74.6%), monophasic *S. typhimurium* 1,4,[5],12:i:- (69.4%) and *S. infantis* (61.9%). Another interesting observation derived from this study was the resistance to colistin which was commonly detected in *S. enteritidis* (67.5%, two member states) and it is thought that could be due to intrinsic resistance in this serovar.

In another study [85], it was reported that over 80% of strains from both human and animal sources that were tested for their antimicrobial resistance, showed that resistance patterns were similar among strains from humans and animals: the commonest phenotype comprised resistance to ampicillin, sulphonamides, streptomycin, chloramphenicol, and tetracycline and was found in 76% of human and 73% of animal strains. Between 1972 and 1974, almost 50,000 *Salmonella* isolates from several sources (humans, animals, animal products, sewage, etc.) were tested for resistance to ampicillin, chloramphenicol, kanamycin and tetracycline in the Netherlands. The incidence of resistance to at least one of the above drugs ranged from 39.2 to 45.6%. An interesting finding was that multidrug-resistant strains of *S. typhimurium* and *S. dublin* were isolated from calves and cattle. A total of 64.4% of all strains of *S. typhimurium* from these animals appeared to be resistant to ampicillin, tetracycline, chloramphenicol and kanamycin, and 25.5% of *S. dublin* were found to be resistant to chloramphenicol and tetracycline in the latest year of the study [86]. In NARMS's last report which presents data for 2013 in the USA [87], *Salmonella*, antimicrobial resistance varies by serotype: 3% (61/2178) of non-typhoidal *Salmonella* isolates were resistant to nalidixic acid. The most common serotypes among the 55 ceftriaxone-resistant isolates were *S. newport, dublin, typhimurium, heidelberg* and *infantis*.

Overall, antimicrobial resistance varies among different serotypes of non-typhoidal *Salmonella*, and in some of them is considerably significant. It is well-recognized that the emergence of antimicrobial resistance in bacteria, which can be transferred to humans, is attributable to antimicrobial use in animals; therefore the effectiveness of antimicrobial drugs for treating human disease has been reduced extensively. The resistance to certain antimicrobials, especially fluoroquinolones and cephalosporins, are of particular concern with major consequences, since therapy of human systemic bacterial infections are critically dependent on their effectiveness. In face of this public health concern, it is highly recommended to follow a very careful prescription of antimicrobial agents during veterinary practice, regardless of the purpose of this prescription (prophylaxis or therapy) and a prudent use of antimicrobial agents after microbiological identification of the causative pathogen. Last but not least, it is very important to highlight that good hygiene practices and, wherever possible, alternative management methods should be sought and used and should not be substituted by the use of any antimicrobial agent.

Author details

Niki Mouttotou[1], Shakeel Ahmad[2], Zahid Kamran[3], and Konstantinos C. Koutoulis[4]*

*Address all correspondence to: kkoutoulis@vet.uth.gr

1 National Reference Laboratory of Salmonella and Antimicrobial Resistance, Ministry of Rural Development and Food, Chalkis, Greece

2 Al-Watania Poultry Institute of Technology, Al-Bukayriyah, Saudi Arabia

3 University College of Veterinary and Animal Sciences, The Islamia University of Bahawalpur, Bahawalpur, Pakistan

4 Department of Poultry Diseases, Faculty of Veterinary Science, School of Health Sciences, University of Thessaly, Karditsa, Greece

References

[1] Coburn B, Grassl GA, Finlay BB. Salmonella, the host and disease: a brief review. Immunol Cell Biol. 2007;**85:**112–118. DOI: 10.1038/sj.icb.7100007

[2] Majowicz S, Musto J, Scallan E, Angulo F, Kirk M, O'Brien S, Jones T, Fazil A, Hoekstra R. The global burden of nontyphoidal *Salmonella* gastroenteritis. Clin Infect Dis. 2010;**50:**882–889.

[3] EFSA. Report of the Task Force on Zoonoses Data Collection on the analysis of the baseline survey on the prevalence of *Salmonella* in turkey flocks, in the EU, 2006–2007. Part A: *Salmonella* prevalence estimates. EFSA J. 2008;**134:**1–91.

[4] Vargas-Galindo Á. Probabilistic inversion in priority setting of food borne pathogens [MSc thesis]. Delft University of Technology: Department of Applied Mathematics and Risk Analysis; 2007

[5] Popoff MY, Le Minor L. Antigenic formulas of the Salmonella serovars, 8th ed. WHO Collaborating Centre for Reference and Research on Salmonella, Institute Pasteur, Paris, France; 2001

[6] Porwollik S, Boyd EF, Choy C, Cheng P, Florea L, Proctor E, McClelland M. Characterization of Salmonella enterica subspecies I genovars by use of microarrays. J Bacteriol. 2004;**186:**5883–5898.

[7] Brenner F, Villar R, Angulo F, Tauxe R, Swaminathan B. *Salmonella* nomenclature. J Clin Microbiol. 2000;**38:**2465–2467.

[8] Jay LS, Davos D, Dundas M, Frankish E, Lightfoot D. Salmonella. In: Hocking AD (ed). Foodborne microorganisms of public health significance. 6th ed, Australian Institute of Food Science and Technology (NSW Branch), Sydney; 2003; pp. 207–266.

[9] Gast RK. Salmonella infections. In: Swayne DE, Glisson JR, McDougald LR, Nolan LK, Suarez DL, Nair VL (eds). Diseases of Poultry. 13th ed, Ames, IA: John Wiley and Sons Inc.; 2013; pp. 677–736. ISBN: 978-0-470-95899-5.

[10] Allison MJ, Dalton HP, Escobar MR, Martin CJ. *Salmonella choleraesuis* infections in man: a report of 19 cases and a critical literature review. South Med J. 1969;**62:**593–596.

[11] EFSA. The European Union summary report on trends and sources of zoonoses, zoonotic agents and food-borne outbreaks in 2013 Scientific Report of EFSA and ECDC. EFSA J. 2015;**13(1):**3991.

[12] Castagna SMF, Schwartz P, Canal CW, Cardoso M. Presence of Salmonella sp. in the intestinal tract and tonsils/mandibular lymph nodes in pigs at slaughter. Arq Brasil Med Veter Zoo. 2004;**56(3):**300–306 DOI: 10.1590/S0102-09352004000300003

[13] Shimoni Z, Pitlik's K, Leibovici L. Nontyphoidal salmonella bacteremia: age-related differences in clinical presentation, bacteriology, and outcome. Clin Infect Dis. 1999;**28:**822–7.

[14] De Jong B, Ekdahl K. Human salmonellosis in travellers is highly correlated to the prevalence of Salmonella in laying hen flocks. Eurosurveillance. 2006;**11:**E060706.1.

[15] Bell C, Kyriakides A. *Salmonella*: a practical approach to the organism and its control in foods. Oxford: Blackwell Science; 2002.

[16] FAO/WHO. Risk assessments of *Salmonella* in eggs and broiler chickens (Microbiological Risk Assessment Series 2). Food and Agriculture Organization of the United Nations/ World Health Organization. 2002. Available from: http://www.who.int/foodsafety/publications/micro/en/salmonella.pdf

[17] CCFH. Food safety risk profile for *Salmonella* species in broiler (young) chickens. Codex Committee on Food Hygiene Working Group on guidelines for control of *Campylobacter* and *Salmonella* species in broiler (young bird) chicken meat. 2007. Available from: http://www.foodsafety.govt.nz/elibrary/industry/Food_Safety_Risk-Compiled_Ccfh.pdf.

[18] Poppe C. *Salmonella* infections in the domestic fowl. In: Wray C, Wray A (eds). *Salmonella* in domestic animals. Oxon, United Kingdom: CABI Publishing; 2000;107–132.

[19] Gast RK, Guraya R, Jones DR, Anderson KE. Persistence of fecal shedding of *Salmonella enteritidis* by experimentally infected laying hens housed in conventional or enriched cages. Poult Sci. 2015;**94:**1650–1656. http://dx.doi.org/10.3382/ps/pev113

[20] Davies RH, Wray C. Persistence of *Salmonella enteritidis* in poultry units and poultry food. Br Poult Sci. 1996;**37(3):**589–96.

[21] Santos RL, Zhang S, Tsolis RM, Baumler AJ, Adams LG. Morphologic and molecular characterization of Salmonella typhimurium infection in neonatal calves. Vet Pathol. 2002;**39:**200–215.

[22] Jones BD. Salmonella invasion gene regulation: a story of environmental awareness. J Microbiol. 2005;**43:**110–117.

[23] Solari CA, Mandarino JR, Panizzutti MHM, Farias RHG. A new serovar and a new serological variant belonging to Salmonella enterica subspecies diarizonae. Mem Inst Oswaldo Cruz. 2003;**98(4)**. http://dx.doi.org/10.1590/S0074-02762003000400013

[24] Hidalgo-Vila J, Díaz-Paniagua C, de Frutos-Escobar C, Jiménez-Martínez C, Pérez-Santigosa N. Salmonella in free living terrestrial and aquatic turtles. Vet Microbiol. 2007;**119:**311–315.

[25] Foster JW, Spector MP. How Salmonella survive against the odds. Annu Rev Microbiol. 1995;**49:**145–74.

[26] Turpin PE, Maycroft KA, Rowlands CL, Wellington EMH. Viable but non-culturable Salmonellas in soil. J Appl Bacteriol. 1993;**74:**421–427.

[27] Mannion C, Lynch PB, Egan J, Leonard FC. Seasonal effects on the survival characteristics of Salmonella Typhimurium and Salmonella Derby in pig slurry during storage. J Appl Microbiol. 2007;**103(5):**1386–1392.

[28] Heaton JC, Jones K. Microbial contamination of fruit and vegetables and the behaviour of enteropathogens in the phyllosphere: a review. J Appl Microbiol. 2008;**104(3):**613–626.

[29] Loewenstein M. An outbreak of salmonellosis propogated by person-to-person transmission on an Indian reservation. Am J Epidemiol. 1974;**102:** 257–262.

[30] Pether J, Scott R. *Salmonella* carriers: are they dangerous? A study to identify finger contamination with *Salmonella* by convalescent carriers. J Infect. 1982;**5:**81–88.

[31] Dryden MS. Asymptomatic foodhandlers as the source of nosocomial salmonellosis. J Hosp Infect. 1994;**28:**195–208.

[32] Stein-Zamir C, Tallen-Gozani E, Abramson N, Shoob H, Yishai R, Agmon V, Reisfeld A, Valinsky L, Marva E. *Salmonella enterica* outbreak in a banqueting hall in Jerusalem: the unseen hand of the epidemiological triangle? Israel Med Assoc J. 2009;**11:**94–97.

[33] Kendall ME, Crim S, Fullerton K, Han PV, Cronquist AB, Shiferaw B. Travel-associated enteric infections diagnosed after return to the United States, Foodborne Diseases Active Surveillance Network (FoodNet), 2004–2009. Clin Infect Dis. 2012;**54(Suppl 5):**S480–S487.

[34] Havelaar AH, Ivarsson S, Löfdahl M, Nauta MJ. Estimating the true incidence of campylobacteriosis and salmonellosis in the European Union, 2009. Epidemiol Infect. 2013;**141(2):**293–302.

[35] Hoffmann S, Maculloch B, Batz M. Economic burden of major foodborne illnesses acquired in the United States. In: Economic Research Service Economic Information Bulletin; Number 140, May 2015; pp.33; United States Department of Agriculture (USDA). Available from: https://www.ers.usda.gov/webdocs/publications/eib140/52806_eib140_summary.pdf

[36] Commission Decision No. 2119/98/EC of the European Parliament and of the Council of 24 September 1998 setting up a network for the epidemiological surveillance and control of communicable diseases in the community. O J L. 1998;268:1–6.

[37] Commission Decision No. 2000/96/EC of 22 December 1999 on the communicable diseases to be progressively covered by the community network under Decision No. 2119/98/EC of the European Parliament and of the Council. O J L. 2000;28:50–53.

[38] Rose N, Beaudeau F, Drouin P, Toux J, Rose V, Colin P. Risk factors for *Salmonella enterica* subsp. *enterica* contamination in French broiler-chicken flocks at the end of the rearing period. Prevent Vet Med. 1999;**39:**265–277.

[39] Marin C, Balasch S, Vega S, Lainez M. Sources of Salmonella contamination during broiler production in Eastern Spain. Prevent Vet Med. 2011;**98:**39–45.

[40] Arsenault J, Letellier A, Quessy S, Normand V, Boulianne M. Prevalence and risk factors for Salmonella spp. and Campylobacter spp. caecal colonization in broiler chicken and turkey flocks slaughtered in Quebec, Canada. Prevent Vet Med. 2007;**81:**250–264.

[41] Denagamage T, Jayarao B, Patterson P, Wallner-Pendleton E, Kariyawasam S. Risk factors associated with Salmonella in laying hen farms: systematic review of observational studies. Avian Dis. 2015;**59(2):**291–302. DOI: 10.1637/10997-120214-Reg

[42] EFSA. Scientific opinion on microbiological risk assessment in feeding stuffs for food-producing animals. Scientific opinion of the panel on biological hazards. EFSA J. 2008;**720:**1–84.

[43] Directive 2003/99/EC of the European Parliament and of the Council of 17 November 2003 on the monitoring of zoonoses and zoonotic agents, amending Council Decision 90/424/EEC and repealing Council Directive 92/117/EEC. O J L. 2003;325:31–40.

[44] Fernanda DC, Cole DJ, Hofacre C, Zamperini K, Mathis D, Doyle MP, Lee MD, Maurer JJ. Effect of *Salmonella* vaccination of breeder chickens on contamination of broiler chicken carcasses in integrated poultry operations. Appl Environ Microbiol. 2010;**76(23):**7820–7825. DOI:10.1128/AEM.01320-10 DOI:10.1128%2FAEM.01320-10#pmc_ext

[45] Papatsiros VG, Katsoulos PD, Koutoulis KC, Karatzia M, Dedousi A, Christodoulopoulos G. Alternatives to antibiotics for farm animals. CAB Rev. 2013;**8:**32

[46] Roth N. The use of acidifiers in controlling Salmonella. Poultry World. 2012; Dec 31. Available from: http://www.poultryworld.net/Health/Articles/2012/12/The-use-of-acidifiers-in-controlling-Salmonella-1136075W/

[47] Young I, Rajic A, Wilhelm BJ, Waddell L, Parker S, McEwen SA. Comparison of the prevalence of bacterial enteropathogens, potentially zoonotic bacteria and bacterial resistance to antimicrobials in organic and conventional poultry, swine and beef production: a systematic review and meta-analysis. Epidemiol Infect. 2009;**137:**1217–1232.

[48] Mulder RWAW. Impact of transport and related stresses on the incidence and extent of human pathogens in pigmeat and poultry. J Food Safety. 1995;**15(3):**239–246.

[49] Corry JEL, Allen VM, Hudson WR, Breslin MF, Davies RH. Sources of *Salmonella* on broiler carcasses during transportation and processing: modes of contamination and methods of control. J Appl Microbiol. 2002;**92(3):**424–432.

[50] Marin C, Lainez M. *Salmonella* detection in feces during broiler rearing and after live transport to the slaughterhouse. Poult Sci. 2009;**88(9):**1999–2005.

[51] Lillard H. The impact of commercial processing procedures on the bacterial contamination and cross-contamination of broiler carcasses. J Food Protect. 1990;**53(3):**202–204.

[52] Lake R, Hudson A, Cressey P, Bayne G, Turner N. Quantitative risk model: *Salmonella* spp. in the poultry food chain. In: ESR Client Report FW0546. ESR, Christchurch; 2005.

[53] EFSA. Scientific opinion on the public health risks related to the maintenance of the cold chain during storage and transport of meat. Part 2 (minced meat from all species). EFSA Panel on Biological Hazards (BIOHAZ). EFSA J . 2014;**12(7):**3783.

[54] ICMSF. Microorganisms in Foods 6: Microbial Ecology of Food Commodities. 2nd edition. International Commission on Microbiological Specifications for Foods (ICMSF). New York: Kluwer Academic & Plenum Publishers; 2005; pp108. ISBN: 0-306-48675-X.

[55] Abu Ruwaida AS, Sawaya WN, Baroon ZH, Murad M, Terry WR. Shelf life and microbiological quality of eviscerated broiler carcasses in the State of Kuwait. Arab Gulf J Sci Res. 1996;**14:**363–381.

[56] King N, Wong T. Feasibility study: trace back of fresh poultry portions sold at retail. In: ESR Client Report FW10056. Christchurch: ESR; 2010.

[57] Dominguez SA, Schaffner DW. Survival of *Salmonella* in processed chicken products during frozen storage. J Food Protect. 2009;**72:**2088–2092.

[58] Gilbert S, Bayne G, Wong T, Lake R, Whyte R. Domestic food practices in New Zealand. 2005–2006 project report. In: ESR Client Report FW0640. Christchurch: ESR; 2006.

[59] Gilbert S, Whyte R, Bayne G, Paulin S, Lake R, van der Logt P. Survey of domestic food handling practices in New Zealand. Int J Food Microbiol. 2007;**117:**306–311.

[60] McIntyre L, Bayne G, Gilbert S, Lake R. Domestic food practices in New Zealand. Freezer survey. In: ESR Client Report FW0735. Christchurch: ESR; 2007. Available from: http://foodsafety.govt.nz/elibrary/industry/Domestic_Food_Practices-Baseline_Information.pdf

[61] CAC. Report of the forty-second session of the Codex Committee on Food Hygiene, Kampala, Uganda, 29 November–3 December 2010. Codex Alimentarius Commission. Available from: https://ec.europa.eu/food/sites/food/files/safety/docs/codex_ccfh_42_agenda-item_04.pdf

[62] Anonymous. Outbreak of *Salmonella* Enteritidis 9a, Auckland, April-May 2005 (an internal report provided by Public Health Services).

[63] Hess IM, Neville LM, McCarthy R, Shadbolt CT, McAnulty JM. A Salmonella Typhimurium 197 outbreak linked to the consumption of lambs' liver in Sydney, NSW. Epidemiol Infect. 2008;**136(4):**461–467.

[64] Jansen A, Frank C, Stark K. Pork and pork products as a source for human salmonellosis in Germany. Berliner und Münchener tierärztliche Wochenschrift. 2007;**120(7-8):**340–346.

[65] Luzzi I, Galetta P, Massari M, Rizzo C, Dionisi AM, Filetici E, Cawthorne A, Tozzi A, Argentieri M, Bilei S, Busani L, Gnesivo C, Pendenza A, Piccoli A, Napoli P, Loffredo L, Trinito MO, Santarelli E, Ciofi degli Atti ML. An Easter outbreak of Salmonella Typhimurium DT 104A associated with traditional pork salami in Italy. Euro Surveill. 2007;**12(4):**11–12.

[66] Haeghebaert S, Duché L, Gilles C, Masini B, Dubreuil M, Minet JC, Bouvet P, Grimont F, Delarocque Astagneau E, Vaillant V. Minced beef and human salmonellosis: review of the investigation of three outbreaks in France. Euro Surveill. 2001;**6(2):**21–26

[67] Little CL, Richardson JF, Owen RJ, de Pinna E, Threlfall EJ. Campylobacter and Salmonella in raw red meats in the United Kingdom: prevalence, characterization and antimicrobial resistance pattern, 2003–2005. Food Microbiol. 2008;**25(3):**538–543.

[68] EFSA. Panels on Biological Hazards (BIOHAZ), on Contaminants in the Food Chain (CONTAM) and on Animal Health and Welfare (AHAW), 2012. Scientific Opinion on the public health hazards to be covered by inspection of meat (poultry). EFSA J. 2012;**10(6):**2741 (179 pp.). DOI:10.2903/j.efsa.2012.2741

[69] EFSA (European Food Safety Authority) and ECDC (European Centre for Disease Prevention and Control). The European Union summary report on trends and sources of zoonoses, zoonotic agents and food-borne outbreaks in 2012. EFSA J. 2014;**12(2)**:3547 (312 pp.). DOI:10.2903/j.efsa.2013.3129

[70] EFSA. Panel on Biological Hazards (BIOHAZ). Scientific opinion on an estimation of the public health impact of setting a new target for the reduction of Salmonella in turkeys. EFSA J. 2012;**10(4)**:2616 (89 pp). DOI: 10.2903/j.efsa.2012.2616

[71] Scanga JA, Grona AD, Belk KE, Sofos JN, Bellinger GR, Smith GC. Microbiological contamination of raw beef trimmings and ground beef. Meat Sci. 2000;**56**:145–152.

[72] James C, James S. Quantification of the controls that should be placed on meat prior to mincing. FSA (Food Standards Agency) Project: M01054. 2012; Available from: http://www.foodbase.org.uk//admintools/reportdocuments/876-1-1619_M01054.pdf

[73] Unicomb LE, Simmons G, Merritt T, Gregory J, Nicol C, Jelfs P, Kirk M, Tan A, Thomson R, Adamopoulos J, Little CL, Currie A, Dalton CB. Sesame seed products contaminated with Salmonella: three outbreaks associated with tahini. Epidemiol Infect. 2005;**133**:1065–1072.

[74] Kretsinger K, Noviello S, Moll M. Tomatoes sicken hundreds: multistate outbreak of Salmonella Newport. In: Proceedings of the 52nd Annual Epidemic Intelligence Service Conference; 2003; Atlanta, Georgia, USA.

[75] CDC. National antimicrobial resistance monitoring system for enteric bacteria (NARMS): human isolates final report, 2007. Atlanta, GA: U.S. Department of Health and Human Services, CDC, 2009. Available from: http://www.cdc.gov/narms/annual/2007/NARMSAnnualReport2007.pdf

[76] Greene SK, Daly ER, Talbot EA, Demma LJ, Holzbauer S, Patel NJ, Hill TA, Walderhaug MO, Hoekstra RM, Lynch MF, Painter JA. Recurrent multistate outbreak of Salmonella Newport associated with tomatoes from contaminated fields, 2005. Epidemiol Infect. 2008;**136(2)**:157–165.

[77] Jain S, Bidol SA, Austin JL, Berl E, Elson F, Lemaile-Williams M, Deasy M 3rd, Moll ME, Rea V, Vojdani JD, Yu PA, Hoekstra RM, Braden CR, Lynch MF. Multistate outbreak of Salmonella Typhimurium and Saintpaul infections associated with unpasteurized orange juice—United States, 2005. Clin Infect Dis. 2009;**48(8)**:1065–1071.

[78] Vojdani JD, Beuchat LR, Tauxe RV. Juice-associated outbreaks of human illness in the United States, 1995 through 2005. J Food Prot. 2008;**71(2)**:356–364.

[79] Nygård K, Lassen J, Vold L, Andersson Y, Fisher I, Löfdahl S, Threlfall J, Luzzi I, Peters T, Hampton M, Torpdahl M, Kapperud G, Aavitsland P. Outbreak of Salmonella Thompson infections linked to imported rucola lettuce. Foodborne Pathog Dis. 2008;**5(2)**:165–173.

[80] Little CL, Gillespie IA. Prepared salads and public health. J Appl Microbiol. 2008;**105(6)**:1729–1743. DOI: 10.1111/j.1365-2672.2008.03801.x. Epub 2008 Apr 4.

[81] EFSA. The European Union summary report on antimicrobial resistance in zoonotic and indicator bacteria from humans, animals and food. EFSA J. 2016;**14(2):**4380.

[82] European Centre for Disease Prevention and Control (ECDC), European Food Safety Authority (EFSA), European Drugs Agency (EMEA), Scientific Committee on Emerging and Newly Identified Health Risks (SCENIHR). Joint opinion on antimicrobial resistance (AMR) focused on zoonotic infections. EFSA J. 2009;**7(11):**1372. Available from: http://www.ema.europa.eu/docs/en_GB/document_library/Other/2009/11/WC500015452.pdf

[83] Chen S,Zhao S, White DG, Schroeder CM, Lu R, Yang H, McDermott PF, Ayers S, Meng J. Characterization of multiple-antimicrobial-resistant *Salmonella* serovars isolated from retail meats. Appl Environ Microbiol. 2004;**70(1):**1–7. DOI:10.1128/AEM.70.1.1-7.2004 DOI:10.1128%2FAEM.70.1.1-7.2004#pmc_ext

[84] Le Hello S, Bekhit A, Granier SA, Barua H, Beutlich J, Zając M, Münch S, Sintchenko V, Bouchrif B, Fashae K, Pinsard JL, Sontag L, Fabre L, Garnier M, Guibert V, Howard P, Hendriksen RS, Christensen JP, Biswas PK, Cloeckaert A, Rabsch W, Wasyl D, Doublet B, Weill FX. The global establishment of a highly-fluoroquinolone resistant Salmonella enterica serotype Kentucky ST198 strain. Front Microbiol. 2013;**4:**395. DOI:10.3389/fmicb.2013.00395

[85] Brisabois A, Cazin I, Breuil J, Collatz E. Surveillance of antibiotic resistance in Salmonella. Euro Surveill. 1997;2(3):pii=181. Available online: http://www.eurosurveillance.org/ViewArticle.aspx?ArticleId=181

[86] Voogd CE, van Leeuwen WJ, Guinée PA, Manten A, Valkenburg JJ. Incidence of resistance to ampicillin, chloramphenicol, kanamycin and tetracycline among Salmonella species isolated in the Netherlands in 1972, 1973 and 1974. Antonie van Leeuwenhoek. 1977;**43(3–4):**269–281.

[87] NARMS report for human isolates final report. National Center for Emerging and Zoonotic Infectious Disease; 2013.

Chapter 13

Effects of Environment and Socioeconomics on *Salmonella* Infections

Hafiz Anwar Ahmad and Luma Akil

Additional information is available at the end of the chapter

http://dx.doi.org/10.5772/67501

Abstract

Objectives: *Salmonella* is a major public health concern particularly in areas of low socioeconomic status (SES) and high temperature. In this chapter, we examined several socioeconomic and environmental factors that may increase the spread of *Salmonella* in the southern states of the USA.

Methods: In our recent studies, relevant US-southern states data of foodborne illnesses, from 2002 to 2011, were collected and used in various analytical models. The associations among low socioeconomic status, climatic variables and *Salmonella* infections were determined using several software packages.

Results: Our studies showed a significant increase in *Salmonella* outbreaks in Mississippi during the observed periods with regional and district variations. Regression and neural network models revealed a moderate correlation between *Salmonella* infection rates and low socioeconomic factors. A seasonal trend was observed for *Salmonella* infections. In one of our study, an increase of 1°F (0.556°C) was shown to result in four new cases of *Salmonella* infection in Mississippi.

Conclusions: Geographic location besides socioeconomic status may contribute to the high rates of *Salmonella* outbreaks. There are consistent evidence that gastrointestinal infections with bacterial pathogens are positively correlated with ambient temperature. Warming trends in the USA may further increase rates of *Salmonella* infections.

Keywords: *Salmonella* infection, socioeconomic status, climate change, global warming

1. Introduction

Salmonella is a serious foodborne pathogen with an estimated 94 million human cases of gastroenteritis and 155,000 deaths around the world each year [1]. It causes around 1.4 million human cases with 15,000 hospitalizations and more than 400 deaths in the USA annually [2].

Contaminated eggs and poultry meat are common source of human salmonellosis. Wide range of domestic and wild animals, such as poultry and swine, can act as reservoirs for *Salmonella*. Institutions such as schools and nursing homes have often been linked to *Salmonella* outbreaks with devastating effects [3].

Salmonella rates in USA fluctuate considerably by geographic regions, with particularly higher rates in the Mid-Atlantic and New England States. This variation may be partly attributed to reporting differences. Salmonellosis rates between geographically and socio-economically similar to USA have been documented with as much as 200% differences between neighbouring states [1]. Southern USA, due to its socioeconomic status (SES), climatic changes and agricultural practices, is more vulnerable to increased outbreaks of foodborne illnesses compared to other parts of the country.

Emergence or resurgence of numerous infectious diseases is strongly influenced by environmental factors, such as climate or land use change [4]. Climate, weather, topology, hydrology and other geographical characteristics of the crop-growing site may influence the magnitude and frequency of transfer of pathogenic microorganisms from environmental sources [5].

2. Geographical variation and socioeconomic status effects

Socioeconomic status (SES) is an important predictor of diseases. SES is frequently measured based on individual and community-level education, income, wealth, employment and family background when compared with other individuals or groups. Low SES is generally associated with greater morbidity and mortality of diseases [6]. Socioeconomic and demographic indicators can be used to predict the individuals and communities that are at an increased risk of acquiring infections. Generally, low socioeconomic status is an important predictor of several poor health outcomes including chronic diseases, mental illnesses and mortality.

In our previous study [7], we examined the extent of *Salmonella* infections in Mississippi and compared it with other southern states and with two referenced northern states of the USA (**Figure 1**) to determine the infections' correlation with socioeconomic status. Several analytical modelling approaches including geographical information system (GIS) and neural network (NN) were employed. Laboratory confirmed data of *Salmonella* cases, from 2002 to 2011, were collected for Mississippi, Alabama, Tennessee, Louisiana, Montana and Michigan. Southern states including Alabama, Tennessee and Louisiana were selected as neighbouring states of Mississippi, while Montana and MI were selected as reference states based on their geographical and climatic conditions. Monthly *Salmonella* outbreak cases were grouped by year and districts. Data sources for this study included the US Centers for Disease Control and

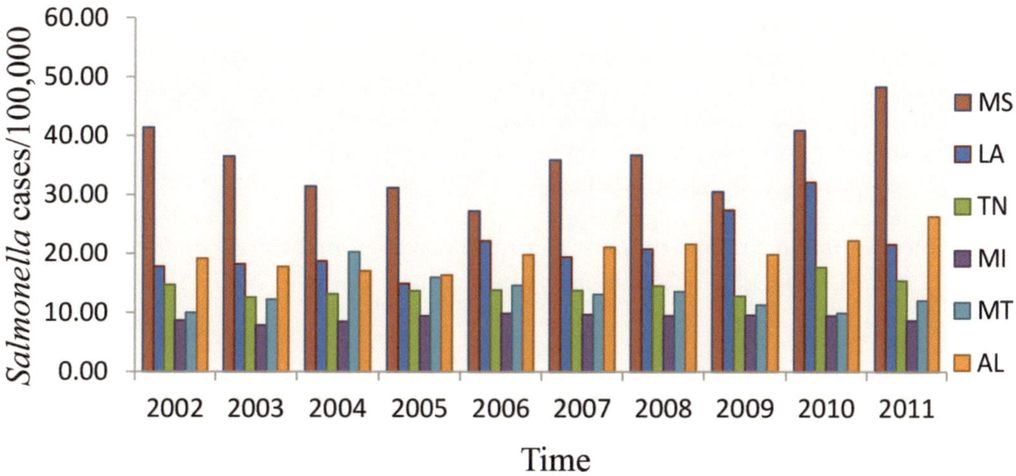

Figure 1. *Salmonella* Rates in Selected US States. MS-Mississippi; LA-Louisiana; TN-Tennessee; MI-Michigan; MT-Montana; AL-Alabama.

Prevention (CDC) and the respective States Department of health and Epidemiology [8–11]. Data were adjusted to 100,000 of population [12]. In addition to *Salmonella* infections, data for Mississippi, socioeconomic variables for its various counties, categorised by public health districts, for the year 2010–2011, were also retrieved [13]. The selected variables included poverty, uninsured, unemployment and primary care providers' rates.

Results of the study showed mostly positive correlation between low socioeconomic variables and increased rates of *Salmonella* infections; however, poverty rates were negatively correlated with *Salmonella* outbreaks.

Results of this study also revealed *Salmonella* rates in Mississippi to be twice than the average US *Salmonella* rates (36 cases/100,000 vs. 16.42 cases/100,000, respectively) [14]. Substantial regional differences in the incidence of *Salmonella* infections have also been reported previously [15]. A significant variation was observed in *Salmonella* outbreaks among the Mississippi districts through GIS mapping, regression analysis and NN models.

2.1. Poverty, education and unemployment

Underreporting of enteric infections is a critical issue in disease surveillance systems. Generally, patients with severe symptoms tend to visit the doctor and are subsequently notified to health authorities. As of 2011, almost 23% of Mississippi populations are living under poverty with average per-capita income of $32,000, although rural per-capita income lagged at $29,550, according to the USDA Economic Research Service. There are 96 hospitals in Mississippi, 163 Rural Health Clinics, and 21 Federally Qualified Health Canters that provide services at 170 sites in the state. An average of 19% of Mississippi residents lacks health insurance [12, 13].

The west-central region of Mississippi showed higher rates of *Salmonella* infections and lower poverty rates (36%), when compared to the Delta region of high poverty. However, more medical facilities are available in west-central region, resulting in higher identification and reporting of diseases. In 2011, 20% of the populations in west-central region were college graduate, with 10% unemployment rate, while only 14% of populations in Delta region were college graduate and 13% were unemployed. Lower rates of shigellosis and salmonellosis in communities with high rates of unemployment were identified. It was speculated that the reduced access to health care due to lack of employment may lead to under-detection of a disease among the unemployed individuals [16].

Geographical variations in poverty rates were also observed in different districts of the state (**Figure 2**). In the Delta region of Mississippi, the poverty rate was 44.2%. The lowest *Salmonella*

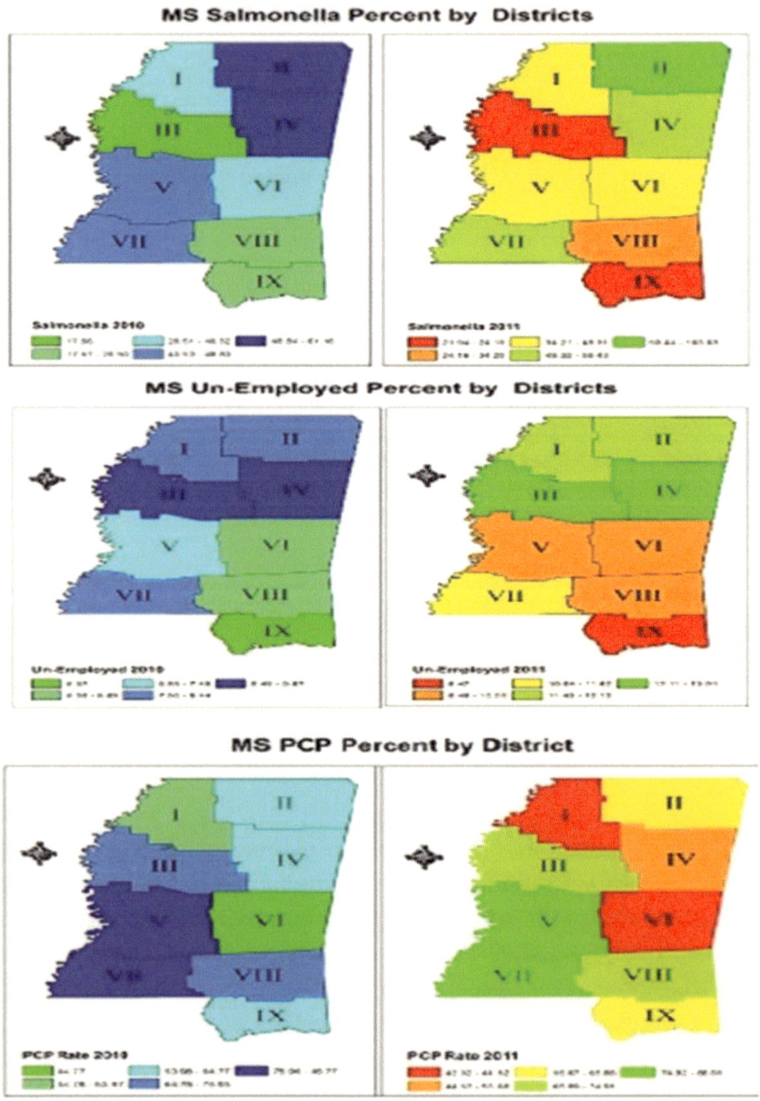

Figure 2. Geographical variations in *Salmonella* rates and socioeconomic factors in Mississippi.

rates were observed in this region as well. With high rates of poverty, many individuals cannot afford to seek medical care, which suggested underreporting of the disease.

The northern region of the state including northeast, northwest, Tombigbee and Delta district had the highest rates of unemployment. An average of 42% increase in unemployment rate was observed in the region in 2011. Primary care provider rate was the lowest in the northwest and east-central regions of Mississippi. An average of 17% decrease in primary care provider rates was observed in these regions. On the other hand, highest rates of primary care providers were found in west-central and southeast regions of the state, with 2% increase from 2010 to 2011.

Our results are different from reported individual level epidemiologic studies that had found higher levels of foodborne infections among low education and low-income groups. Studies suggested that high socioeconomic status (HSES) groups may be overrepresented in incidence statistics. It is possible that lower socioeconomic status (LSES) groups tend not to have health insurance or do not seek medical care when needed due to financial constraints. Access to health care may be an important influence on rates of reported bacterial infections. In an economy without universal health care coverage, tendency to seek care for GI infection has been associated with having health insurance [17, 18]. However, the Affordable Care Act (ACA) is expected to expand insurance coverage to millions of people in the USA. As a result, rates of reported cases of diseases and infections are expected to increase. In future projects, we will try to understand the impact of Affordable Care Act of 2010 on diseases reporting, especially among minority and LSES groups.

It is quite possible that various SES groups have different exposures because of dietary differences, or differences in food safety behaviours [8]. Behavioural studies have revealed that high SES groups are more likely to eat undercooked foods, such as raw oysters and rare beef [9, 12]; while low SES groups are less likely to have adequately cool refrigerators [4].

Other studies had similarly utilised GIS to examine the relationships between area-based socioeconomic measures and incidence of salmonellosis [18, 19]. The results showed higher incidences of salmonellosis in groups with high education compared to the less educated groups suggesting the role of education in health-seeking behaviour and the predisposition for *Salmonella* infections at the population level [19].

Neural network modelling was shown to be a useful tool in this study to predict the correlation between socioeconomic factors and *Salmonella* outbreaks. A moderate correlation between actual and network predicted output was observed at 41%, a reasonable level considering the biological system. Artificial neural networks (ANNs) are non-linear mapping structures comparable to human brain. They have been shown to be universal and highly flexible function to approximate any data. ANNs were developed initially to model biological functions [20–23]. Neural network melding has been used previously for prediction of T-Cell epitopes [24], prediction of cancer using gene expression profiling [25], temperature prediction [26], diabetes prediction [21], poultry growth modelling [27], egg price forecasting [28], in addition to predicting the relation between obesity and high blood pressure [23].

In the USA, Mississippi ranked 50th among all the states for health care, according to the Commonwealth Fund, a non-profit foundation working to advance performance of the health care system. For the past 3 years, obese populations were accounted for more than 30% of Mississippi's residents and 22.8 % of the state's children. On top of obesity, Mississippi had the highest rates in the nation for high blood pressure, diabetes and adult inactivity [24].

Social and economic conditions underpin poverty and can directly or indirectly affect health status and health outcomes. Major epidemics emerge and chronic conditions cluster persist wherever poverty is widespread [5].

3. Effects of climatic variables

3.1. Temperature

Diseases associated with climate change are estimated to comprise 4.6% of all environmental risks and hazards. Climate change, in the year 2000, contributed to about 2.4% of all diarrhoea outbreaks in the world, 6% of malaria outbreaks in certain developing countries and 7% of the episodes of dengue fever in some industrial countries. In total, the estimates showed that climate change related mortalities were 0.3%, whereas the related burden of disease was 0.4% [29].

Global average temperature, from 1906 to 2005, has warmed by 0.74°C; and since 1961, sea level has risen on average by 2 mm per year. On the other hand, Arctic sea ice has declined by 7.4% per decade while snow cover and glaciers have diminished in both hemispheres [4]. The climate change rate is faster now than in any other period during the last 1000 years. According to the United Nations Intergovernmental Panel on Climate Change, average global temperatures will increase between 1.8 and 4.0°C in next 90 years along with sea level rise of 18–59 cm [30, 31].

Changes in expected weather patterns can lead to the transfer of microbial contaminants to leafy vegetables and herbs. Dry periods can cause dust storms that settle dust particles on leafy vegetables. The rate of microbial growth was shown to increase with rise in temperature. It influences the population of insects and pests found in and around farms that transfer human pathogens to leafy vegetables as well. Relative humidity has been shown to have an effect on survival of human pathogens [32]. Climate change scenarios predict a change distribution of infectious diseases with warming temperature and changes in outbreaks associated with weather extremes, such as flooding and droughts.

Several infectious agents, vector organisms, non-human reservoir species, and rate of pathogen replication are sensitive to climatic conditions. Both *Salmonella* and *Vibrio cholera*, for example, proliferate more rapidly at higher temperatures, *Salmonella* in animal gut and food, cholera in water. In regions where low temperature, low rainfall, or absence of vector habitat restrict transmission of vector-borne disease, climatic changes could tip the ecological balance and trigger epidemics [31]. Furthermore, strong linear associations have been noted between temperature and notifications of Salmonellosis in European countries and Australia [31]. The USA is likely to experience increases in extreme heat, extreme cold, hurricanes, floods, wildfires, droughts, tornadoes and severe storms [33]. The health impacts of global climate change are expected to be widespread, geographically myriad and profoundly influenced by pre-existing social and economic disparities [34].

The southern states, including Mississippi's climate, has been fluctuating with extreme patterns. The average temperatures in Mississippi have varied significantly over the past century, with an average of 1°F increase, since the late 1960s. Extreme rainfall events, primarily thunderstorms, have increased as well. While rainfall totals have changed little, seasonal trends are apparent, summers have become slightly drier and winters slightly wetter [33]. On an average, 29 tornadoes are reported annually in Mississippi; the highest number was in 2008 with 109 tornadoes. In addition, during the past decade, Mississippi had experienced multiple hits by hurricanes including the devastating Katrina in 2005 [33].

Global warming and the climate change have contributed to the spread of several foodborne pathogens [5, 30]. In our previous research, we determined the extent of *Salmonella* infections in Mississippi along with its correlation to climate variations [35]. Monthly data of *Salmonella* outbreaks from 2001 to 2011 were obtained from Mississippi State Department of Health and Department of Epidemiology. In addition, meteorological data, including average air temperatures, minimum and maximum, and total precipitation for the selected station across the state were collected from the Southeast Regional Climate Center, available at: http://www.sercc.com/climateinfo/monthly_seasonal.html.

Analysis of variance was performed to determine the seasonal change in *Salmonella* outbreaks during the study period. Time series analysis, including the Mann-Kendall test and a Seasonal trend test, was applied to quantify the relationships between the temperature and the number of notified cases of *Salmonella*.

Our results indicated an increase in temperature is positively correlated with *Salmonella* infections. A seasonal trend was also observed in this study with the highest outbreaks during the summer to early fall (**Figure 3**).

The positive relationship between temperature and *Salmonella* infections, observed in our study, using regression and NN models, was similar to recent findings from Australia, Europe, North America and Asia with similar trends [36–38]. Endemic regions for *Salmonella* outbreaks include developing countries in South Central and South East Asia; and many parts of Africa, Middle East and Latin America. In the same study, we found that an increase of 1°F (0.556°C) in Mississippi was shown to result in four new cases of *Salmonella* (**Figure 4**). Studies also found that weekly counts of enteric bacterial disease cases generally increased with weekly temperature after adjusting for seasonal and long-term trends [37, 39]. Another study [40] had suggested that a potential 1°C rise in mean weekly maximum temperature may be associated with an 8.8% increase in the weekly number of cases, and a 1°C rise in mean weekly minimum temperature may lead to a 5.8% increase in the weekly number of cases.

The US-southern states climate is generally warm and wet, with mild and humid winters. The average annual temperatures in the region have increased by about 2°F since 1970, and the average annual temperatures in the region are projected to increase by 4 to 9°F by 2080 [41].

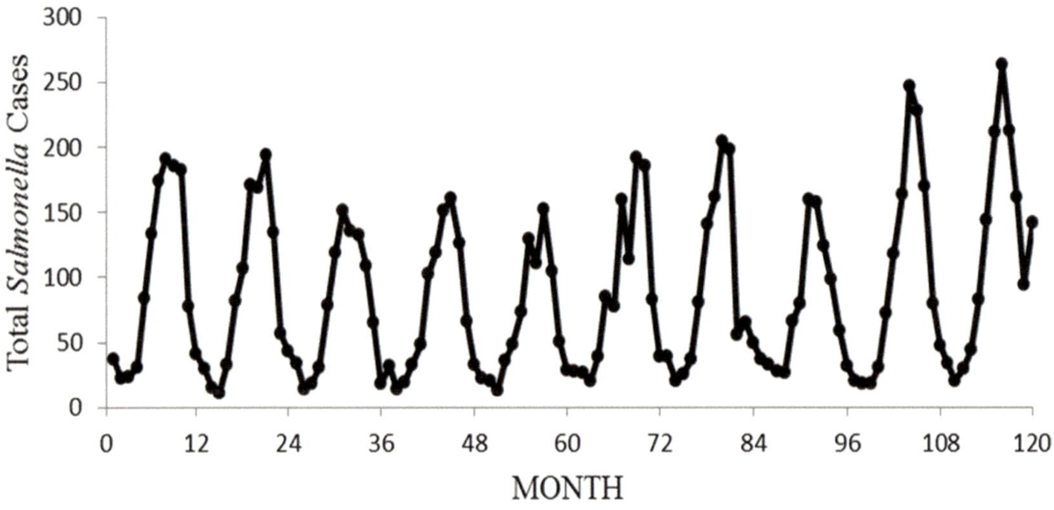

Figure 3. Seasonal trend in *Salmonella* cases.

Climate change and extreme events may increase the spread of foodborne diseases in this region, particularly in the disadvantaged states, such as Mississippi.

Increased growth *of Salmonella* at higher temperatures leads to higher concentration of *Salmonella* in the food supply, particularly during the warmer months. Poor cooking practices are also more common during these summer months (picnics, barbecues, etc.). Temperature

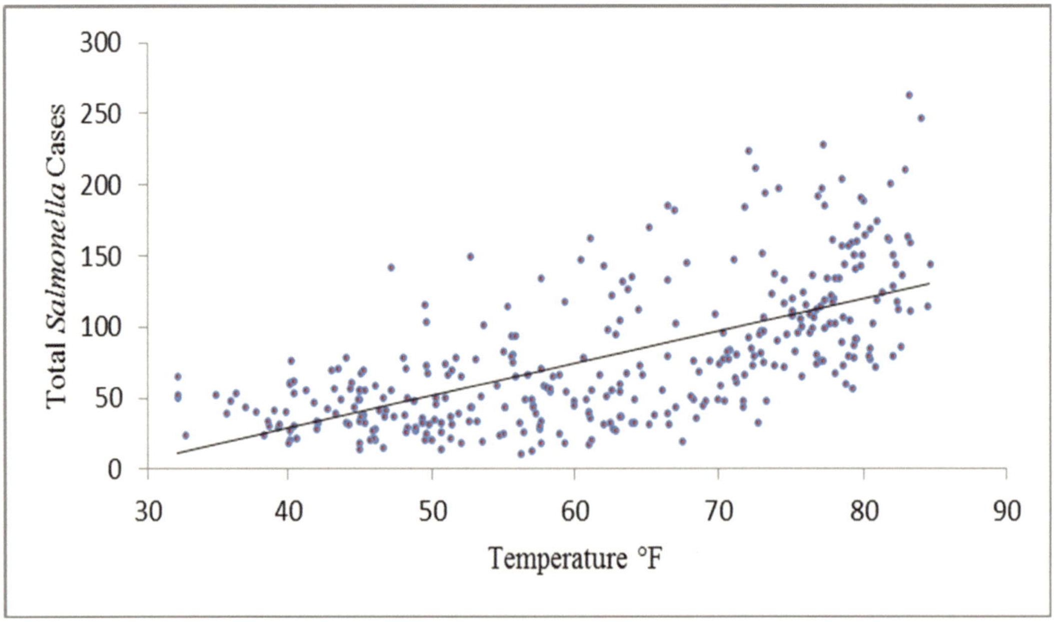

Figure 4. Correlation between *Salmonella* outbreaks and increase in temperature.

may affect the transmission of *Salmonella* infections via several causal pathways, such as direct effects on bacterial proliferation and indirect effects on eating habits during hot days. The optimum temperature for the growth of *Salmonellae* is between 35 and 37°C. The growth is greatly decreased at less than 15°C. Ambient temperature influences the development of *Salmonella* at various stages in the food chain, including bacterial loads on raw food production, transport and inappropriate storage [37, 42].

Studies showed that an increase in the ambient temperature correlated positively with an increase in human *Salmonella* with a delay of approximately five weeks. *Salmonella* has the ability to multiply itself within 20 min at ambient temperatures; this growth rate however, is increased at 30°C or higher temperature. Additionally, cross-contamination and undercooking of meat during barbecuing is more likely to occur during summer months [43].

There is consistent evidence that gastrointestinal infection with bacterial pathogens is positively correlated with ambient temperature, as warmer temperatures enable rapid replications of pathogens. *Salmonella* notifications peak in summer and the rate of notifications has been shown to be positively and linearly correlated with the mean temperature of the previous month or week [44, 45]. Some of this increase in summer months may be due to changed eating behaviours (more 'eating out' while on holidays and attending outdoor functions such as barbecues). Ambient temperatures contribute directly to pathogen multiplication in foods and thus the likelihood of infection. Furthermore, it was noted that enteric diseases in temperate latitudes have a seasonal pattern, with the highest incidence of illnesses during the summer months. A study of foodborne illnesses in the UK found a relationship between the incidence of disease and the temperature in the month preceding the illness [46]. It is believed that the survival and growth of certain enteric pathogens are, within limits, positively correlated with ambient temperature [39].

Rates of *Salmonella* are expected to increase in the future as climate change causes ambient temperatures to rise above the average, contributing to around 1000 extra cases annually. This links to an annual difference of approximately 1200 lost workdays and $120,000 in the cost of health care and surveillance by 2050 [44]. By considering a suite of future climate scenarios, the UN-Intergovernmental Panel on Climate Change projected global surface temperature increases between 1.1 and 6.4°C over the next century. Studies had shown that the main health risks caused by climate change include health impacts of weather disasters, health impacts of temperature extremes, including heat waves, mosquito-borne infectious diseases, foodborne infectious diseases (including those due to *Salmonella, Campylobacter* and many other microbes), water-borne infectious diseases and other health risks from poor water quality. In addition, diminished food availability, costs/affordability, nutritional consequences, and increases in urban air pollution are also reported as health risks from climate change [44, 47, 48].

Higher ambient temperatures are main concerns on farm and during food processing and should be considered as an early warning for increased numbers of foodborne infections with 4–6-week lag time. Heightened surveillance during such times may act as a mitigation and enhance the preventive measures. Proper hygiene during slaughter, processing, wholesale and retail sale should be carefully implemented and monitored for further safeguards.

More importantly, active consumer education through mass media and other sources regarding the potential danger of consuming contaminated food with *Salmonella* or *Campylobacter*, especially during the summer months should be properly disseminated to mitigate the increased infection rates of *Salmonella*.

3.2. Precipitation effect

In our previous study [35], no correlation between monthly average precipitation rate and *Salmonella* was observed. A better association with *Salmonella* outbreaks was noted in studies using daily or weekly rates of precipitation. Other studies, however, indicated that maximum and minimum temperatures, relative humidity and rainfall were positively correlated with the number of cases of *Salmonella* with a lag time of 2–8 weeks. It was reported that rainfall, especially heavy rainfall events, may affect the frequency and level of contamination of drinking water, and consequently enteric infection. A strong association between drinking water quality, precipitation and gastroenteritis was reported [49].

A study by Jiang *et al.* [50] suggested that extreme temperature and precipitation events are associated with salmonellosis. It was shown that the frequency and intensity of such extreme events are increasing and will continue to do so in the coming decades as a result of changing climate [50]. The influence of precipitation on salmonellosis is not always immediate but most often delayed by 2–4 weeks [51]. Precipitation likely increases salmonellosis incidence shortly after a rainfall event by increasing pathogen loads in household rainwater tanks through runoff. The delayed effect of rainfall on salmonellosis is also likely to be through increased pathogen loads in surface water which is then used to irrigate or process fresh produce that later may be consumed raw [51].

Climatic changes impact the emergence or re-emergence of infectious disease agents. There are some general principles of pathogen emergence, which are associated with changes in ecology and agriculture, technology and industry, globalization, human behaviour and demographics, epidemiological surveillance and microbial adaptation [52, 53]. It is important to recognise that pathogen emergence usually occurs as a consequence of a combination of two or more specific factors [54].

4. Modelling approaches

4.1. Regression analysis

Multiple regression analysis were carried out to test the relationship between *Salmonella* rates and socioeconomic factors, including poverty, uninsured, unemployment and primary care providers' rates. Socioeconomic factors were used as classification variables and *Salmonella* infection rate as a response variable. Regression analysis was also performed for climate factors, where temperature and precipitation were used as independent (classification) variables and *Salmonella* outbreaks as dependent (response) variable.

4.2. Neural network modelling of *Salmonella* and temperature

Neural network models for temperature effects on *Salmonella* outbreaks were developed using @RISK and NeuroShell2 software packages. NeuroShell2 is a program that mimics the human brain's ability to classify patterns or to make predictions or decisions based upon past experience. The network is exposed to the problem being predicted or classified, and the software will 'learn' the patterns from training data and will make its own classifications, predictions or decisions when presented with new data. NN models are particularly useful when there are implicit interactions and complex relationships in the data.

Over the last few years, artificial neural networks, as nonlinear modelling techniques, had been proposed for use in predictive microbiology [55–61]. In our study, two neural network models, General Regression Neural Network (GRNN) model and Polynomial Net model, were used to predict the effects of temperature on *Salmonella* outbreaks in Mississippi. Several architectures of neural network models were developed to establish the best fitting models. Both of the reported models showed a significant correlation between temperature and *Salmonella* outbreak. GRNN model and Monte Carlo simulation for predicting survival and growth of *Salmonella* on raw chicken skin, as a function of serotype, temperature and time, were used in previous studies as well [62].

Monthly data for temperature and *Salmonella* data in Mississippi from 2001 to 2011 were used to build these models. Temperature was used as an input while *Salmonella* outbreaks as output variables (**Figure 5**). A General Regression Neural Network Model and Polynomial Net Models were selected from the software design architecture. Twenty per cent of the data were extracted for testing, and 80% were used for training the NN models. A test data file was applied to previously saved trained NN models and outputs were generated. Results were exported to Excel, and graphs were created to show the association between actual data and the predicted model.

Salmonella outbreaks and socioeconomic data for Mississippi districts were used for NN models. Mean and Standard deviation were calculated for each variable, including *Salmonella*, poverty, uninsured and unemployment and primary care providers' rates. Those means and SD were subsequently used to generate data with 500 iterations using @RISK in Risk Normal distribution. The simulated data were then used as training examples for the NN models, while the original data were used for testing with NeuroShell2 software.

Advanced NNs were selected and the simulated data files were imported. The network was built by defining input variables as poverty, uninsured, unemployment and primary care providers' rates, while *Salmonella* outbreaks as output. A General Regression Neural Network (GRNN) model was selected from the software design architecture. This model was trained with the simulated data. The test file containing the original data was imported to the system and applied to previously saved trained NN models. Results were exported to Excel where graphs were created to show the association between actual data and the predicted model.

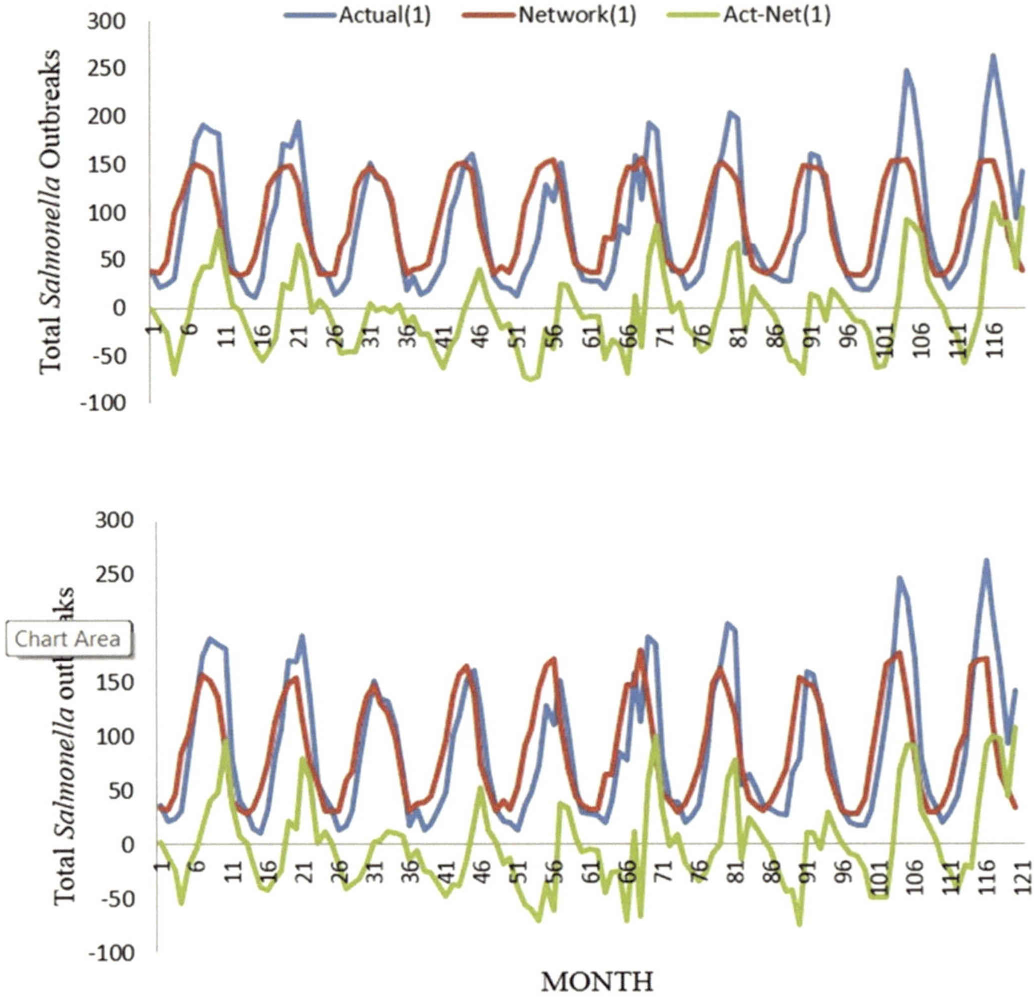

Figure 5. Neural network models for *Salmonella* and temperature correlation.

4.3. GIS mapping

A GIS incorporates hardware, software and data for capturing, managing, analysing and displaying all forms of geographically referenced information.

Study area for GIS map: Mississippi (32.9906° N, 89.5261° W) is located in the southern USA. It is bordered by TN on the north, Gulf of Mexico on the south, AL on the east and Arkansas and LA on the west. It covers a total area of 47,689 square miles. GIS allows for the integration and analysis of geographic data, such as coordinates and area perimeters, and tabular data (i.e., attributes of geographic data points). Data are imported into mapping software in layers, where each layer represents a different visual component of the map. Shape files are layers which provide visual output of coordinates and area perimeters on the map.

http://dx.doi.org/10.5772/67501

Mississippi counties' data were grouped by public health districts. Background map was obtained from ESRI ArcGIS online resources. Maps' layers for *Salmonella*, unemployment and primary care providers' rates were created for the years 2010 and 2011, to visually analyse areas with higher disease rates and socioeconomic status (**Figure 2**).

5. Conclusions

Human foodborne illnesses are significant public health concerns. Socioeconomic status and climate changes contribute to the increased rates of *Salmonella*. A significant correlation between increase in outbreaks of *Salmonella* and the lower socioeconomic status was observed in several studies. Understanding the geographical and economic relation with infectious diseases will help to determine effective methods to reduce outbreaks within these communities. Climate changes in the USA are likely to increase the severity, frequency, timing and duration of extreme weather events, which consecutively will increase the associated health risks. The transmission of *Salmonella* to humans is a complex ecological process; warmer temperatures in combination with differences in eating pattern, may contribute to enteric infections.

Modelling approaches, such as neural network were shown to be a useful tool to model and predict outbreaks. Neural network models accounting for non-linearity may predict better association than regression models. Geographical information system mapping was also shown to be a very useful instrument to map and visualise the areas and districts of highest *Salmonella* outbreaks in addition to socioeconomic status.

Regression and neural network models were used to determine the correlation between increase in temperature and increase in *Salmonella* outbreaks. Considering the seasonal variation, neural network models turned out to be better predictor models.

Acknowledgements

The reported research work is funded by the National Institute on Minority Health and Health Disparities of the National Institutes of Health under Award Number G12MD007581. The content is solely the responsibility of the authors and does not represent in any form or shape the official views of the National Institutes of Health.

Author details

Hafiz Anwar Ahmad* and Luma Akil

*Address all correspondence to: hafiz.a.ahmad@jsums.edu

1 Department of Biology-Environmental Science, Jackson State University, Jackson, MS, USA

2 Department of Behavioral and Environmental Health, Jackson State University, Jackson, MS, USA

References

[1] Hoelzer K., Isabel A., Switt M. and Wiedmann M. "Animal Contact as a Source of Human Non-typhoidal Salmonellosis". Vet Res 42 (2011): 34.

[2] Callaway T.R., Edrington T.S, Anderson R.C., Byrd J.A. and Nisbet D.J. "Gastrointestinal Microbial Ecology and the Safety of Our Food Supply as Related to Salmonella". J Anim Sci 86 no. 14 Suppl (2008): E163–E172.

[3] Brichta-Harhay D.M., Arthur T.M., Bosilevac J.M., Kalchayanand N., Shackelford S.D., Wheeler T.L. and Koohmaraie M. "Diversity of Multidrug-Resistant *Salmonella enterica* Strains Associated with Cattle at Harvest in the United States". Appl Environ Microbiol 77 no. 5 (2011): 1783–1796.

[4] Mills, J. N., Gage, K. L., & Khan, A. S. (2010). Potential influence of climate change on vector-borne and zoonotic diseases: a review and proposed research plan. *Environmental health perspectives, 118*(11), 1507.

[5] World Health Organization. Food Safety. (2009) Available at: http://www.who.int/foodsafety/en/last access 2009

[6] Newman K.L., Leon J.S., Rebolledo P.A. and Scallan E. "The Impact of Socioeconomic Status on Foodborne Illness in High-Income Countries: A Systematic Review". Epidemiol Infect 143 no. 12 (2015): 2473–2485.

[7] Akil L. and Ahmad H.A. "Salmonella Infections Modelling in Mississippi Using Neural Network and Geographical Information System (GIS)". BMJ Open 6 no. 3 (2016): e009255.

[8] TN Department of Health. Communicable Disease Interactive Data. Available at: http://health.state.tn.us/ceds/WebAim/WEBAim_criteria.aspx Last Accessed 8/15/2016

[9] State of Louisiana Department of Health and Hospitals. Infectious Diseases Reports. Available at: http://new.dhh.louisiana.gov/index.cfm/newsroom/archives/64 Last Accessed 8/15/2016

[10] Montana Department of Public Health and Human Services Surveillance. Available at: http://www.dphhs.mt.gov/publichealth/cdepi/surveillance/index.shtml Last Accessed 8/15/2016

[11] Division of Communicable Disease, Bureau of Epidemiology, Michigan Department of Community Health. Reportable Infectious Diseases in Michigan 2002–2011 Summaries. Available at: http://www.michigan.gov/documents/mdch/2005_CD_Epi_Profile_177917_7.pdf http://www.michigan.gov/documents/mdch/2009_CDEpiProfile_337815_7.pdf http://www.michigan.gov/documents/mdch/2011_CDEpiProfile_400563_7.pdf Last Accessed 8/15/2016

[12] United States Census Bureau. Available at: www.Census.gov Last Accessed 8/15/2016

[13] MSDH, County Health Ranking Mississippi. Available at: http://msdh.ms.gov/msdhsite/_static/31,0,211.html Last Accessed 8/15/2016

[14] Centers for Disease Control and Prevention. Food Safety. Retrieved 15 March 2014, from http://www.cdc.gov/foodsafety/ Last Accessed 8/15/2016

[15] Chai S.J., White P.L., Lathrop S.L., Solghan S.M. and Medus C. "*Salmonella enterica* Serotype Enteritidis: Increasing Incidence of Domestically Acquired Infections." Clin Infect Dis 54 (2012): S488–S497.

[16] Chang M., Groseclose S.L., Zaidi A.A. and Braden C.R. "An Ecological Analysis of Sociodemographic Factors Associated with the Incidence of *Salmonellosis, Shigellosis*, and *E. coli* O157:H7 Infections in US Counties." Epidemiol Infect 137 no. 6 (2009): 810–820.

[17] Scallan, E., Hoekstra, R. M., Angulo, F. J., Tauxe, R. V., Widdowson, M. A., Roy, S. L., & Griffin, P. M. (2011). Foodborne illness acquired in the United States—major pathogens. *Emerg Infect Dis, 17*(1).

[18] Darcey, V. L. (2010). *GIS mapping of retail food access to assess risks of (chronic and acute) illness in populations of different socioeconomic status* (Doctoral dissertation, Drexel University).

[19] Younus M., Edward H., Azfar A.S., Wilkins M., Davies H.D., Rahbar M., Funk J. and Saeed M. "The Role of Neighbourhood Level Socioeconomic Characteristics in Salmonella Infections in Michigan (1997–2007): Assessment Using Geographic Information System." Int J Health Geogr 6 (2007): 56.

[20] Lin B. "Resilience in Agriculture Through Crop Diversification: Adaptive Management for Environmental Change." BioScience 61 no. 3 (2011): 183–193.

[21] Park J. and Edington D.W. "A Sequential Neural Network Model for Diabetes Prediction." Artif Intell Med 23 no. 3 (2001): 277–293.

[22] Sovan L. and Guegan J.F. "Artificial Neural Network as a Tool in Ecological Modeling, an Introduction." Ecol Model 120 (1999): 65–73.

[23] Akil L. and Ahmad H.A. "Relationships Between Obesity and Cardiovascular." J Health Care Poor Underserved 22 (2011): 61–72.

[24] Nielsen M., Lundegaard C. and Worning P. "Reliable Prediction of T-cell Epitopes Using Neural Network with Novel Sequence Representations." Protein Sci 12 no. 5 (2003): 1007–1017.

[25] Khan J., Wei J.S. and Ringner M. "Classification and Diagnostic Prediction of Cancers Using Gene Expression Profiling and Artificial Neural Networks". Nat Med 7 no. 6 (2001): 673–679.

[26] Smith B.A., Hougenboom G. and McClendon R.W. "Artificial Neural Network for Automated Year-Round Temperature Prediction." Comp Electron Agric 68 no. 1 (2009): 52–61.

[27] Ahmad H.A. "Poultry Growth Modeling Using Neural Networks and Simulated Data." J Appl Poult Res. 18 (2009): 440–446.

[28] Ahmad H.A. and Mariano M. "Comparison of Forecasting Methodologies Using Egg Price as a Test Case." Poultry Sci 85 no. 4 (2006): 798–807.

[29] Kendrovski, Vladimir, and Dragan Gjorgjev. *Climate Change: Implication for Food-Borne Diseases (Salmonella and Food Poisoning Among Humans in R. Macedonia).* INTECH Open Access Publisher, 2012.

[30] Patz J.A., Olson S.H., Uejio C.K. and Gibbs H.K. "Disease Emergence from Global Climate and Land Use Change". Med Clin N Am 92 (2008): 1473–1491.

[31] McMichael A.J., Woodruff R.E. and Hales S. "Climate Change and Human Health: Present and Future Risks." Lancet 367 (2006): 859–869.

[32] Hunter PR. Climate change and waterborne and vector-borne disease. Journal of applied microbiology. 2003 May 1; 94(s1):37-46.

[33] National Oceanic and Atmospheric Administration: U.S. Climate Extremes Index. Available at: http://www.ncdc.noaa.gov/extremes/cei/retrieved Last Accessed 4/20/2012

[34] Sheffield P.E. and Landrigan P.J. "Global Climate Change and Children's Health: Threats and Strategies for Prevention". Environ Health Perspect 119 no. 3 (2011): 291–298.

[35] Akil L., Reddy R.S. and Ahmad H.A. "Effects of Climate Change on Salmonella Infections". Foodborne Pathog Dis 11 no. 12 (2014): 974–980. doi:10.1089/fpd.2014.1802.

[36] D'Souza R.M. "Climatic Factors Association with Hospitalization and Emergency Room Presentations of Diarrhea". Epidemiology 16 (2005): S60.

[37] Zhang Ying, Bi Peng and Hiller Janet E. "Climate Variations and Salmonella Infection in Australian Subtropical and Tropical Regions". Sci Total Environ 408 (2010): 524–530.

[38] Taylor E., Kastner J. and Renter D. "Challenges Involved in the Salmonella Saintpaul Outbreak and Lessons Learned". (2009). Retrieved from http://krex.k-state.edu

[39] Fleury Manon, Charron Dominique F., Holt John D., Allen O. Brian and Maarouf Abdel R. "A Time Series Analysis of the Relationship of Ambient Temperature and Common Bacterial Enteric Infections in Two Canadian Provinces." Int J Biometeorol 50 no. 6 (2006): 385–391.

[40] Zhang G., Brown E.W. and González-Escalona N. "Comparison of Real-Time PCR, Reverse Transcriptase Real-Time PCR, Loop-Mediated Isothermal Amplification, and the FDA Conventional Microbiological Method for the Detection of Salmonella spp. in Produce." Appl Environ Microbiol 77 no. 18 (2011): 6495–6501.

[41] Karl T.R., Melillo J.M. and Peterson T.C. (Eds.). USGCRP. Global Climate Change Impacts in the United States. United States Global Change Research Program. Cambridge University Press, New York (2009).

[42] Junejaa Vijay K., Melendresb Martin Valenzuela, Huanga Lihan, Gumudavellic Vinod, Subbiahc Jeyamkondan and Thippareddi Harshavardhan. "Modeling the Effect of Temperature on Growth of Salmonella in Chicken". Food Microbiol 24 (2007): 328–335.

[43] Milazzo A., et al. "The Effect of Temperature on Different Salmonella Serotypes During Warm Seasons in a Mediterranean Climate City, Adelaide, Australia." Epidemiol Infect 144 no. 6 (2016): 1231–1240.

[44] Bambrick, Hilary, Keith Dear, Rosalie Woodruff, Ivan Hanigan, and Anthony McMichael. "The impacts of climate change on three health outcomes: temperature-related mortality and hospitalisations, salmonellosis and other bacterial gastroenteritis, and population at risk from dengue." *Garnaut climate change review* 26 (2008): 2010.

[45] Russell R., Paterson M. and Lima Nelson. "How Will Climate Change Affect Mycotoxins in Food?" Food Res Int 43 (2010): 1902–1914.

[46] Bentham Graham and Langford I.H. "Environmental Temperatures and the Incidence of Food Poisoning in England and Wales." Int J Biometeorol 45 no. 1 (2001): 22–26.

[47] Petrescu C., Suciu O., Ionovici R., Herbarth O., Franck U. and Schlink U. "Respiratory Health Effects of Air Pollution with Particles and Modification Due to Climate Parameters in an Exposed Population: Long and Short Term Study." Int J Energy Environ 1 no. 5 (2011): 102–112.

[48] Semenza Jan C. and Bettina M. "Climate Change and Infectious Diseases in Europe." Lancet Infect Dis 9 (2009): 365–375.

[49] Zhang Y., Bi P. and Hiller J. "Climate Variations and Salmonellosis Transmission in Adelaide, South Australia: A Comparison Between Regression Models". Int J Biometeorol 52 no. 3 (2008): 179–187.

[50] Jiang, Chengsheng, Kristi S. Shaw, Crystal R. Upperman, David Blythe, Clifford Mitchell, Raghu Murtugudde, Amy R. Sapkota, and Amir Sapkota. "Climate change, extreme events and increased risk of salmonellosis in Maryland, USA: Evidence for coastal vulnerability." *Environment international* 83 (2015): 58-62.

[51] Stephen D.M. and Barnett A.G. "Effect of Temperature and Precipitation on Salmonellosis Cases in South-East Queensland, Australia: An Observational Study". BMJ Open 6 no. 2 (2016): e010204.

[52] Tauxe R.V. "Emerging Foodborne Pathogens." Int J Food Microbiol 78 no. 1–2 (2002): 31–41.

[53] Rose J.B., Epstein P.R., Lipp E.K., Sherman B.H., Bernard S.M. and Patz J.A. "Climate Variability and Change in the United States: Potential Impacts on Water and Foodborne Diseases Caused by Microbiologic Agents". Environ Health Perspect 109 no. 2 (2001): 211–220.

[54] Jaykus, L.-A., Woolridge M., Frank J.M., Miraglia M., McQuatters-Gollop A., Tirado C., Clarke R. and Friel M. "Climate Change: Implications for Food Safety. "FAO Rep (2011) Available @ https://health2016.globalchange.gov/food-safety-nutrition-and-distribution/content/food-safety.

[55] Garcíaa-Gimeno R.M., Hervás-Martíanez C., Barco-Alcalá E., Zurera-Cosano G. and Sanz-Tapi E. "An Artificial Neural Network Approach to *Escherichia Coli* O157:H7 Growth Estimation." J Food Sci 68 no. 2 (2003): 639–645.

[56] Ibarra, Juan G., and Yang Tao. "Estimation of internal temperature in chicken meat by means of mid-infrared imaging and neural networks." In *Photonics East (ISAM, VVDC, IEMB)*, pp. 24-31. International Society for Optics and Photonics, 1999.

[57] Valero A., Hervás C., García-Gimeno R.M. and Zurera G. "Product Unit Neural Network Models for Predicting the Growth Limits of Listeria Monocytogene." Food Microbiol 24 no. 5 (2007): 452–464.

[58] McKee K.T., Shields T.M., Jenkins P.R., Zenilman J.M. and Glass G.E. "Application of a Geographic Information System to the Tracking and Control of an Outbreak of Shigellosis." Clin Infect Dis 31 (2000): 728–733.

[59] Hervás C., Martínez J.A., Zurera G., García R.M. and Martínez J.A. "Optimization of Computational Neural Network for Its Application in the Prediction of Microbial Growth in Food." Food Sci Technol Int 7 (2001): 159.

[60] Khanzadi S., Gharibzadeh S., Raoufy M.R., Razavilar V., Khaksar R. and Radmehr B. "Application of Artificial Neural Networks to Predict Clostridium Botulinum Growth as a Function of Zataria Multiflora Essential Oil, Ph, Nacl and Temperature." J Food Saf 30 no. 2 (2010): 490–505.

[61] Jacoboni I., Martelli P.L., Fariselli P., De Pinto V. and Casadio R. "Prediction of the Transmembrane Regions of β-Barrel Membrane Proteins with a Neural Network-Based Predictor." Protein Sci 10 no. 4 (2001): 779–787.

[62] Oscar T.P. "A Quantitative Risk Assessment Model for Salmonella and Whole Chickens." Int J Food Microbiol 93 (2004): 231–247.

Chapter 14

Application of Ionizing Radiation for Control of *Salmonella* in Food

Małgorzata E. Szczawińska

Additional information is available at the end of the chapter

http://dx.doi.org/10.5772/67408

Abstract

Ionizing radiation (gamma rays from the radionuclides cobalt-60 or cesium-137, e-beams) is an effective, nonthermal method to reduce or eliminate food-borne pathogens, including *Salmonella* spp. both in raw and in cooked meats, poultry, fish, and shellfish. Irradiation treatment, applied as the final processing step, seems to be particularly promising in the case of packed food products, including ready-to-eat food. Final packaged food products can be contaminated from post-lethality exposure, that is, after heat treatment and before packaging. The application of ionizing radiation after packaging can eliminate or considerably reduce both saprophytic and pathogenic microflora in final products. It is of particular importance in the case of ready-to-eat food which is not subjected to heat treatment before consumption. According to hurdle concept technology, the combination of existing and novel preservation methods can ensure safety of food by applying all treatments as mild as possible. Irradiation treatment can be combined with the use of natural antibacterial compounds, such as extracts of spices and herbs, or various packaging systems. Doses of ionizing radiation required for the inactivation of *Salmonella* spp. in fish and seafood are lower than those used for meats and poultry.

Keywords: *Salmonella*, radiation, meat, poultry, fish

1. Introduction

In the last years, the great consumer interest in "natural" or "fresh" foods, nonprocessed or only minimally processed, has caused an increasing interest in nonthermal preservation methods, that is, ionizing radiation, ultraviolet radiation, high-pressure processing (HPP), pulsed electric field (PEF), high-pressure carbon dioxide (HPCD), the use of natural antibacterial compounds, such as extracts of spices and herbs, or the application of various packaging systems. However, at the same time consumer demand for ensuring food safety has to be met. Those two ideas are very often tough to reconcile in practice.

A great number of studies have shown that ionizing radiation improve the safety of various foods of animal as well as plant origin. Food irradiation is a process which can be used to inactivate both food-borne pathogens and microorganisms causing spoilage of food, thus extending storage of foods such as red meats, poultry, fish, and so on. It can also extend the storage of vegetables by prevention of sprouting (potatoes, onions, and garlic) or fruits by the delay of ripening. At present time, this technology may be used not only to raw foods but also as post-lethality treatment. The product may be exposed to the post-lethality processing environment into which the product is routed after having been subjected to an initial lethality treatment. The foodstuffs may be exposed to the environment in the area of establishment as a result of, for example, slicing, peeling, and re-bagging, or other procedures. Hotdog products are examples of ready-to-eat (RTE) meat and poultry products that receive a lethality treatment to eliminate pathogens (core temperatures of +70° to +72°C must be reached due to cooking) and they are subsequently exposed to the environment during peeling, slicing, and repackaging operations. Then, the technology of irradiation, used as an intervention step, can be applied to the final product or sealed package of product in order to reduce or eliminate the level of pathogens resulting from contamination from post-lethality exposure. Thus, for example, vacuum-packaged ready-to-eat (RTE) meat products may be subjected to irradiation to reduce or eliminate dangerous food-borne pathogens such as *Salmonella* spp. and *Listeria monocytogenes* in a final food product. According to hurdle concept technology, the combination of existing and novel preservation methods can ensure safety of food by applying all treatments as mild as possible [1, 2].

A good example of such combination of preservation methods (low-dose irradiation and modified atmosphere packaging (MAP)) is the work of Chouliara et al. [3] who investigated the combined effect of gamma irradiation (2 and 4 kGy) and modified atmosphere (MA) packaging (30% CO_2/70% N_2 and 70% CO_2/30% N_2) on shelf-life extension of fresh chicken meat stored under refrigeration. The authors noted the reduction of the number of various groups of bacteria (from 1 to 5 logs), including Enterobacteriaceae family. Sensory evaluation showed that the combination of irradiation at 4 kGy and MAP (70% CO_2/30% N_2) resulted in the highest shelf-life extension by 12 days compared to the air-packaged samples. A study of Grant and Patterson [4] is another good example of hurdle concept technology: mild heating combined with low-dose irradiation. In this study, thermal treatment (70, 65, or 60°C) was applied alone, directly post 0.8 kGy irradiation or post irradiation combined with refrigerated storage on inactivation of *L. monocytogenes* and *Salmonella typhimurium* inoculated into beef and gravy. The researchers observed heat sensitization of *S. typhimurium* at 60°C, but not at either 65 or 70°C like in the case of *L. monocytogenes*. In another study [5], the influence of heating and low-dose irradiation *S. typhimurium* in MDCM (mechanically deboned chicken meat) was examined. The researchers noted that salmonellae irradiated with 0.9 kGy were more heat sensitive; this effect was maintained during 6 weeks of refrigerated storage.

Those readers who want to deepen their knowledge of the subject can find an extensive description of microbiological issues associated with all muscle foods, their specific spoilage, safety issues, and their control for meat, poultry, and seafood in the work provided by Sofos et al. [6].

Thermal treatment is a very effective method for eliminating *Salmonella* spp. in foods. This organism is rather sensitive to pasteurization temperatures used in meat processing. Properly conducted heat treatment in industrial food processing should cause complete inactivation of these bacteria in meat and meat products; however, recontamination of ready-to-eat meat products with *Salmonella* spp. after cooking, as well as subsequent storage at abuse temperatures at food establishments or at a consumer's home, can cause a significant risk to human health. Szczawińska et al. [7] inoculated commercial, smoked, cured, and cooked ham with *Salmonella* enteritidis and stored the samples at abused temperature (15°C). Lag time for *S.* enteritidis was at that temperature only 139.08 h, that is, less than 6 days [7]. Usually, the length of time for storage of such product recommended by the food manufacturer is much longer than the time mentioned above. It means that a consumer can contract food-borne salmonellosis during the recommended length of storage time for such ready-to-eat meat product if it was recontaminated with *Salmonella*. Thus, due to beneficial effects of ionizing radiation treatment of final packaged food product (RTE), we can expect that *Salmonella* (and other vegetative bacterial pathogens which show similar radiation resistance, e.g., *L. monocytogenes*) will be significantly reduced or eliminated.

2. The use of ionizing radiation

According to the Codex General Standard for Irradiated Foods [8], the following sources of ionizing radiation can be used:

(a) Radionuclides, such as Cobalt-60 and Cesium-137, which emit gamma rays (γ-rays)

(b) Machines that produced high-energy electron beams (an energy level up to 10 MeV)

(c) X-rays machines (an energy level up to 5 MeV).

Compared to γ-rays, e-beams are characterized by a low penetrative capacity; therefore, e-beam irradiation is particularly useful for products which can be processed in thin layers or surface-contaminated products.

The dose of radiation received is commonly measured in grays. One gray is a derived unit of ionizing radiation. It is defined as the absorption of one joule of radiation energy in a mass of one kilogram (1 Gy = 1 J/kg). The gray has superseded the older unit—the rad (1 Gy = 100 rad). The **gray** (symbol: **Gy**) is used as a measure of absorbed dose.

According to several objectives for food (fresh or processed meats, poultry, and seafood) irradiation, the following terms are used [9]:

(a) Radicidation is the elimination of bacterial pathogens, non-spore formers; doses range 2.5–10 kGy.

(b) Radurization is the significant reduction of the number of saprophytic microorganisms ensuring shelf-life extension of foods; doses range 0.75–2.5 kGy.

(c) **Radappertization** is based on a similar concept ("botulinum cook") like in canning industry. It should ensure complete elimination of spore formers in foods, thus significant shelf-life extension (years) and botulism food safety; doses range 30–40 kGy. The term was established to honor Nicolas Appert who invented the method of preserving food from spoilage by placing it in hermetically sealed containers and then sterilized by heat treatment.

In this review, special attention will be paid to **radicidation**. In case of this technology, one of the most important pathogens, *Salmonella* spp., public health problem, has been the main target for control, particularly in meat and poultry products (i.e., for example, see Ref. [10]). The most recent European Food Safety Authority (EFSA) summary report has informed us that the total number of food-borne outbreaks in Europe was 5251, including water-borne outbreaks [11]. *Salmonella* caused 20.0% of all reported food-borne outbreaks in European Union (EU) and it was the second most frequent cause of outbreaks; the largest number of reported food-borne outbreaks was caused by viruses (20.4% of all outbreaks) [11]. High level of noncompliance was noted for poultry meat [11]. Monitoring activities and control programs for *Salmonella* in fresh broiler meat are based on sampling at the slaughterhouse and/or at processing or cutting plants and at retail. In 2014, *Salmonella* was found in 0.6% of the 2263 units of RTE broiler meat products tested at retail or at processing (0.4% of single samples and 1.7% of batches) [11].

As in previous years, the two most commonly reported *Salmonella* serovars in 2014 were *S. enteritidis* and *S. typhimurium*, representing 44.4% and 17.4%, respectively, of all reported serovars in confirmed human cases [11]. Generally, there was no major change as regards *Salmonella*-contaminated foodstuffs compared with previous years. *Salmonella* was most frequently detected in fresh turkey meat (3.5%), fresh broiler (2.2%), pig (0.5%), and bovine meat (0.1%) [11]. It should be emphasized that according to the European legislation on microbiological criteria for foodstuffs [12] *Salmonella* spp. is currently included both in food safety as well as food hygiene criteria.

The main reason for the use of food irradiation is the ability of ionizing radiation to inactivate populations of microorganisms including pathogenic bacteria, parasites, and viruses. Depending on irradiation dose, food-borne pathogens can be injured or killed due to DNA damage. Radiation sensitivity depends on many factors such as species of microorganisms, age of cells, and their number. It is also affected by the environment (buffer solution, laboratory medium, or real food product). Thus, the effect of radiation on microorganisms is dependent on intrinsic and extrinsic factors which include temperature, water activity, pH, chemical composition, and structure of food and gaseous environment. Radiation resistance of bacteria is much higher at freezing temperatures than at chill temperatures; however, irradiation of frozen food offers much better results in some foods because it significantly reduces or eliminates some negative sensory changes caused by, for example, lipid oxidation. D10 values (D10 value is defined as decimal reduction dose or the dose of ionizing radiation required for a 90% inactivation of viable colony-forming unit (CFU) or by one logarithmic cycle) are higher in foods with a low water activity because the lack of water means that there are less OH radicals available to cause DNA damage. Hence, higher doses of ionizing radiation have to be used to ensure the elimination of pathogenic bacteria in dry foods such as spices [13].

Some authors observed different effects of meat irradiation depending on radiation source. Rajkowski et al. [14] discovered in their study that D10 values for *S. typhimurium* DT 104 irradiated in ground pork with gamma rays were 0.56–0.62 kGy, whereas D10 values for the same organism treated with e-beams ranged from 0.42 to 0.43 kGy.

However, Miyahara and Miyahara [15] concluded that both gamma rays and e-beams were similarly effective while irradiating ground beef patties inoculated with *S. enteritidis*.

The use of ionizing radiation as a means of reducing the risk to human health from food-borne pathogens, including *Salmonella* spp., is being extensively researched. It seems that the application of ionizing radiation to preserve food or eliminate pathogenic bacteria from food has been so intensively studied like not any other scientific field, because of consumer concerns, particularly associated with fear of nuclear energy and very often occurring confusion between terms, for example, radiation, radioactive contamination, or radioactivity. In general, consumer is rather reluctant to this technology due to well-known nuclear accidents (e.g., Chernobyl and Fukushima) believing that the process of food irradiation can make food radioactive, thus unsafe. Interestingly, there is much less consumer resistance to the high-pressure-processing technology which is used to treat wide range of foods including those of animal origin, for example, RTE products. To date, health and safety authorities in over 60 countries worldwide, for example, the United States, France, Belgium, the Netherlands, Canada, Australia, and New Zealand, granted clearances for irradiation of more than 60 different foods [16]. Frog legs are the most often irradiated food items [17].

Currently, the International Atomic Energy Agency (IAEA) is responsible for updating and maintaining various irradiation databases as resources for researchers, government officials, and the general public. European Food Safety Authority [18] summarized and evaluated an opinion on the efficacy and microbiological safety of irradiation of food taking into consideration recommendations from the two panels: BIOHAZ (the EFSA Panel on Biological Hazards) and CEF (the EFSA Panel on Food Contact Materials, Enzymes, Flavourings and Processing Aids).

EFSA emphasizes its standpoint that food irradiation should only be used in conjunction with an integrated food safety management program. With regard to efficacy and microbiological safety, the BIOHAZ Panel recommended that the application of food irradiation should be based on risk assessment and on the desired risk reduction rather than on predefined food classes/commodities and doses [18]). Concerning the safety assessment of irradiation of food, according to the BIOHAZ Panel, there are no microbiological risks for the consumer linked to the use of food irradiation and its consequences on the food microflora. EFSA's experts conclude that the irradiation dose needed to inactivate food-borne pathogens depends on the targeted pathogen, on the reduction required, and on the physical state of the food, **regardless of the food classes** as previously proposed [18].

2.1. Reducing *Salmonella* spp. in red meats and poultry

Vegetative food-borne bacteria, such as *Salmonella* spp. and *L. monocytogenes*, are moderately sensitive to ionizing radiation. The medium-dose irradiation processes reduce their populations by several logs. As previously mentioned, various factors influence radiation sensitivity of bacterial cells. The presence of proteins can exert a protective effect on microorganisms subjected to radiation treatment. Maxcy and Tiwari [19] studied the effect of fat content in beef on radioresistance of *S. enteritidis*. They found D10 value higher in beef with lower level of fat (0.70 kGy) compared to lower D10 value obtained for salmonellae irradiated in beef with higher content of fat (0.49 kGy). Assuming that the low fat level in the meat is correlated with a higher protein content and because the proteins have the properties of free radicals scavenging, it can be suggested that the higher content of protein in meat protects more the bacteria against the damaging effects of radiation treatment.

There have been frequently voiced concerns that the reduction of the competitive microflora by radiation treatment could facilitate growth of pathogens contaminating the food after irradiation or that food pathogens which survived irradiation can grow better than the indigenous, competitive microflora. Dickson and Olson [20] studied the first problem; ground beef was irradiated at 0, 2, or 4 kGy, thus reducing the number of saprophytic microorganisms which cause food spoilage, and then inoculated with a mixture of four serotypes of salmonellae. The meat was stored at 4°C, temperature proper for storage, and at two abused temperatures 15 and 25°C. Bacterial growth was monitored during storage. The authors observed that there was no significant difference in lag-phase duration or generation time, irrespective of the dose to which the ground beef had previously been exposed. This suggests that, although irradiation eliminates a significant portion of the spoilage microflora in ground beef, the absence of this microflora provides no competitive advantage to the growth of salmonellae in ground beef [20]. Szczawińska [21] studied the effect of irradiation on the survival rate of non-sporing bacteria (*Staphylococcus aureus, S. typhimurium, Escherichia coli, Pseudomonas fluorescens*) during conventional methods of meat preservation (heating, chilling, freezing, salting, curing, and smoking). On the basis of the conducted experiments, it can be concluded that irradiated bacteria stored under conditions preventing their growth die faster compared to unirradiated bacteria or their survival rate is almost identical like unirradiated ones; those organisms which are stored under conditions that allow their growth show a worse adaptability to the environment and begin to grow after a certain delay [21]. In another work, Szczawińska et al. [22] studied the growth of salmonellae in mechanically deboned chicken meat (MDCM), which was irradiated at 0, 1.25, and 2.5 kGy and inoculated with *S. dublin, S. enteritidis*, and *S. typhimurium*. Subsequently, the inoculated MDCM was stored at 5, 10, or 20°C and bacterial numbers were determined over storage time. The results of the study suggested that there was no greater risk from the same number of *Salmonella* cells contaminating irradiated MDCM compared to unirradiated one. In the same study, irradiated indigenous microflora had dose-related increased lag phases and decreased rates of multiplication compared with that of the indigenous microflora in the unirradiated control [22]. Kim and Thayer [23] discovered that the gamma-injured *S. typhimurium* cells on mechanically deboned chicken meat were much more sensitive to heat than the nonirradiated cells, which implies that any cells surviving the irradiation process were unlikely to survive cooking. This increased sensitivity of the salmonellae to gamma radiation was retained during refrigerated storage of the irradiated chicken. Kim and Thayer [23] explained the mechanism of the heat sensitivity of *S. typhimurium* subjected to ionizing radiation. The results proved that combined effects of irradiation and heating were always beneficial in regard to food safety due to synergistic (when heating is applied after irradiation) or additive (when heating is applied before irradiation) effects depending on the order of both treatments. Therefore, on the basis of these studies it can be concluded that any microorganisms which survive irradiation are more sensitive to intrinsic or extrinsic factors, such as temperature, water activity, pH, and so on, compared to unirradiated organisms.

Irradiation of fresh meat up to an overall average dose of 2 kGy was proposed by the SCF in 1986 [24]. Implication of meat in food-borne salmonellosis still remains a concern, particularly in the countries or regions where traditional dishes are served and consumed as raw and cold. In the Netherlands, Belgium, such meat product is "filet américain" composed of raw beef meat, and often raw egg. Kampelmacher [25] reported that a dose of only 1 kGy decreased *Salmonella* number in such a product by two log cycles. Rajkowski et al. [14] examined the effect of e-beam and gamma rays irradiation on the mixture of *S. typhimurium* DT104 strains inoculated into three ground pork products containing various fat contents and obtained D10 values for salmonellae from 0.42 to 0.62 kGy. The data prove that the content of fat had no effect on radiation resistance of salmonellae. The D10 values are similar to the values reported by Szczawińska [26] for *S. typhimurium* strains inoculated into poultry meat. Clavero et al. [27] subjected raw ground beef patties inoculated with mixture of serovars of *S. dublin, S. typhimurium,* and *S. enteritidis* to gamma irradiation (60°C) treatment. The influence of two levels of fat (8–14% (low fat) and 27–28% (high fat)) and temperature (frozen (−17 to −15°C) and refrigerated (3–5°C)) on the inactivation of pathogens by irradiation was investigated. D10 values for salmonellae in beef patties ranged from 0.618 to 0.800 kGy. The authors discovered that temperature did not have a significant effect when salmonellae were irradiated in high-fat ground beef.

D10 values for *Salmonella* spp. have been reported [28] to range from 0.38 to 0.77 kGy at 2°C in mechanically deboned chicken; sensitivity of *Salmonella* spp. to ionizing radiation has been found to be highly dependent on serovars. Similarly, the D10 values were reported by Szczawińska [26] for *S. typhimurium* strains inoculated into poultry meat, whereas a D10 value of 0.57 kGy has been observed for the pathogen in ground beef treated at 18–20°C [29].

In another work by Thayer et al. [30], *Musculus longissimus dorsi* from beef, pork, and lamb and turkey breast and leg meats were inoculated with *Salmonella* spp., and the gamma radiation resistance of the pathogens was determined at 5°C under identical conditions. The authors concluded that the *D*-value for a mixture of *Salmonella* spp. was significantly lower on pork than on beef, lamb, turkey breast, and turkey leg meats; however, all *D*-values were within expected ranges. Thayer et al. [31] studied the survival of salmonellae in vacuum-canned, commercial MDCM. The MDCM was challenged with *S. enteritidis* (ca 10^4 CFU/g of meat) followed by irradiation to 0, 1.5, and 3.0 kGy and storage at 5°C for 0, 2, and 4 weeks. The researchers reported that the number of salmonellae in unirradiated MDCM decreased about one log cycle after 1 month of storage; however, in meat irradiated with 3.0 kGy dose the presence of this pathogen was not detected at the very beginning of storage. Thayer and Boyd also found that *S. typhimurium* was more resistant to gamma radiation when vacuum packaged than when air was present during irradiation [32]. The final equations predict a reduction in the number of surviving *Salmonella* in mechanically deboned chicken meat. If MDCM is irradiated at −20°C with a dose of 1.50 kGy in air then the expected reduction of this pathogen is 2.53 and 2.12 logs in vacuum. After 3.0 kGy dose, at −20°C in air the level of bacteria will be lower by 4.78 and 4.29 logs in vacuum [32].

Bacteria are more resistant when irradiated at frozen temperatures compared to chill or ambient temperatures; Szczawińska [26] reported that the mean D_{10} value for 13 *Salmonella* strains irradiated in chicken meat using gamma rays at 4°C amounted to 0.575 kGy, whereas for samples irradiated in a frozen state (at −18°C) the mean D_{10} value amounted to 0.687 kGy.

Gamma-irradiated broiler halves packed in polyethylene pouches with the dose of 2.5 kGy should ensure *Salmonella* reduction adequate to eliminate naturally occurring contamination. In frozen poultry meat, similar effects can be expected after a dose of 3.5 kGy [26]. In the same work, Szczawińska [26] discovered that the packaging material exerted a very strong effect on radiation resistance of *S. typhimurium*. Two strains of *S. typhimurium* were irradiated in ground chicken meat at temperatures +4 and −18°C. D10 values obtained for salmonellae irradiated at +4 and packed in PE pouches were 0.194 and 0.210 kGy, whereas D10 values obtained for salmonellae packed in PA/PE laminate pouches at the same temperature were 0.424 and 0.533 kGy. D10 values obtained for salmonellae irradiated at -18°C and packed in PE pouches were 0.412 and 0.633 kGy, whereas D10 values obtained for salmonellae packed in PA/PE laminate pouches at the same temperature were 0.538 and 0.721 kGy. Thus, the contribution of food-packaging material and packaging system is a very important issue in this technology. Irradiation was also combined with curing salts. The combined effects of 1-kGy irradiation dose and curing salts ($NaNO_2$ and NaCl) on the survival of *S. typhimurium, S. agona, and S. cholerasuis* in pork meat were studied by Szczawiński et al. [33]. Salmonellae were inoculated in ground *M. longissimus dorsi*, and irradiated at 1 kGy dose. The three experimental groups were designed. The meat was treated with 100 mg $NaNO_2$, 200 mg $NaNO_2$, and 200 mg $NaNO_2$ plus 3% NaCl. Meat samples were stored at 0–2°C for 3 weeks or at 20°C for 7 days. The authors reported that irradiation at 1 kGy dose reduced *Salmonella* number by 1.2–2 logs and that an additive effect of curing salts and irradiation was observed at low temperature of storage, and that synergistic effect of irradiation and curing salts was observed at temperature abuse [33].

Poultry, as already mentioned, as regards the radicidation, has been recognized as one of the best candidates for irradiation aiming a reduction or elimination of food-borne pathogenic bacteria such as *Salmonella* spp. and *Campylobacter* spp. Irradiation of poultry up to an overall average dose of 7 kGy was proposed by the Scientific Committee on Food [24] with the purpose to improve microbiological safety.

Salmonella caused 38.18%, the highest number of outbreaks and human cases among all causative agents according to data of EFSA for 2014 [34]. Raw poultry meat and poultry products are vehicles of those two food-borne pathogenic bacteria. In the EU, in 2013 [34], *Salmonella* was detected in 3.5% of the broiler meat. At retail, the overall proportion of *Salmonella*-positive samples was 7.5%, higher than at slaughterhouse (4.9%) and at the processing plant (2.6%) level [34]. Since December 2011, a *Salmonella* criterion for *S. enteritidis* and *S. typhimurium* in raw poultry entered into force [35].

In 2013, EFSA [34] reported that *Salmonella* was found in 0.3% of the 4776 samples of RTE broiler meat products tested at retail or at processing (0.1% of single samples and 1.9% of batches). Of the 2100 tested units of RTE products from turkey meat, only 0.1% in total were found to be *Salmonella*-positive [34].

Kudra et al. [36] studied the survival of *S. typhimurium* subjected to irradiation combined with high-CO_2 + CO MAP in chicken meat product. The authors did not find significant difference between D10 values for bacteria irradiated in vacuum (0.55 kGy) or in high-CO_2 + CO MAP (0.54 kGy). The dose of 1.5 kGy decreased the number of salmonellae by three logs. *Salmonella* presence was detected in both packaging systems during cold storage. During storage of this meat product at temperature abuse (25°C), *Salmonella* was able to grow in both packaging systems. The authors concluded that low-dose irradiation is a suitable method for destruction of this pathogen; however, packaging system did not exert significant influence on *Salmonella* number during storage at low temperature. The authors concluded that if the initial contamination of these pathogens is high, cross-contamination of ready-to-eat food at temperature abuse of the product is likely to continue to be a food safety concern regardless of irradiation treatment doses or packaging treatments.

Szczawińska [26] reported that the mean D_{10} value for 13 *Salmonella* strains irradiated in chicken meat using gamma rays at 4°C amounted to 0.575 kGy, whereas for samples irradiated in a frozen state (at −18° C) the mean D_{10} value amounted to 0.687 kGy. Gamma-irradiated broiler halves packed in polyethylene pouches with the dose of 2.5 kGy should ensure *Salmonella* reduction adequate to eliminate naturally occurring contamination; in frozen poultry meat, similar effects can be expected after a dose of 3.5 kGy [26].

Nassar et al. [37] evaluated the survival of *Salmonella virchow* inoculated into raw chicken carcasses as a result of radiation treatment (dose range of 2–7 kGy) or disinfection with three chemical substances. The presence of salmonellae in chicken meat was not detected after 7 kGy dose; however, after chemical disinfection this pathogen was still present.

On the basis of the various published data, it seems that the dose up to 7 kGy for frozen poultry and about 3.5 kGy for unfrozen meat can be recommended to reduce the most radioresistant vegetative pathogenic bacteria by five logs [18].

Thayer et al. [38] compared gamma radiation resistance of a mixture of salmonellae (*S. dublin, S. enteritidis, S. newport, S. senftenberg, and S. typhimurium*) in the so-called "exotic" meats such as ground bison, ostrich, alligator, and caiman meats at 5°C. The type of meat did not significantly alter the radiation resistance of salmonellae, and the *D*-value of 0.53 ± 0.02 kGy for *Salmonella* spp. was obtained. In the conclusions, authors emphasized that the efficacy of the radiation treatment in elimination of *Salmonella* spp. in exotic meats and non-exotic meats (e.g., poultry) is similar, thus similar control measures can be applied to ensure exotic meat safety. When considering cooked chilled and other ready-to-eat poultry meat products, the food-borne pathogens of higher concern are represented by *L. monocytogenes* and *Salmonella* spp. Hence, stricter microbiological criteria for poultry meat products intended to be eaten cooked, as amended by the Commission Regulation (EU) No 365/2010, which enhance food safety, must be respected by EU members [39]. Another (EC) regulation [40], which lays down general rules for food business operators on the hygiene of foodstuffs, requires food business operators to comply with microbiological criteria for foodstuffs. Regulation (EC) No 853/2005 [41], which sets specific hygiene rules for foods of animal origin, also requires that food business operators ensure compliance with microbiological criteria.

Radiation sensitivity of *L. monocytogenes* was determined by many authors (i.e., for example, see Ref. [42]). Reported D10 values for *L. monocytogenes* in cooked turkey nuggets were about 0.70 kGy, making *L. monocytogenes* generally more radiation-resistant than *Campylobacter* and *Salmonella*. Taking into consideration similar radiation sensitivity of *L. monocytogenes* and *Salmonella* spp., it can be assumed that doses of ionizing radiation effective for the inactivation of *L. monocytogenes* will be sufficient to inactivate salmonellae.

2.2. Reducing of *Salmonella* spp. in ready-to-eat foods

Ready-to-eat foods deserve special interest. Very often, they contain not only cooked poultry or other meats and cooked seafoods but also raw meats which are consumed without heat treatment (e.g., "filet américain" composed of raw beef meat). Thus, those complex RTE foods may represent an individual specific hazard to consumers since they are often composed of a mixture of several types of ingredients. RTE foods vary by country and may include, for example, dried meat (beef jerky), uncooked and fermented minced meat products (salami), cooked offal or minced meat products (chicken liver pâté or luncheon sausage), and cooked whole meat products (ham) [43]. Gormley et al. [44] conducted a wide study on microbiological quality of ready-to-eat specialty meats (2359 samples of continental sausages, cured/fermented, and dried meats) and reported that 0.4% were unacceptable due to the presence of *Salmonella* spp. or *L. monocytogenes* (>10(2) CFU/g). These unacceptable meats were all prepacked prior to supply to retail premises indicating that contamination with bacterial pathogens occurred earlier in the production chain; the authors emphasize how important it is to prevent food contamination before final packaging and to control conditions of storage.

Song et al. [45] investigated the efficacy of radiation treatment and fumaric acid on the reduction of *L. monocytogenes* and *S. typhimurium* inoculated into sliced ham. The authors noted the decrease of number of listeriae and salmonellae by 2.42 and 3.78 logs, respectively, after irradiation of this ready-to-eat product while the decrease of only one log for both organisms was found after acid treatment.

The US Food and Drug Administration (FDA) is currently evaluating a petition to allow irradiation of RTE meats in the United States including deli turkey, ham, pastrami, beef bologna, bacon bits, and pepperoni. The basis for the petition is data reported by Sommers and Mackay [46].

The authors observed in their study that irradiation of food-borne pathogenic bacteria with a dose of 3.75 kGy on ready-to-eat meats caused reduction of bacteria comparable to that obtained due to pasteurization, that is, minimum of five logs.

Sommers and Boyd [47] discovered that doses in the range of 2–4 kGy eliminate *Salmonella* spp. in many RTE foods.

The ability of ionizing radiation to inactivate *E. coli* O157:H7, *Salmonella, L. monocytogenes*, and *S. aureus* inoculated onto a frankfurter on a roll product containing the antimicrobials sodium diacetate and potassium lactate in the presence of an MA (100% N_2, 50% N_2 plus 50% CO_2, or 100% CO_2) was investigated. The authors reported that the radiation resistance (D10 values) for *Salmonella* in frankfurter on a roll product was from 0.61 to 0.71 kGy. MA had no effect on the radiation resistance of the pathogens. During a 2-week storage period under mild temperature abuse (10°C), both salmonellae and other pathogens were not able to proliferate on the frankfurter on a roll product, regardless of the MA used. Although the pathogens were unable to proliferate on the frankfurter on a roll product during the storage period, the application of a postpackaging intervention step was needed to actually inactivate the food-borne pathogens. The authors concluded that, when applied as a terminal intervention as part of a HACCP plan, food irradiation could reduce the risk of food-borne pathogens on complex ready-to-eat foods such as sandwiches. It seems that intervention technologies including ionizing radiation, antimicrobials, and modified atmospheres (MAs) can be used to inhibit the growth of or inactivate food-borne pathogens on complex ready-to-eat foods such as sandwiches. Cárcel et al. [48] in their study elaborated mathematical model for the most efficient elimination of *Salmonella* spp. from two poultry products taking into consideration shelf life and sensory attributes. It was concluded that in the case of hamburgers, the optimum calculated dose was 2.04 kGy, which guaranteed the safety of the product and provided the best combination of sensory and instrumental attributes. As regards the steaks, the optimum assessed dose was 1.11 kGy, significantly lower than for hamburgers.

According to the data of a research project of a joint Food and Agriculture Organization/International Academy of Engineering (FAO/IAE), the application of ionizing radiation combined with other methods used for food preservation offers improved safety of many various prepared meals and longer shelf life [49].

Kang et al. [50] studied the efficacy of radiation treatment combined with leek (*Allium tuberosum* R.) extract on the survival of several food-borne pathogens inoculated in pork jerky. The authors used doses in the range of 0.5–4 kGy. The D_{10}-value for *S. typhimurium* irradiated with leek extract was 0.32 kGy and without this extract 0.39 kGy. The results prove that this combination strengthens both microbiological safety and shelf life of this meat.

2.3. Reducing *Salmonella* spp. in fish and shellfish

Raw fish and shellfish can be contaminated with pathogenic bacteria such as *Salmonella, Shigella, Vibrio parahaemolyticus, vulnificus, Vibrio cholerae, S. aureus*, and viruses.

According to the data delivered by the United States Department of Agriculture (USDA) [51], *Salmonella* was found in 21% of 153 aquaculture catfish collected from aquaculture ponds and retail markets. The U.S. Food and Drug Administration data from 1998 to 2004 on examination of seafood import refusal identified *Salmonella* contamination to be the most frequent violation in catfish (41.91% of violation categories). Hatha and Laksmanaperumalsamy [52] found *Salmonella* spp. in 14–25% of fish belonging to 18 families. On the basis of the data presented in the literature, along with outbreak data and FDA import refusal data, it can be concluded that the highest microbial hazard associated with catfish consumption is *Salmonella* spp. Raw finfish might contain *V. parahaemolyticus, Salmonella* spp., or *L. monocytogenes* [53]. According to the report of USDA, nontyphoidal *Salmonella* spp. in raw and RTE catfish are considered as higher priority microbial hazards [51]. In terms of risk assessment related to catfish consumption, USDA estimated that the mean reduction of *Salmonella* per catfish serving caused by frying is about two logs, and caused by baking is about three logs [51]. Thus, it seems that such reduction of *Salmonella* spp. number, taking into consideration that naturally contaminated foods contain usually low levels of salmonellae, may significantly lower the risk of food-borne disease due to consumption of contaminated catfish. These findings could partially explain the differences between a significant contamination of raw finfish by pathogenic bacteria and relatively small number of outbreaks in which etiologic agent is *Salmonella* spp.

The monthly data on import refusal published in the USA prove that 1/10 of the refused products are seafood products and that second in terms of rejection reason is the detection of *Salmonella* spp. [54]. Risk analysis conducted in New Zealand by Reed [55] for fillet meat of *Pangasius* spp. fish from Vietnam considered that contamination of fillets with water not of a suitable purity could result in the presence of exotic strains of *Corynebacterium diphtheriae, E. coli, Salmonella* spp., *V. cholerae,* and *Cryptosporidia* spp., which is a risk to human health. Shabarinath et al. [56] studied the prevalence of *Salmonella* in seafood samples by conventional culture and by a DNA-based molecular technique, polymerase chain reaction (PCR). Using PCR, which was considered to be better method, they isolated *Salmonella* spp. from over 50% of seafood samples collected from the southwest coast of India; 14 of 19 isolates belonged to serovar *Salmonella enterica* Weltevreden.

The FAO experts in their report, after thorough evaluation of *Salmonella* spp. problem related to seafood, concluded that good hygienic practices during aquaculture production and biosecurity measures can minimize but not eliminate *Salmonella* in products of aquaculture [57].

Among various seafood, shrimp as the largest single seafood commodity in value terms (at around 15% of the total value of internationally traded fishery products in 2012) mainly produced in developing countries such as South and East Asia and Latin America deserves special attention [58] particularly that the consumption of this commodity consumption has been trending upward.

Norhana et al. [59] in their comprehensive review paper on prevalence, persistence, and control of *Salmonella* and *Listeria* in shrimp and shrimp products indicated that the continued reporting of the presence of these bacteria in fresh and frozen shrimps, and even in the lightly preserved and ready-to-eat products, shows that the existing hygienic practices in fishery industry are insufficient to eliminate these pathogens which have been isolated from shrimps and shrimp products on a regular basis since the 1980s. Shrimp is frequently imported from tropical and subtropical areas and reports indicate that the product does not always meet the microbiological standards set for EU-producing countries or USA, because of either contaminated production sites or unhygienic processing conditions.

Salmonella bacteria are associated with pond water, sediment, and shrimp throughout the culture cycle, including the pre-stocking period, farming phase, and harvest. Untreated chicken manure used to fertilize ponds and droppings from aquatic birds are significant sources of *Salmonella*. The survival rate of the microorganism is enhanced by nutrients, manure, and feed present in the pond system and by the favorable interaction of various biological and physical factors [60]. Shrimps are usually eaten fully cooked. The major health hazards with these products are contamination during or after processing.

Pinu et al. [61] evaluated the microbiological condition of the frozen shrimps found in the local markets and departmental chain shops of Dhaka city. Pathogenic bacterial load was found greater in the samples of departmental shops rather than that of local markets. The researchers found *Salmonella* spp., *Vibrio* spp., and *Shigella* spp. in shrimps' samples and discovered that the samples collected from local markets and departmental shops were heavily contaminated and were of special concern for human consumption.

Asai et al. [62] reported that the examination of 353 samples of 29 types of seafood revealed that *S. enterica* serotype Weltevreden was isolated from two of 47 black tiger prawn samples. The contamination levels of *Salmonella* were in a range of <30–40 most probable number per 100 g. Asai concluded that these results indicate the possibility that shrimp and prawns contribute to food-borne infections.

In recent years, safety risks are associated to the consumption of raw or subjected to mild heat treatment fish and shellfish; molluscan shellfish (oysters, clams, mussels, and scallops) are often consumed whole and raw. Huss et al. [54] and Olgunoglu [63] in his comprehensive review on *Salmonella* in fish and fishery products show that the pathogens of concern in this seafood include both bacteria (e.g., *Vibrio* spp., *Salmonella* spp., *L. monocytogenes, Shigella* spp., *C. jejuni*), viruses (e.g., hepatitis A virus and norovirus), and parasites. Molluscan shellfish feed on phytoplankton and zooplankton. They are passive feeders that filter and concentrate pathogens present in harvest area. Their environment, particularly near-shore harvest water, is contaminated from sewage, which may contain pathogens from both human and animal fecal sources (e.g., *V. cholerae* O1 and O139, *Salmonella* spp.). Also, poor sanitary practices on the harvest vessel, poor aquacultural practices, and transportation can cause contamination of fishery products.

As observed in previous years, the food category with the highest level of non-compliance at processing was RTE fishery products (4.7% of single samples and 10.8% of batches), mainly in smoked fish [34].

Distribution of strong-evidence outbreaks by food vehicle in the EU in 2014 indicated that crustaceans, shellfish, molluscs, and products thereof were responsible for 8.1% of outbreaks with strong evidence (data from 592 outbreaks with strong evidence) [34]. Taking the above-mentioned data into consideration, health authorities in many countries including European Community emphasized that the increasing trend in raw fish consumption (sushi, sashimi, salmon, etc.) has been identified as a risk to human health. Oysters and mussels can cause food-borne illness. Consumer can contract food-borne salmonellosis due to consumption of raw oysters.

It is generally known that the best method of controlling pathogens is to use a postharvest treatment. Some treatments, such as thermal treatment, ionizing radiation, and high hydrostatic pressure processing, reduce the number of pathogenic microorganisms (bacteria and viruses) while the long-term freezing most widely used method of food preservation is mainly effective in controlling parasites.

Brands et al. [64] reported that *Salmonella* was isolated from oysters from each coast of the United States, and 7.4% of all oysters tested contained *Salmonella*. Isolation tended to be bay specific. The vast majority (78/101) of *Salmonella* isolates from oysters were *S. enterica* serovar Newport, a major human pathogen, confirming the human health hazard of raw oyster consumption. Bakr et al. [65] showed that out of the 150 seafood samples examined, collected from 11 localities in Alexandria, Egypt, Salmonella was isolated from 10% of samples (shrimp, oyster, and mussel). In 1986, the Scientific Committee for Foods [24] recommended that fish and shellfish could be irradiated at doses up to 3 kGy. In the United States, FDA has approved the use of ionizing radiation for the control of *V. parahaemolyticus* and *V. vulnificus* and other food-borne pathogens in fresh or frozen molluscan shellfish. Irradiation of fresh and frozen molluscan shellfish may not exceed an absorbed dose of 5.5 kGy [53]. Also, FDA proposes radiation treatment for the control of food-borne bacteria in crustaceans with a dose of 6.0 kGy. The D10 values cited in the published literature for several *Salmonella* serotypes in grass prawns and shrimp homogenate ranged from 0.30 to 0.59 kGy. Thus, irradiation of crustaceans at a maximum absorbed dose of 6.0 kGy would be effective at controlling pertinent pathogens. The petitioner requested a maximum absorbed dose of 6.0 kGy to achieve a six-log reduction of *L. monocytogenes*. It can be expected that this dose should also eliminate majority of non-sporing pathogenic bacteria including *Salmonella*. Irradiation of fish and shellfish is intended, similarly like in the case of other foods to extend shelf life, reduce pathogen load, and inactivate parasites. Irradiation has been applied to fresh, frozen, as well as dried fish, fish products, and shellfish [18]. As for other foods, pathogenic bacteria are more resistant to irradiation in frozen state compared to chilled one. Most studies indicate that irradiation at doses recommended by the SCF (3 kGy) should yield two to five logs reduction of pathogenic, non-spore-forming bacteria for the majority of fish and fish products. Sommers and Rajkowski [66] determined the radiation D10 values for *Salmonella* inoculated onto seafood samples (scallops, lobster meat, blue crab, swordfish, octopus, and squid). The samples were frozen and irradiated in the frozen state (−20°C); D10 values for *Salmonella* ranged from 0.47 to 0.70 kGy. By contrast, the radiation D10 value for *Salmonella* suspended on frozen pork was 1.18 kGy. They concluded that radiation dose needed to inactivate these food-borne pathogens on frozen seafood is significantly lower than that for frozen meat or frozen vegetables. *Salmonella* spp. and other primary pathogens of concern can also be introduced after pasteurization. Some fishery products are cooked before they are packaged; therefore, they are at risk for recontamination between cooking and packaging (e.g., vacuum packaging, modified atmosphere packaging). Kamat and Thomas [67] evaluated the effect of fat content in fish on radiation sensitivity of *L. monocytogenes, Bacillus cereus, S. typhimurium*, and *Yersinia enterocolitica*. The radiation response of all those pathogens was examined in sardine with high fat and golden anchovy with low fat. The results clearly suggest that regardless of the level of lipid in fish, the application of a 3 kGy dose at refrigeration temperature would effectively decontaminate approximately 10^5 CFU g^{-1} of all the organisms tested, except spores of *B. cereus*. The authors concluded that the studies revealed a lack of influence of lipid levels in fish on radiation resistance of four food-borne bacterial pathogens.

Jakabi et al. [68] studied the survival of *S. enteritidis* and *S. infantis* inoculated into oysters and sensory properties as the result of irradiation with doses in the dose range of 0.5–3.0 kGy. The number of those both *Salmonella* populations decreased after a 3.0 kGy dose by five to six logs. The authors also discovered that oysters irradiated with the highest dose were still alive and concluded that a dose of 3.0 kGy could be considered effective in inactivating *Salmonella* in oysters without changing their odor, flavor, or appearance.

The SCF [24] recommended that shrimps could be irradiated at doses of 5 kGy which is considered to be an effective decontamination method. Ito et al. [69] reported that the dose of gamma irradiation necessary to reduce both *S. typhimurium* and *L. monocytogenes* in frozen shrimps at a level of below 10^{-4} per gram was about 3.5 kGy. Sinanoglou et al. [70] irradiated using a cobalt-60 gamma source frozen molluscs (squid, octopuses, and cuttlefish) and crustaceans (shrimp) with different doses. The authors noted the substantial decrease of mesophiles number in shrimp irradiated with the dose of 2.5 kGy, whereas after the dose of 4.7 kGy the presence of those bacteria in squid was not detected. Shrimp is considered separately from fish and shellfish given that certain pathogens (i.e., *L. monocytogenes*) require doses about 3 kGy for several log10 reduction. Sommers et al. [71] evaluated the effect of cryogenic freezing (−82°C, 3 min), and gamma irradiation on the survival of mixture of *Salmonella* spp. (*S. schwarzengrund, S. bahrenfeld, S. weltevreden,* and *S. panama* isolated from seafood, including shrimp), on raw frozen shrimp. D10 values for salmonellae irradiated in shrimp were about 0.56 kGy. The authors observed the decrease of *Salmonella* spp. number after cryogenic freezing and irradiation with a dose of 2.25 kGy by over five logs and that this effect persisted during 3 months storage at −20°C. The authors conclude that radiation treatment combined with cryogenic freezing offers big benefits in regard to frozen shrimp.

Nerkar and Bandekar [72] studied radiation resistance of *S. typhimurium* and *S. enteritidis* inoculated at 1×10^8 cells/ml in shrimp homogenate and they determined that the D10 value was in the range from 0.30 to 0.40 kGy. Finally, they concluded that a dose of 4.0 kGy could be used to completely eliminate *Salmonella* in frozen prepackaged shrimp.

Luo et al. [73] studied radioresistance of non-spore-forming and spore-forming pathogenic microorganisms inoculated into shelf-stable foods, semi-dried pork, and fish which have been vacuum-packaged. The water activity (aw) of semi-dried food products ranged between 0.930 and 0.940 for pork, and 0.852 and 0.895 for fish. The authors observed that *S. enteritidis* was eliminated at a dose of 2.5 kGy in semi-dried fish, and the minimum irradiation dose required to inactivate this pathogen in pork was 5 kGy.

2.4. Reducing *Salmonella* spp. in frog's legs

The skin of frogs and their internal organs are often contaminated with *Salmonella* spp. and other pathogens, such as *E. coli* and *S. aureus*. Although frog's legs are cooked before consumption, there is a risk for cross-contamination.

The highest radiation dose for frog's legs suggested by the Scientific Committee for Foods is 5 kGy [18]. The most important hazard arises from contamination with *Salmonella* and other fecal pathogens occurring in frog's legs at the time of deep-freezing. *E. coli* and *S. aureus* have been also found in frog's legs. Tambunan's [74] studies showed that irradiating frog legs artificially contaminated with *Salmonella* up to 10^6/g before freezing a dose of 3 kGy and above resulted in no detection of the bacteria. If irradiation was carried out after freezing, a dose of 4 kGy and above has to be used. The latter procedure appears to be more feasible commercially than the former one. It was concluded that a combination of chlorination, freezing, and irradiation with a dose ranging from 3 to 6 kGy should provide sufficient conditions for the elimination of *Salmonella* in the product.

3. Concluding remarks

Ionizing radiation in industry can be used to reduce the level of *Salmonella* spp. in both raw and cooked meats, poultry, and seafood. This intervention technology can be regarded as a Critical Control Point in the HACCP plan. Irradiation treatment, applied as the final processing step, seems to be of particular importance in the case of packed food products, including ready-to-eat food. In the USA, FDA [75] proposes radiation treatment with the maximum dose of 4.5 kGy for a variety of raw meats and meat products for the improvement of microbial safety and for shelf-life extension.

The data from literature prove that the *D*-values for *L. monocytogenes* are similar to those reported for *Salmonella* spp. irradiated under similar conditions. Thus, *Salmonella* spp. in meats, poultry, and fish and shellfish including ready-to-eat foods may be controlled by the same dose required for *L. monocytogenes*.

It should be noted, however, that dose range used for radicidation (2.5–10 kGy) is not sufficient to sterilize foods. Thus, all additional control measures (e.g., an unbroken cold chain, appropriate handling of raw meat, and procedures for cleaning disinfection and waste disposal, etc.) should maintain or even increase the beneficial effects of radiation treatment.

Referring to irradiation facilities, electron beams are much more useful for packs of relatively thin cooked, sliced meats, and other ready-to-eat products while gamma radiation is more suited for treating whole carcasses [76].

Author details

Małgorzata E. Szczawińska

Address all correspondence to: malgorzata_szczawinska@sggw.pl

Warsaw University of Life Sciences – SGGW, Faculty of Veterinary Medicine, Department of Food Hygiene and Public Health Protection, Warsaw, Poland

References

[1] Leistner L., Gorris L.G.M.: Food preservation by hurdle technology. Trends in Food Science and Technology. 1995;6:41–46.

[2] Farkas J.: Combination of irradiation with mild heat treatment. Food Control. 1990;1: 223–229.

[3] Chouliara E., Badeka A., Savvaidis I., Kontaminas MG.: Combined effect of irradiation and modified atmosphere packaging on shelf-life extension of chicken breast meat: microbiological, chemical and sensory changes. European Food Research and Technology. 2008;226:877–888. DOI: 10.1007/s00217-007-0610-3.

[4] Grant I.R., Patterson M.F.: Combined effect of gamma radiation and heating on the destruction of *Listeria monocytogenes* and *Salmonella typhimurium* in cook-chill roast beef and gravy. International Journal of Food Microbiology. 1995;27:117–128. DOI: 10.1016/0168-1605(94)00156-Z.

[5] Thayer D.W., Songprasertchai S., Boyd G.: Effects of heat and ionizing radiation on *Salmonella typhimurium* in mechanically deboned chicken meat. J. Food Prot. 1991;54: 718–724.

[6] Sofos J., Flick G., Nychas G., O'Bryan C., Ricke S., Crandall P. Meat, Poultry, and Seafood, p 111-167. In: Doyle M, Buchanan R (ed), Food Microbiology. ASM Press, Washington, DC. 4th ed. 2013. DOI: 10.1128/9781555818463.ch6.

[7] Szczawińska M.E., Szczawiński J., Łobacz A.: Effect of temperature on the growth kinetics of *Salmonella* enteritidis in cooked ham. Bulletin of the Veterinary Institute in Pulawy. 2014;58:47–56. DOI: 10.2478/bvip-2014-0008.

[8] Anonymous: CODEX STAN 106-1983, REV.1-2003 Revised Codex General Standard for Irradiated Foods, 1–10.

[9] Goresline H.E., Ingram M., Macuch P., Mocquot G., Mossell D.A.A., Niven C.F., Thatcher F.S.: Tentative classification of food irradiation processes with microbiological objectives. Nature 1964;204:237–238.

[10] Mulder R.W.A.W.: *Salmonella* radicidation of poultry carcasses [thesis]. Spelderholt Institute for Poultry Research, Beekbergen, The Netherlands. Report 363. 1982.

[11] European Food Safety Authority: The European Union summary report on trends and sources of zoonoses, zoonotic agents and food-borne outbreaks in 2014. European Food Safety Authority, European Centre for Disease Prevention and Control. EFSA Journal 2015;13(12):4329 AMENDED: 4 February 2016.

[12] Anonymous: Commission Regulation (EC) No 2073/2005 of 15 November 2005 on microbiological criteria for foodstuffs. OJ, L338,22.12.2005, p. 1.

[13] Farkas J.: Radiation processing of dry food ingredients. Radiation Physics and Chemistry. 1985;25:271–280.

[14] Rajkowski K.T., Niebuhr S.E., Dickson J.: Effect of gamma or beta radiation on *Salmonella* DT 104 in ground pork. Journal of Food Protection. 2006;69:1430–1433.

[15] Miyahara M., Miyahara M.: Effects of gamma ray and electron-beam irradiations on survival of anaerobic and facultatively anaerobic bacteria. Kokuritsu Iyakuhin Shokuhin Eisei Kenkyusho Hokoku. 2002; 120: 75–80.

[16] Webpage IAEA Clearance of Irradiated Foods Database at http://nucleus.iaea.org/NUCLEUS/nucleus/Content/Applications/FICdb/FoodIrradiationClearances.jsp?module=cif) Internet. Available from http://nucleus.iaea.org.

[17] Anonymous: European Commission: Report From The Commission To The European Parliament And The Council On Food And Food Ingredients Treated With Ionising Radiation For The Year 2014. Brussels, 17.12.2015 COM(2015) 665 final. EUR-Lex-52015DC0665.

[18] European Food Safety Authority: Statement summarising the Conclusions and Recommendations from the Opinions on the safety of Irradiation of Food adopted by the BIOHAZ and CEF Panels. EFSA Journal 2011; 9(4): 2107 [155 pp.]. DOI: 10.2903/j.efsa.2011. 2107.

[19] Maxcy R.B., Tiwari N.P.: Irradiation of meats for public health protection. In: Radiation Preservation of Food. IAEA, Vienna, 1973, pp. 491–504.

[20] Dickson J.S., Olson D.G.: Growth rates of *Salmonella* and *Escherichia coli* O157:H7 in irradiated beef. Journal of Food Protection 2001;64:1828–1831.

[21] Szczawińska M., Szczawiński J., Szulc M.: The survival of irradiated bacteria during conventional methods of meat preservation. Archiv fur Lebensmittelhygiene 1983;34:53–58.

[22] Szczawińska M.E., Thayer D.W., Phillips J.G.: Fate of unirradiated *Salmonella* in irradiated mechanically deboned chicken meat. International Journal of Food Microbiology. 1991;14:313–324.

[23] Kim A.Y., Thayer D.W.: Mechanism by which gamma irradiation increases the sensitivity of *Salmonella typhimurium* ATCC 14028 to heat. Applied and Environmental Microbiology. 1996; 62:1759–1763.

[24] SCF (Scientific Committee on Food). Food - Science and Techniques. Reports of the Scientific Committee for Food (Eighteenth Series). 1986.

[25] Kampelmacher E.H.: Irradiation of food: a new technology for preserving and ensuring the hygiene of foods. Fleischwirtschaft 1984;64:322–327.

[26] Szczawińska M.: Prospects for elimination of salmonellae from poultry by irradiation in Poland. Food Irradiation in the Middle East and Europe. Proceedings of the Final Coordination Meeting of an FAO/IAEA Coordinated Research Programme organized by the Joint FAO/IAEA Division of Nuclear Techniques in Food and Agriculture and held in Cadarache, France, 8–12 March 1993. IAEA-TECDOC-754, pp. 77–96, July 1994.

[27] Clavero M.R., Monk J.D., Beuchat L.R., Doyle M.P., Brackett R.E.: Inactivation of Escherichia coli O157:H7, salmonellae, and Campylobacter jejuni in raw ground beef by gamma irradiation. Applied and Environmental Microbiology. 1994;60:2069–2075.

[28] Thayer D.W., Boyd G., Muller W.S., Lipson C.A., Hayne W.C., Baer S.H. Radiation resistance of *Salmonella.* Journal of Industrial Microbiology. 1990;5:383–390.

[29] Tarkowski J.A., Beumer R.R., Kampelmacher E.H.: Low gamma irradiation of raw meat. International Journal of Food Microbiology. 1984;1:25–31.

[30] Thayer D.W., Boyd G., Fox I. B., Ir., Lakritz L., Hampson I.W.: Variations in radiation sensitivity of foodborne pathogens associated with the suspending meat. I. Food Science. 1995a;60:63–67.

[31] Thayer D.W., Boyd G., Huhtanen C.N.: Effects of ionizing-radiation and anaerobic refrigerated storage on indigenous microflora, *Salmonella,* and *Clostridium botulinum* type-A and type-B in vacuum-canned, mechanically deboned chicken meat. Journal of Food Protection. 1995;58:752–757.

[32] Thayer D.W., Boyd G.: Survival of *Salmonella typhimurium* ATCC 14028 on the surface of chicken legs or in mechanically deboned chicken meat gamma irradiated in air or vacuum at temperatures of -20 to +20 degree. Poultry Science. 1991:70:1026–1033.

[33] Szczawiński J., Szczawińska M., Szulc M.: Combined effects of irradiation and curing salts ($NaNO_2$ and NaCl) upon the behaviour of salmonellae in meat. Archiv fur Lebensmittelhygiene. 1985;36:(3):55–58.

[34] EFSA: SCIENTIFIC REPORT OF EFSA AND ECDC The European Union summary report on trends and sources of zoonoses, zoonotic agents and food-borne outbreaks in 2013 European Food Safety Authority, European Centre for Disease Prevention and Control European Food Safety Authority (EFSA), Parma, Italy European Centre for Disease Prevention and Control (ECDC), Stockholm, Sweden: EFSA Journal. 2015;13(1):3991.

[35] COMMISSION REGULATION (EU) No 1086/2011of 27 October 2011 amending Annex II to Regulation (EC) No 2160/2003 of the European Parliament and of the Council and Annex I to Commission Regulation (EC) No 2073/2005 as regards *salmonella* in fresh poultry meat.

[36] Kudra L.L., Sebranek J.G., Dickson J.S., Mendonca A.F., Zhang Q., Jackson-Davis A., Prusa K.J.: 2011. Control of *Salmonella* enterica Typhimurium in chicken breast meat by irradiation combined with modified atmosphere packaging. Journal of Food Protection. 2011 Nov;74(11):1833–1839. DOI: 10.4315/0362-028X.JFP-11-195.

[37] Nassar T.J., al-Mashhadi A.S., Fawal A.K., Shalhat A.F.: Decontamination of chicken carcasses artificially contaminated with *Salmonella*. Revue Scientifique et Technique. 1997;16:891–897.

[38] Thayer D.W., Boyd G., Fox J.B. Jr., Lakritz L.: Elimination by gamma irradiation of *Salmonella* spp. and strains of *Staphylococcus aureus* inoculated in bison, ostrich, alligator, and caiman meat. Journal of Food Protection. 1997;60:756–760.

[39] Commission Regulation (EU) No 365/2010 of 28 April 2010 amending Regulation (EC) No 2073/2005 on microbiological criteria for foodstuffs as regards Enterobacteriaceae in pasteurised milk and other pasteurised liquid dairy products and Listeria monocytogenes in food grade salt. OJ L 107, 29 April 2010, pp. 9–11.

[40] Regulation (EC) No 852/2004 of the European Parliament and of the Council of 29 April 2004 laying down specific hygiene rules for on the hygiene of foodstuffs. OJ L 139, 30.4.2004.

[41] Regulation (EC) No 853/2005 of the European Parliament and of the Council of 29 April 2004 laying down specific hygiene rules for on the hygiene of food of animal origin. OJ L 139, 30.4.2004.

[42] Thayer D.W., Boyd G., Kim A., Fox J.B., Jr., Farrell H.M., Jr.: Fate of gamma-irradiated *Listeria monocytogenes* during refrigerated storage on raw or cooked turkey breast meat. Journal of Food Protection. 1998;61:979–987.

[43] Responsibilities in relation to producing and handling ready-to-eat (RTE) meats in Queensland. Available from: http://www.safefood.qld.gov.au/images/PDF/meat_meat_products/Responsibilities%20for%20RTE%20Meats.PDF.

[44] Gormley F.J., Little C.L., Grant K.A., de Pinna E., McLauchlin J.: The microbiological safety of ready-to-eat specialty meats from markets and specialty food shops: a UK wide study with a focus on *Salmonella* and *Listeria monocytogenes*. Food Microbiology. 2010;27:243–249. Doi: 10.1016/j.fm.2009.10.009. Epub 2009 Oct 21.

[45] Song H.J., Lee J.H., Song K.B.: Effects of irradiation and fumaric acid treatment on the inactivation of *Listeria monocytogenes* and *Salmonella typhimurium* inoculated on sliced ham. Radiation Physics and Chemistry. 2011. Doi:10.1016/j.radphyschem.2011.06.012.

[46] Sommers C.H., Mackay W.J.: Irradiation of Ready-To-Eat Meat Products. In: Institute of Food Technologist Series: Food Irradiation Research and Technology, 2nd ed. Fan X and Sommers CH., editors. 2012. DOI: 10.1002/9781118422557.ch11. This edition first published 2013 © 2013 Blackwell Publishing and the Institute of Food Technologists.

[47] Sommers C.H., Boyd G.: Radiation sensitivity and postirradiation growth of foodborne pathogens on a ready-to-eat frankfurter on a roll product in the presence of modified atmosphere and antimicrobials. Journal of Food Protection. 2006;69:2436–2440.

[48] Cárcel J.A., Benedito J., Cambero M.I., Cabeza M.C., Ordóñez J.A.: Modeling and optimization of the E-beam treatment of chicken steaks and hamburgers, considering food safety, shelf-life, and sensory quality. Food and Bioproducts Processing. 2015;96:133–144. DOI: http://dx.doi.org/10.1016/j.fbp.2015.07.006

[49] IAEA (International Atomic Energy Agency), Vienna, Irradiation to Ensure the Safety and Quality of Prepared Meals. STI/PUB/1365. 2009. ISBN 978-92-0-111108-1.

[50] Kang M., Kim H.-J., Jayasena D.D., Bae S.Y., Yong I.H., Lee M., Jo C.: Effects of combined treatments of electron-beam irradiation and addition of Leek (Allium tuberosum) extract on reduction of pathogens in pork jerky. Foodborne Pathogens and Disease. 2012;9:1083–1087. DOI: 10.1089/fpd.2012.1249.

[51] Bauer N., Cook V., Disney T., Ebel E., Guo C., Johnston J., La Barre D., Lee J., McCoy E., Morrison J., Schlosser W., Williams M.: DRAFT Risk Assessment of the Potential Human Health Effect of Applying Continuous Inspection to Catfish, Prepared by the Risk Assessment Division Office of Public Health Science Food Safety and Inspection Service United States Department of Agriculture. December, 2010.

[52] Hatha AAM and Laksmanaperumalsamy P.: Prevalence of *Salmonella* in fish and crustaceans from markets in Coimbatore, South India. Food Microbiology.1997;14:111–116.

[53] FDA Guidance for the Industry: Fish and Fishery Products Hazards and Controls Guidance Department Of Health And Human Services Public Health Service Food and Drug Administration Center For Food Safety And Applied Nutrition Office Of Food Safety. Fourth Edition – APRIL 2011.

[54] Huss H.H., Ababouch L., Gram L.: Assessment and management of seafood safety and quality. FAO Fisheries Technical Paper. No. 444. Rome, FAO. 2004.

[55] Reed C.: Import risk analysis: Frozen, skinless and boneless fillet meat of *Pangasius* spp. fish from Vietnam for human consumption MAF Biosecurity New Zealand, 2008.

[56] Shabarinath S., Kumar H.S., Khushiramani R., Karunasagar I.: Detection and characterization of *Salmonella* associated with tropical seafood. International Journal of Food Microbiology. 2007;114:227–233. DOI: 10.1016/j.ijfoodmicro.2006.09.012.

[57] FAO: Report of the FAO Expert Workshop on The Application Of Biosecurity Measures To Control *Salmonella* Contamination In Sustainable Aquaculture. FAO. Mangalore, India, 19–21 January 2010. Fisheries and Aquaculture Report No. 937 FIPM/R937 (En).

[58] Dent F.: Fishery Industry Officer, Fish Products, Trade & Marketing Branch (FIPM): Global Outlook for Shrimp Markets and Demand, 2013, at www.globefish.org.

[59] Norhana M.N.W., Poole S.E., Deeth H.C., Dykes G.A.: Prevalence, persistence and control of *Salmonella* and *Listeria* in shrimp and shrimp products: a review. Food Control. 2010;21:343–361. http://dx.doi.org/10.1016/j.foodcont.2009.06.020.

[60] Flick G.J., Jr., Granata L.A.: Biological Safety of Fresh and Processed Shellfish. Southern Regional Aquaculture Center (SRAC) SRAC Publication No. 4901, April 2010.

[61] Pinu F.R., Yeasmin S., Bar B.L., Rahman M.M.: Microbiological conditions of frozen shrimp in different food markets of Dhaka City. Food Science and Technology Research. 2007;13:362–365. DOI: 10.3136/fstr.13.362.

[62] Asai Y., Kaneko M., Ohtsuka K., Morita Y., Kaneko S., Noda H., Furukawa I., Takatori K., Hara-Kudo Y.: *Salmonella* prevalence in seafood imported into Japan. Journal of Food Protection. 2008;71:1460–1464. PMID: 18680947.

[63] Olgunoglu I.A.: Salmonella in Fish and Fishery Products. 2012. In: Salmonella - A Dangerous Foodborne Pathogen, Dr. Dr. Barakat S M Mahmoud (Ed.), ISBN:978-953-307-782-6, Rijaka, Croatia, InTech, Available from: http://www.intechopen.com/books/salmonella-a-dangerous-foodborne-pathogen/salmonella-in-fish-and-fishery-products.

[64] Brands D.A., Inman A.E., Gerba C.P., Maré C.J., Billington S.J., Saif L.A., Levine J.F., Joens L.A.: Prevalence of *Salmonella* spp. in Oysters in the United States. Applied and Environmental Microbiology. 2005;71:893–897. DOI: 10.1128/AEM.71.2.893-897.2005. PMCID: PMC546685

[65] Bakr Wafaa M.K., Hazzah Walaa A., Abaza Amani F.: Detection of *Salmonella* and *Vibrio* species in some seafood in Alexandria. Journal of American Science. 2011;7:663–668.

[66] Sommers C.H., Rajkowski K.T.: Radiation inactivation of foodborne pathogens on frozen seafood products. Journal of Food Protection. 2011;74:641–644. Doi: 10.4315/0362-028X.JFP-10-419.

[67] Kamat A., Thomas P.: Radiation inactivation of some food-borne pathogens in fish as influenced by fat levels. Journal of Applied Microbiology. 1998;84:478–484.

[68] Jakabi M., Gelli D.S., Torre J.C., Rodas M.A., Franco B.D., Destro M.T., Landgrafi M.: Inactivation by ionizing radiation of *Salmonella* Enteritidis, *Salmonella* Infantis, and *Vibrio parahaemolyticus* in oysters (*Crassostrea brasiliana*). Journal of Food Protection. 2003;66:1025–9.

[69] Hitoshi I., Harun Or R., Naruemon S., Pitaya A., Pongpen R., Isao I.: Effect of gamma-irradiation on frozen shrimps for decontamination of pathogenic bacteria. Radiation Physics and Chemistry 1993;42:279–282. DOI: 10.1016/0969-806X(93)90249-T.

[70] Sinanoglou V.J., Batrinou A., Konteles S., Sflomos K.: Microbial population, physico-chemical quality, and allergenicity of molluscs and shrimp treated with cobalt-60 gamma radiation. Journal of Food Protection. 2007;70:958–966.

[71] Sommers C.H., Rajkowski K.T., Sheen S., Samer C., Bender E.: The effect of cryogenic freezing followed by gamma radiation on the survival of *Salmonella* spp. on frozen shrimp. Journal of Food Processing & Technology2011;S8. http://dx.doi.org/10.4172/2157-7110.S8-001

[72] Nerkar D.P., Bandekar J.R.: Elimination of *Salmonella* from frozen shrimp by gamma radiation. Journal of Food Safety, 1990;10(3):175–180.

[73] Luo X., Cui S., Li Y., Jiang T.: A Study On The Use Of Irradiation In Combination With Vacuum Packaging To Produce Non-Sterile Shelf-Stable Food, Semi-Dried Meat, Seafood And Vegetables. In: Radiation Processing For Safe, Shelf-Stable And Ready-To-Eat Food. Proceedings of a final Research Co-ordination Meeting held in Montreal, Canada, 10–14 July 2000. IAEA, VIENNA, 2003 IAEA-TECDOC-1337 ISBN 92–0–100703–5 ISSN 1011–4289, p.194-198.

[74] Tambunan P.R.: Elimination of *Salmonella* in frog legs by irradiation. Final Report to the International Atomic Energy Agency on Contract No 2711/R1/RB. Central Research Institute for Fisheries, Indonesia. 1984.

[75] Federal Register: Irradiation in the Production, Processing and Handling of Food, A Rule by the Food and Drug Administration on 11/30/2012 Fed Regist. 2012 Nov 30;77(231):71312–71316.

[76] Farkas J.: Irradiation of poultry meat. In: Food Safety Control in the Poultry Industry. G. Mead. Cambridge, 2005:433–452.